Opium Slavery

Civil War America

Caroline E. Janney and Aaron Sheehan-Dean, editors

This landmark series interprets broadly the history and culture of the Civil War era through the long nineteenth century and beyond. Drawing on diverse approaches and methods, the series publishes historical works that explore all aspects of the war, biographies of leading commanders, and tactical and campaign studies, along with select editions of primary sources. Together, these books shed new light on an era that remains central to our understanding of American and world history.

A complete list of books published in Civil War America is available at https://uncpress.org/series/civil-war-america.

Opium Slavery

Civil War Veterans and America's First Opioid Crisis

JONATHAN S. JONES

The University of North Carolina Press
Chapel Hill

© 2025 The University of North Carolina Press
All rights reserved

Manufactured in the United States of America
Set in Minion Pro by Jamie McKee, MacKey Composition

Cover art courtesy of Stanley B. Burns, MD, Historic Medical Photography Collection, Medical Historical Library, Harvey Cushing / John Hay Whitney Medical Library, Yale University, New Haven, CT.

Library of Congress Cataloging-in-Publication Data
Names: Jones, Jonathan S. (Historian) author
Title: Opium slavery : Civil War veterans and America's first opioid crisis / Jonathan S. Jones.
Other titles: Civil War America (Series)
Description: Chapel Hill : University of North Carolina Press, [2025] | Series: Civil War America | Includes bibliographical references and index.
Identifiers: LCCN 2025015422 | ISBN 9781469689524 cloth alk. paper | ISBN 9781469689531 paperback alk. paper | ISBN 9781469686622 epub | ISBN 9781469689548 pdf
Subjects: LCSH: Opium abuse—United States—History—19th century | Morphine abuse—United States—History—19th century | Opioid abuse—United States—History—19th century | Drug abuse—Treatment—United States—History—19th century | Drug abuse—Social aspects—United States—History—19th century | United States—History—Civil War, 1861–1865—Veterans—Drug use | BISAC: HISTORY / United States / Civil War Period (1850-1877) | PSYCHOLOGY / Psychopathology / Addiction
Classification: LCC HV5825 .J645 2025 | DDC 362.29/30973—dc23/eng/20250609
LC record available at https://lccn.loc.gov/2025015422

Portions of this work appeared earlier, in somewhat different form, in Jonathan S. Jones, "Buying and Selling Health and Manhood: Civil War Veterans and Opiate Addiction 'Cures,'" in *Buying and Selling Civil War Memory in Gilded Age America*, ed. Caroline E. Janney and James Marten (Athens: University of Georgia Press, 2021), 31–47; and "Opium Slavery: Civil War Veterans and Opiate Addiction," *Journal of the Civil War Era* 10, no. 2 (June 2020): 185–212.

For product safety concerns under the European Union's General Product Safety Regulation (EU GPSR), please contact gpsr@mare-nostrum.co.uk or write to the University of North Carolina Press and Mare Nostrum Group B.V., Mauritskade 21D, 1091 GC Amsterdam, The Netherlands.

For Bethany, Mom, Dad, and Bubba

Contents

List of Figures, ix

Acknowledgments, xi

Abbreviations, xv

Introduction, 1

PART I Origins

Chapter 1 The Magnum Dei Donum of the Materia Medica, 19
  The Rise of Opiates in Antebellum American Medicine

Chapter 2 So Dreadful an Evil, 40
  The Cultural Construction of Addiction in Antebellum America

Chapter 3 The Drs. Put Me on Morphine, 60
  Civil War Medicine and Addiction

PART II Experiences

Chapter 4 Opium Slavery, 107
  Veterans and the Experience of Addiction

Chapter 5 Opium Mania, 147
  Addiction as Mental Illness

Chapter 6 Vicious Habits, 177
  Addiction and Military Entitlements

PART III Reactions

Chapter 7 Buying and Selling the Cure, 209
  Veterans and Patent Medicine Remedies for Addiction

Chapter 8 The Revolt against Opium, 234
  Physicians React to Mass Addiction

Epilogue The Army Disease, 277
    *Remembering Addicted Veterans in the Twentieth-
    and Twenty-First-Century United States*

Notes, 285

Bibliography, 341

Index, 381

Figures

1.1. Frontispiece from Samuel DuBois medical thesis, 1855, 28
3.1. Tin of opium pills, 66
3.2. Andersonville prison, Georgia, 1864, 72
3.3. Civil War–era hypodermic syringe kit, 78
4.1. Civil War veteran about to receive a morphine injection, 116
4.2. "Result of Subcutaneous Injection," 119
4.3. The ideal Gilded Age male physique, 122
4.4. Solomon Sivils mugshot, ca. 1904, 123
4.5. Frances B. Goolrick, 128
4.6. John Tackett Goolrick and President Warren G. Harding, 1921, 128
5.1. Edward Sylvester Matthews, ca. 1864, 165
6.1. Examiners of pension office preparing claims for action, undated, 182
6.2. Surgeon's report, January 4, 1893, Samuel M. Martin pension application, 188
7.1. Advertisement for Samuel B. Collins's Painless Opium Antidote, 1879, 216
8.1. Silas Weir Mitchell examines a Civil War veteran, Philadelphia Orthopaedic Hospital and Infirmary for Nervous Diseases, 1902, 249

Acknowledgments

They say a book is not a solo project, and believe me, they are right. So I have many people to thank without whom this project would never have come to fruition.

At the University of North Carolina Press, Mark Simpson-Vos took this project under his wing, gave terrific advice on how to streamline the arguments and prose, and was helpfully flexible on deadlines. Thomas Bedenbaugh, Mary Carley Caviness, Nancy Raynor, and Cristian Roberto Walk guided me through the editing and publication process and saved me from countless errors. The late Peter Carmichael initially solicited the project for UNC and served as a peer reviewer, and his thoughtful reading helped clarify and hone the book's arguments. I also am grateful for the continued support of series editors Caroline E. Janney and Aaron Sheehan-Dean. I want to give special thanks to the anonymous reader for their attentiveness to detail and for so closely engaging with multiple drafts of the manuscript. Their feedback pushed me to carefully consider and articulate evidence. They also helped me situate what started out as a Civil War book within a broader historiography of drugs and addiction.

A number of institutions generously supported this project at various stages through grants and fellowships, including the History Department and Institute for Advanced Studies in the Humanities (IASH) at Binghamton University; Virginia Military Institute; James Madison University; The College of Physicians of Philadelphia; the Consortium for History of Science, Technology and Medicine; Duke University Libraries; Louis Round Wilson Special Collections Library at the University of North Carolina at Chapel Hill; the Medical Historical Library at Yale University's Harvey Cushing/John Hay Whitney Medical Library; the Huntington Library; New York State Archives; New-York Historical Society; the North Caroliniana Society; Virginia Historical Society; and the Special Collections Research Center at William & Mary. Scholars at meetings of the Society of Civil War Historians, the Southern Historical Association, the Southern Association for Women Historians, and several other organizations asked thoughtful questions that shaped my analysis.

Numerous individuals shared source material that appears throughout the book. Sarah Handley-Cousins and James Marten provided crucial sources related to Grover Cleveland, soldiers' homes, and Leslie E. Keeley. Judith Giesberg and Susannah J. Ural read early versions of key sections and provided feedback that grew the project by leaps and bounds. Early conversations with David T. Courtwright and John Harley Warner informed my research questions and guided me toward key primary sources. Patrick Foley helped me understand the pharmacology of opioids, and Daniel Goldstein helped decipher arcane pharmacy symbols. Jonathan W. White, Lonnie Drayer, Kate Daly, Michelle Krowl, Cornelia King, Anna-Morgan Leonards, Marcy Sacks, Sarah Gardener, Amy Laurel Fluker, Janet Olson, Glenn Falgoust, Frank Jastrzembski, Mary Beth Henley, Laurie Snyder, Jonathan Tracey, William S. Cossins, and Peter Thompson shared key information and sources about some of the men whose stories are told in the book. Beth M. Lander and Caitlin Angelone at The College of Physicians of Philadelphia—my favorite archive—enthusiastically guided me through the college's inimitable collection of nineteenth-century medical daybooks, hospital records, and the papers of Silas Weir Mitchell, leading to several key discoveries. Melissa Grafe and Christopher Zollo at Yale's Medical Historical Library introduced me to the medical records of Jacob Mendes Da Costa's post–Civil War medical clinic in Philadelphia. Matthew Turi at UNC–Chapel Hill's Wilson Library steered me toward the records of the Dorothea Dix Hospital in Raleigh. Anna-Morgan Leonards and Catie White helped digitize sources during a crucial phase of research. A special thanks to the resourceful Interlibrary Loan staff of Binghamton University, Cornell Law School, Penn State, VMI, and JMU. Jim Downs, Catherine Clinton, Shauna Devine, Jane Turner Censer, and Shae Smith Cox have been generous with their time, advice, and encouragement. Megan Kate Nelson and Judkin Browning gave invaluable professional advice for an early career scholar. Mike Williams, David Stricklin, Greg Kelm, Don Brown, and Jack Goodyear at Dallas Baptist University nurtured my interest in history and gave support during a hard season; without their mentoring, I would not have gone on to graduate school.

Colleagues at Virginia Military Institute provided great company during the early phase of this book, especially M. Houston Johnson, Turk McCleskey, Mark Boonshoft, Deneise P. Shafer, Liz Elizondo Schroepfer, Madeleine Forrest Ramsey, and Geoffrey Jensen. Colleagues at James Madison University kindly welcomed me into the History Department and gave support and advice, especially Eva Carrara, Andrew Witmer, Rebecca Brannon, Steven Reich, Maura Hametz, Kevin Borg, Shah Mahmoud Hanifi, Colleen Moore, Philip Herrington, Alison Sandman, Evan Friss, Michael Gubser, Kevin Hardwick, and Meg Mulrooney. Colleagues at the George and Ann Richards Civil War Era Center at Penn State nurtured this project while I was a postdoc there in 2020–21. I am especially grateful to Rachel Shelden, Matthew Isham, Barby Singer, Cathleen Cahill, Amy S. Greenberg, Amira Rose Davis, Christina Snyder, Christopher Heaney, Dara Walker, and Moyra Williams Eaton for engaging with the manuscript and sharing sage advice. Deirdre Cooper Owens and

LeeAnn Whites read an early version of the manuscript during a workshop at the Richards Center, and their advice helped me reframe the project. Caroline E. Janney, Brian Neumann, and Elizabeth R. Varon at the Nau Civil War Center at the University of Virginia kindly welcomed me to Charlottesville. Scholars and participants at the National Museum of Civil War Medicine, the American Civil War Museum, UNC-Chapel Hill's Wilson Library, Virginia Tech's Virginia Center for Civil War Studies, and Shenandoah University's McCormick Civil War Institute asked insightful questions and shared great source leads at various stages of my research. Cadets and students at VMI, JMU, and McKinney Boyd High School were always curious about my research and asked really, really good questions. Decklan Wilkerson, my first teaching assistant at JMU, made work flow smoothly.

At Binghamton University, I was fortunate to learn from the best teachers and historians I know. My doctoral adviser, Diane Miller Sommerville, bet on me as a graduate student, and I am forever grateful she did. Diane supervised this project in dissertation form and in the process taught me how to be a historian. I can't bring to words how much her support has meant over the years. I can only wish that every student would be blessed with such an amazing adviser! Robert Parkinson encouraged me to "go big," which saved me from several pitfalls and deeply shaped my choices in the book. The late Gerald Kutcher introduced me to the history of medicine and shepherded early versions of this project. Stephen Ortiz grounded me in the early twentieth-century world of veterans and was always willing to lend an ear. Meg Leja and Alex Chase-Levenson gave comments on early versions of the project and provided candid advice on navigating the academic job market, and for that, I'm especially grateful. Bat-Ami Bar On and Wendy Wall gave crucial support while I wrapped up the dissertation. Jason Tercha, Stephen Sutherland, Melissa Franson, and Matthew Hollis laughed and commiserated, and Scott Martin and Matthew Fosheim helped keep me in good spirits during visits home to Texas.

I am grateful to my family for their support. Each one of them has shaped this book. My mom and dad, Terry Jones-Smith and Scott Jones, modeled perseverance and hard work in all circumstances, encouraged me to ask questions about anything and everything, took me to historical places, kept a constant stream of books in front of me, and above all loved and supported me. My sisters Audrey, Taylor, and Samantha, sister-in-law Saralyn, brother-in-law Eddie, and nephews Max and Alex have been the best friends I could ask for and always kept me laughing. Roy Smith has enthusiastically supported me, and I am thankful for him. I am so very thankful for Bill Meier, "Bubba," who helped raise my sisters and I, made us smart, taught us patience, and modeled unfailing generosity. Sandra Glasgow, "Tanti," gave love and kindness, and her memory is a blessing. My in-laws Chris and Maria Adkins and Marshall and

Janella Martin welcomed me into the family and have always, always been in my corner with love and encouragement. I can't express how much they have meant to me. Mogli (cat) and Chloe (dog) literally kept me on my toes, which I needed.

Most important, I owe my biggest thanks to Bethany, my wife, who has done more to support me than anybody. She believed in the project when I didn't, and her true grit has kept me going more times than I can count. Words can't say how thankful I am for her unfailing love and encouragement.

Abbreviations

AASCI   American Association for the Study and Cure of Inebriety
AMA   American Medical Association
BMSJ *Boston Medical and Surgical Journal*
GAR   Grand Army of the Republic
NHDVS   National Home for Disabled Volunteer Soldiers
QJI   *Quarterly Journal of Inebriety*
WCTU   Woman's Christian Temperance Union

Opium Slavery

Introduction

In the wake of the Civil War, thousands of Union and Confederate veterans became addicted to opiates, a tragic outcome of the war's health conditions and medical practices. Opium, morphine, and laudanum were among the war's most common medicines. Used to treat pain, diarrhea, anxiety, and more, these drugs were "important to the surgeon, as gunpower to the ordnance."[1] Opiate use was meant to mitigate the war's misery but often had disastrous, unintended consequences. An epidemic of addiction brought terrible suffering for veterans and a reckoning for American medicine. Families, doctors, government officials, and even presidents looked on in horror as "slavery" to opium—contemporary shorthand for addiction—appeared to ruin veterans' health and bodies; undermine their manhood, reputations, and whiteness; and ostensibly drive men mad. Long-term opiate use often proved unhealthy and dangerous, but even more harmful was the perception that addiction violated ideals of manhood, morality, and sanity. A culture of victim blaming meant that addicted veterans were denied pensions, ejected from soldiers' homes, and ended up in asylums, jails, and morgues.

The Civil War was far from the only cause of opiate addiction in the 1860s–90s, a period that scholars have described as witnessing America's first opioid crisis.[2] But the war helped bring addiction into focus as an epidemic. The visibility of "opium slavery" among veterans drew attention to the issue of mass addiction and raised unsettling questions about doctors' culpability as well as the government's obligation to veterans. Reactionary measures—like policing drug use through the withholding of military entitlements, the institutionalization of users, the sale of controversial patent medicine addiction "cures," and a medical "revolt" against opiates—were sometimes intended to alleviate the addiction crisis but were just as often wielded as cudgels against veterans.

Investigating opiate addiction among Civil War veterans illuminates the war's tragic human costs and provides fresh insight into its haunting legacies for American society and medicine. Reconstructing veterans' experiences of addiction also presents an unusually rich and complex portrait of opiate use in the nineteenth century, underscoring how the Civil War era was a formative period in drug history. The veterans who suffered, the families who grieved for them, the doctors who agonized over them, and the bureaucrats who punished them never fully got over or moved on from the war. Four years of slaughter and sickness left an indelible, permanent impression on many survivors' day-to-day lives and had cascading effects on postwar American society and medicine. Lingering traces of the veterans' addiction epidemic continue to ripple throughout US drug policy today.

Historians have long recognized that some Civil War veterans became addicted to opiates. In an influential 1978 essay, the pioneering drug historian David T. Courtwright convincingly argued that opiate addiction was a common, if unintended, consequence of Civil War medical care, settling a contemporary debate among historians about the causative link between the war and addiction. To date, Courtwright's essay remains the authoritative account of the phenomenon and was "for a number of years the most-cited work on any form of disability among Civil War veterans," according to James Marten.[3] In *Dark Paradise*, his foundational 1982 book, Courtwright contextualized the Civil War within the broader history of opiates in the nineteenth century.[4] These studies broke new historiographical ground but also gave voice to existing murmurs and echoes of the addiction crisis. For more than a century, references to opiate addiction have been staples in histories of the Civil War.[5]

Yet historians have not picked up where Courtwright left off by investigating the lived experiences of opiate addiction for veterans or the ways that their addictions affected postwar medicine or society. Consequently, we know next to nothing about the phenomenon beyond merely recognizing that addiction occurred. This lacuna is remarkable, considering that the Civil War era is perhaps the best-documented and most studied period in American history, with more books published about the war than the number of days elapsed since Lee's surrender at Appomattox.[6] Addiction has been oft cited but rarely analyzed in the scholarship of the Civil War era. The phenomenon first emerged as the "army disease" (sometimes "soldier's disease") in Progressive Era social-science literature on drug use before slowly bleeding into historiography of the Civil War during the twentieth century. Nods to opiate use and addiction have consistently appeared in scholarship on Civil War medicine and veterans ever since. Along the way, the morphine-addicted veteran has also become a recurring character in popular depictions of Civil War medicine. Debuting in novels during the 1860s and continuing over the next century and a half, addicted veterans resurfaced everywhere from World War I–era newspapers to 1960s medical textbooks, the 1970s television show *Little House on the Prairie*, and even congressional hearings about drug policy in the 1910s and 2010s.[7] Yet in historical scholarship, addicted veterans are almost always relegated to footnotes. A macabre Civil War curio, drug addiction among veterans has never been thoroughly investigated.

Current scholarly trends in Civil War studies, drug history, and the ongoing opioid crisis in the United States demand a fresh look. What did Americans know about opiate addiction before the Civil War? How exactly did veterans become addicted, and could military surgeons have predicted the crisis? How prevalent was addiction among survivors of the war? What were the health and personal consequences of addiction for veterans and their families, and how did they seek to mitigate those costs? Did veterans' experiences vary by race and region? And how did the lives of addicted Civil War veterans—who came from the best-documented demographic of nineteenth-century Americans and had a special place in postwar American society—compare with those of other cohorts of nineteenth-century drug users, such as white women and Chinese immigrant opium smokers? How did cultural ideas about manhood, race, and disability inflect and inform contemporary labels for addiction such as "opium slavery," and how did the ideas conveyed in these labels affect veterans' lived experiences? In what ways did the addiction crisis reflect on American physicians, whose protocols and prescriptions played a major role in causing the epidemic? How did the American medical community, society, and the growing Gilded Age state respond? Finally, what was the long-term impact of opiate addiction in the Civil War era on US drug policy, as seen through the lives of veterans and the memory of the crisis after they died? The continuing opioid crisis in the United States adds urgency to these as yet unanswered questions about the Civil War's tortured legacy of opiate addiction. In *Opium Slavery* I ask and answer these questions, reconstructing America's Civil War–era opiate epidemic in greater detail than ever before.

Until the recent mass digitization of many Civil War records, investigating the experiences and outcomes of opiate addiction for veterans was methodologically impractical, one explanation for the lack of research following up on Courtwright's landmark work. Sifting through traditional manuscript sources—handwritten letters, diaries, pension applications, and census records—takes much time, institutional resources, and serendipity. To study Civil War veterans before the age of mass digitization, historians had to travel back and forth between various state and federal archives that store such documents. Identifying even a handful of cases of addiction was akin to finding the proverbial needle in a haystack that spans tens of thousands of cubic feet in archives spread across multiple regions. This methodological approach was practical if researching a handful of men at a time but not for the kind of large-scale studies that must be undertaken to broadly and deeply survey an epidemic.[8] Thus, until recently, a fulsome investigation of the experiences of opiate-addicted Civil War veterans was unfeasible.

Utilizing newly digitized nineteenth-century medical journals, monographs, advertisements, pamphlets, newspapers, novels, coroners' inquests, military service records, census, and soldiers' home registers in conjunction with manuscript archival sources such as letters, lunacy inquests, pension applications, and rare mental asylum patient records, I identified a large sample of 200 Civil War veterans who suffered from opiate addiction in their postwar lives. Many of these individuals self-identified as being addicted. Other men were described or diagnosed as such by contemporary doctors, families, and community members. Seeking to understand the lived experiences and outcomes of opiate addiction, I investigated these veterans' military careers, postwar lives, and deaths, creating a composite portrait of addiction. Tracking these men across a spectrum of sources—for example, identifying a veteran in a mental asylum admissions log or a patent medicine testimonial, then working backward to illuminate his military experience and postwar life through service records, pension applications, registers of soldiers' homes, census data, letters, and obituaries—enables an investigation that is both granular in scale and wide-ranging in scope. This methodology allowed me to explore diverse individual stories in depth while also grappling with a broad spectrum of outcomes.

A history of opiate addiction among Civil War veterans is especially salient considering the recent burst of studies that reconstruct the traumatic experiences endured by so many survivors.[9] Although the Civil War occurred in a cultural context that lionized individual suffering—which had deep religious roots in a heavily Christian culture and offered a means of humanizing the conflict's mass anonymous killing—not all veterans relished their war days.[10] "Neo-revisionist" historians have shown that many soldiers returned home with broken bodies, hearts, and minds. War survivors exhibited seemingly aberrant behaviors and committed acts of violence to a degree that alarmed their families and communities. Some men even experienced psychological trauma akin to what is today called post-traumatic stress disorder (PTSD), although most Civil War historians do not use this modern label.[11] *Opium Slavery* builds on scholarship by Eric T. Dean Jr., James Marten, Brian Matthew Jordan, Diane Miller Sommerville, Sarah Handley-Cousins, Jeffrey W. McClurken, David Silkenat, Michael C. C. Adams, Lesley J. Gordon, Gerald F. Linderman, and Dillon J. Carroll. Collectively, these studies have illuminated the Civil War's troubling psychological and emotional legacies, consequences of military service that had long been hiding in historians' plain sight.[12] Documenting veterans' experiences with drug addiction adds chilling evidence to the scholarly interpretation of the Civil War as a conflict that deeply traumatized many people who experienced it. Of course, the majority of veterans did not become "enslaved" to opium or end up in mental asylums. Yet the absence of scholarship on men who did become addicted leaves their tremendous suffering unacknowledged and prevents historians from contextualizing the phenomenon within the broader history of the United States' bloodiest war. Clearly, a connection existed between suffering, substance use, and the Civil War. Megan L. Bever, Lorien Foote, and Andrew Fialka, among other historians, have also produced intimate depictions of alcohol use during and after the Civil War, supplementing the historiography on veterans by calling attention to what they drank, why they drank, and how drink affected them. Intoxication was embedded into the fabric of military life, and camps, depots, and hospitals were positively soddened with alcohol. Substance use in the army caused great anxiety for temperance activists, officers, and courts-martial. After the war, veterans continued imbibing heavily in spaces such as soldiers' homes, where bureaucrats sharply debated how to deal with so-called drunks.[13] The postwar epidemic of opiate addiction did not exist in a vacuum but unfolded within a broader pattern of substance use by military men. Yet some historians insist that so-called dark studies of Civil War soldiers and veterans rely too heavily on modern medical diagnoses to investigate the war's psychological legacy.[14]

Rather than getting bogged down in this now well-worn scholarly debate, *Opium Slavery* builds on the historiography of Civil War veterans by illuminating how these men and other eyewitnesses thought about and experienced addiction as a kind of war trauma.[15] Nineteenth-century medicine posited that, among other explanations, opiate addiction was a form of mental illness, either a symptom or a cause. In many cases, veterans and observers linked addiction directly to medical care for Civil War wounds, injuries, or camp fevers. Contemporary psychiatrists and addiction experts made the causative relationship between the war and addiction especially evident in postwar asylum records and medical studies. Veterans and their families, friends, and communities also used pension applications and letters to link addiction to military service. By interrogating these eyewitness accounts of what doctors sometimes called "opium mania," this book brings to light considerable previously untapped evidence showing how the Civil War generation often attributed insanity and trauma to the war.[16]

Disability history and the history of medicine likewise offer valuable frameworks for understanding the phenomenon of opiate addiction among Civil War veterans. Examining where opiates fit into nineteenth-century medicine helps explain the rise of addiction and allows for a reconstruction of the epidemic's broad contours. Exploring how addiction played out in individual veterans' lives and what they did about it requires a different analytic lens. Among other goals, disability history seeks to uncover the lived experiences of people whom society deemed "disabled" as well as the social construction of disability. Visible disabilities—especially amputations, the Civil War's signature wound—have traditionally attracted more attention from scholars, but *Opium Slavery* joins a growing number of studies on what Sarah Handley-Cousins has called "nonvisible" disabilities, such as gastrointestinal sickness and mental illness.[17]

Uncovering how nineteenth-century Americans understood and experienced addiction calls for situating opiates within the era's medical knowledge and health care systems. Margaret Humphreys has observed that "the American Civil War was the greatest health disaster that this country has ever experienced."[18] Humphreys, Jim Downs, Shauna Devine, and other scholars have documented the war's terribly infectious environment, as well as how doctors, sanitarians, and sufferers responded to mass sickness during the war and after.[19] *Opium Slavery* broadens the Civil War's medical history to include narcotics and extends the narrative chronologically. Addiction represented one of many dreadful health outcomes for survivors. But unlike the explosive epidemics of the 1860s, the postwar opiate crisis represented a slower-moving, longer-term health disaster. Opiate use typically began when soldiers were young men, during or shortly after the Civil War, but addiction often lasted a lifetime, dominating aging veterans' daily lives sometimes well into the twentieth century. Some of the men whose stories appear in *Opium Slavery* spent most of their lives battling addiction that began during the war. Illuminating the addiction epidemic not only helps uncover the traumatic and unpredictable personal costs of the Civil War but also frames the conflict as a prolonged health crisis that lingered into the twentieth century.

Medical historians have been especially concerned with the question of how the Civil War affected American medical knowledge and practices. *Opium Slavery* reconstructs nineteenth-century understandings of opiates, providing an in-depth accounting of what doctors knew (and did not know) about addiction before the modern era. It also traces how the prospect of mass opiate addiction during and after the Civil War helped usher in radical, sweeping therapeutic and conceptual changes that fundamentally altered how American doctors practiced medicine. Civil War veterans, both addicted men and the medical personnel who treated them, became deeply concerned about the addictive and poisonous nature of opiates. When we consider how the phenomenon fits into the broader development of American medicine—which became increasingly professionalized, specialized, and scientific in the late nineteenth century—it becomes clear that addiction was not merely a tangential facet of Civil War medicine. Instead, drug dependence among veterans and the therapeutic "revolt" against opiates that addiction inspired were central to the war's medical legacy. Recounting this history broadens scholars' understanding of how the conflict helped transform American medicine.

Investigating how Civil War veterans experienced and what they thought about opiate addiction also requires situating the phenomenon within the era's gender norms and racial hierarchies. Historians recognize that the war's exigencies—such as the mass departure of white men from the home, the postwar return of disabled veterans in need of support, and emancipation—sparked a broad "crisis in gender," to quote LeeAnn Whites.[20] We cannot hope to understand what addiction felt like or meant to veterans without considering this cultural context. Prevailing ideals of manhood convinced observers and, tragically, many users themselves that chronic opiate use undermined manhood by sapping men's ability to work, altering their physical appearances, and, above all, making them dependent. Addiction thus exacerbated the Civil War's gender crisis and provides a unique vantage into how it rippled throughout American society. The notion that addiction was unmanly predated the Civil War. Thus, tracing the postwar impact of this antebellum idea also shows how the Civil War stressed, but did not always overturn, cultural constructs.[21]

White veterans who became "enslaved" to opium also amplified the racial anxieties of Reconstruction and the Gilded Age. Widespread drug use by white Americans played into cultural and scientific fears about white racial decline in the context of Chinese immigration and Black freedom, providing fodder for the eugenics movement, immigration bans, and racialized drug laws. Even if deeply unsettling, white men's "slavery" to opium nonetheless proved more palatable to contemporary observers than opium smoking among Chinese immigrants, who were demonized despite being far outnumbered by white opium users. The contemporary fixation on white male "opium slaves" and Chinese opium smokers also papered over medical racism, which fostered separate drug protocols for Black Americans. Medical racism meant that enslaved people and, later, Black veterans received subpar medical care with less access to lifesaving, pain-relieving opiates. This discrimination shaped the demographics of addiction for generations.[22]

Although *Opium Slavery* is rooted in the Civil War, it engages with and complements a large body of scholarship on drugs in American society and medicine, especially concerning the late nineteenth and early twentieth centuries. Foundational studies by David T. Courtwright, Arnold Jaffe, Joseph F. Spillane, and Timothy A. Hickman, as well as more recent work by Sarah W. Tracy, Claire D. Clark, David Herzberg, and Kelly Elizabeth Gray, have established that widespread prescribing and consumption of opiates fueled a surge of mass addiction during the 1870s–1890s. These scholars also survey Gilded Age social and cultural origins of the twentieth century's racialized and class-based drug policies, which framed addiction as a "problem" long before criminalization in the early twentieth century. These fruitful studies sketch out a broad framework of responses toward the problem of addiction in the late nineteenth century, including efforts by physicians to curb overprescribing, scrutiny leveled toward patent medicines, and the inebriety movement's struggle to medicalize addiction.[23] To these findings, Susan J. Pearson and Joseph M. Gabriel add that the "new birth of regulation" in the Gilded Age—when state and local governments leveraged police powers to regulate food safety, mandate vaccines and licensure of health care professions, and enforce poison controls—set a precedent for tightly regulating narcotics.[24] Taking cues from this robust historiography, I have found that veterans' experiences with drug use provide a uniquely rich and textured window into the social, medical, and cultural history of drugs in the Gilded Age and Progressive Era.

Opium Slavery also extends historians' knowledge about drugs and addiction backward into the early and mid-nineteenth century, a period that has received less sustained attention from scholars.[25] When I puzzled over why addicted Civil War veterans were treated so harshly, late nineteenth-century developments documented by other historians provided some of the pieces. But I found explanations in the antebellum era too. By deeply investigating opiate addiction in the prewar decades, I learned that Americans developed sophisticated medical and cultural theories of addiction before the Civil War, much earlier than historians have previously realized. Antebellum ideas about addiction—especially the concept of "opium slavery" that was firmly rooted in prewar conventions of gender, race, morality, and disability—presaged the more familiar developments of the late nineteenth and early twentieth centuries. I also discovered that the antebellum decades and the Civil War helped spawn heavy-handed, punitive policies to police addiction through postwar military entitlements and asylums. By documenting this earlier history of opiates, *Opium Slavery* provides crucial context for the history of drugs in the Gilded Age, Progressive Era, and beyond.

Historians have written more about the War on Drugs than on war and drugs. Yet substances and war have gone hand in hand since long before the Civil War. More than a century and a half later, substance use disorders continue to affect American veterans, as documented by a large body of medical and social science studies. Much like their Civil War forebears, modern American veterans have often been negatively stereotyped as drug abusers.[26] Studies by David T. Courtwright, Łukasz Kamieński, and Peter Andreas have illuminated the relationship between drugs and war globally, documenting how opium and other substances have served as a cause for armed conflict and means of enduring it.[27] Yet to date, little historical scholarship exists on the relationship between drugs, war, and veterans in US history. The Civil War provides a compelling case study to fill this gap. Additionally, studies on drugs and war have rarely tracked substance use before, during, and after armed conflicts to probe veterans' outcomes and experiences with drugs. *Opium Slavery* makes such a contribution, following opiates and the men who used them from the antebellum era through the Civil War and into the postwar period. This approach not only shows how war has fueled the consumption of narcotics but also illuminates how substance use has entailed myriad long-term struggles for veterans that often ended in tragedy.

By better documenting addiction in the Civil War era, *Opium Slavery* helps contextualize today's opioid epidemic within the United States' long, tragic history of recurring opioid crises. With record levels of overdose deaths, public and scholarly interest in the origins of the opioid crisis is at an all-time high. *Opium Slavery* underscores how the stigma surrounding addiction today is much older and more deeply rooted than most Americans realize, dating back to the early nineteenth century. Ongoing efforts to reduce overprescribing, broaden access to addiction care, and destigmatize addiction by treating it as a disease instead of a vice are likewise not new. Rather, these modern solutions echo those offered up by addicted people and sympathetic Americans after the Civil War. The media's fixation on white opioid users at the expense of Black Americans likewise reflects patterns established in the Civil War era. Understanding this long, tragic historical context is paramount if we are to respond effectively to mass opioid addiction today or tomorrow.

Why Veterans?

Some readers might wonder, why focus on Civil War veterans? Does an emphasis on veterans, mostly white men, overlook other Americans who used drugs? To the contrary. Investigating veterans' experiences with addiction not only illuminates the human costs and medical legacies of the Civil War, central aims of this book, but also reveals more about addiction among other nineteenth-century Americans than it obscures. Civil War veterans are the best documented group of nineteenth-century Americans. They left a longer, wider paper trail than any other demographic, the product of hulking military bureaucracies and postwar entitlement programs. Indeed, one of the war's unexpected legacies was a boom in recordkeeping to account for the carnage. Simply put, we can know more about Civil War veterans who used opiates than any other group of users. Moreover, veterans came from all regions, classes, ages, and races, representing a cross section of American society, so we can infer that many of the hurdles faced by addicted veterans also affected their civilian neighbors. In fact, because Civil War veterans are so well documented, they have often attracted interdisciplinary attention from economists, medical and scientific researchers, and historians, all seeking to cut through the murkiness that too often shrouds the lives other nineteenth-century Americans.

Far from excluding other subjects, *Opium Slavery* uses the cases of addicted Civil War veterans to produce the most comprehensive portrait of opiate addiction in the nineteenth-century Unites States to date. Rather than overshadowing other addicted people, the uniquely robust documentation surrounding veterans provides an unparalleled window into the history of opiates, enabling scholars to more deeply investigate social history of drugs, addiction treatments, medical debates over culpability, physicians' professional responses to addiction, and the policing of drug use before criminalization, among other topics.

Sources for nonveteran drug users often do not exist. Of course, it goes without saying that using the lives of Civil War veterans (almost all men and mostly white) to study addiction necessitates weighing their experiences against those of other demographics, especially white and Black women as well as Chinese immigrants. *Opium Slavery* takes a comparative approach to paint a fulsome portrait of addiction in the Civil War era.

Organization

Opium Slavery is organized into three roughly chronological sections spanning from the antebellum era into the early twentieth century. Each section includes thematic chapters exploring various facets of opiate addiction that affected veterans' experiences. Part 1 comprises three chapters tracing the origins of the Civil War–era opiate addiction crisis back to its antebellum roots and assessing how opiate use during the war translated to widespread postwar addiction among veterans. To understand how compulsive opiate use affected veterans, it is essential to trace the emergence of addiction in the prewar American medical and cultural consciousness. We cannot comprehend the tragic experience of addiction for veterans without understanding the gendered, moral, and racialized perceptions that branded some opium users as "slaves" or the medical patterns that sparked widespread addiction.

Chapter 1 sets the medical stage for the Civil War's addiction crisis, drawing on medical journals and textbooks, didactic home health guides, prescription records, coroners' inquests, diaries, recipe books, and newspapers to illuminate how opiates became the "magnum Dei donum" of drugs, among the most commonly used and praised substances. Heroic prescribing and self-medication intersected with cheap, accessible imported opium to create conditions ripe for addiction, giving antebellum doctors ample opportunity to observe the phenomenon and articulate facets such as intoxication, tolerance, withdrawal, and overdose. Cases appeared frequently in prewar medical literature, although addiction was far less common than it would become during the postwar decades. Chapter 2 explores how addiction came to be seen as an ailment that chiefly afflicted women, the racial "other," and men with disabilities. Drawing on the rhetoric of slavery as well as the temperance, abolitionist, and missionary movements, antebellum Americans constructed a highly gendered, racialized, and ableist understanding of opium slavery that limited its menace to society by quarantining the phenomenon to marginalized peoples. Prevailing ideas about white womanhood stressed dependence and physical frailty, which in turn explained to observers why white women seemed to become addicted to opiates more often than other demographics. Similarly, observers came to believe that the few men who became "enslaved" by opium were inherently defective. Accounts by missionaries of Chinese opium smokers abroad and lurid stories about disabled male opium eaters, which peppered the medical press and media, explained away male opium use by pointing to alleged racial inferiority or physical disability. The characteristics of dependency, effeminacy, weakness, and racial inferiority became the essential qualities ascribed to opium slavery. Temperance rhetoric also informed the cultural construction of addiction, branding white men who were unmasked as opium users as intemperate sinners culpable for their addictions. Because of medical racism, addiction was infrequent among Black Americans, enslaved or free, foreshadowing the demographics of addiction after the Civil War.

With the medical and cultural stage set, chapter 3 investigates how the Civil War's health conditions and medical practices triggered a massive surge in addiction among white men, far surpassing its extent before the war. Military service records, pension applications, courts-martial files, letters, diaries, newspapers, hospital records, and medical texts tell the Civil War story of opium and morphine. Keeping with antebellum medical knowledge, Union and Confederate surgeons administered opiates in mind-boggling quantities to mitigate pain and diarrhea among the ranks. Soldiers North and South also used opiates to self-medicate for sickness, injuries, anxiety, fatigue, and stress. These medicines were essential to the Union and Confederacy's war efforts. Yet the war's health catastrophe created a perfect storm, ushering in an unprecedented deluge of addiction. Considering the antebellum stigmas surrounding opium slavery, men who habitually used opiates were deemed unpatriotic and cowardly, and were sometimes disciplined, foreshadowing the later struggles of addicted veterans.

Part 2 illuminates the social and cultural history of the postwar addiction crisis. Pension applications, letters, newspapers, records from asylums and hospitals, and medical texts provide chilling insight into addiction. Chapter 4 interrogates the lived experience of addiction for veterans. It shows how opium slavery cost veterans dearly, because of both the physical suffering it engendered and the harsh public reaction to opiate-dependent men. Observers and users widely attributed addiction directly and indirectly to medical care for war-related ailments. This realization might have made veterans seem more sympathetic than some other populations of drug users. Yet most doctors, government authorities, families, and the media nonetheless blamed the victims, reflecting the staying power of antebellum understandings of addiction. In addition to overdose deaths and myriad other poor health outcomes, veterans who became "enslaved" to opiates were widely condemned as unmanly, intemperate, and even insane. Comparing the experiences of women and men, the wealthy and poor, as well as Black, white, and Chinese opium users fleshes out the racial, gendered, and class patterns of the addiction epidemic. Medical racism translated to a lower rate of addiction among Black veterans, shaping the demographics of addiction for generations. Media coverage of Chinese opium smokers muddled the whiteness of addicted veterans in an era of profound racial turmoil and anxiety. Despite the unsettling racial implications of opium slavery for white veterans, whiteness nonetheless shielded them from the harshest social outcomes of opiate use, reserved for Chinese immigrants.

Harmful medical and cultural ideas about opium slavery had tangible costs for veterans. Mining asylum case files, chapter 5 shows how addicted veterans were often institutionalized because of the long-standing notion that excessive opiate use could cause insanity, as evidenced by some users' apparent lack of self-control, deceptiveness, and violent tendencies. Many veterans spent years or even decades trapped in unsanitary, dangerous asylums, where they lost control over their bodies and medical choices, endured lonely separations from loved ones, and were made to work without pay. The asylum records explored at length in chapter 5 also undergird much of the book elsewhere, so this chapter peels back the methodological curtain and probes some of the thorny issues involved with the use of historical asylum records. Chapter 6 uses pension applications and soldiers' home records to investigate addicted veterans' interactions with military entitlement programs. Pensions and soldiers' homes served as a crucial means for the Gilded Age state to police addiction in an era before the criminalization of drugs. Because of the stigma surrounding opium slavery, politicians and bureaucrats went out of their way to block addicted veterans' access to pensions and soldiers' homes, shunting addicted men into jails and mental asylums. Government bureaucrats further stigmatized drug use through rulings and policies designed to ferret out secret opium users, although addicted veterans were not without allies. Some old soldiers spent their entire adult lives fighting for meager pensions, with little to show for it but rejection. Even the widows and children of addicted veterans were excluded from entitlements, sometimes by presidential veto, cutting against the current of the massive expansion of pension programs late in the nineteenth century. Some drug-using veterans had a degree of success in obtaining medical care for addiction at soldiers' homes, suggesting that the nineteenth-century government response to addiction was not monolithic and that self-advocacy could be an effective tool to contest the social harms of addiction.

Part 3 investigates medical responses to opiate addiction and situates this history within broader developments in late nineteenth- and early twentieth-century medicine and drugs. Chapter 7 uses patent medicine advertisements to reconstruct the bustling postwar industry of opiate addiction remedies, cures, and antidotes. Invented by entrepreneurial Civil War veterans with insider knowledge of addiction, patent medicines made some former soldiers filthy rich. Some of these patent medicines might have "worked" in a limited clinical sense; equally important, they provided a means for veterans to contest the stigma of addiction by narrating their stories in product testimonials. Yet many desperate users only grew poorer after gambling small fortunes on these controversial products. The commercial success of patent medicines also invited attacks by skeptical physicians, journalists, and reformers. A considerable backlash against proprietary medicines sought to discredit and squeeze them out of the competitive medical marketplace, helping set the stage for consumer protection laws in the early twentieth century.

Chapter 8 turns to physicians and the medical journals, books, and prescription records they left behind to assess the profession's response to mass addiction, both among Civil War survivors and the many other Americans who used drugs. Veterans and other users vocally blamed doctors as the culprits behind the addiction epidemic. Some physicians took this criticism to heart out of sympathy toward their addicted patients. Other doctors grew alarmed because the commotion threatened the credibility of allopathic medicine and its position in the medical marketplace. Physicians, including several leading former Civil War surgeons who had treated addicted veterans, responded to the epidemic by staging what they called a "revolt" against opium. They embarked on a constellation of reforms during the 1870s–90s intended to stem the tide of addiction and rehabilitate physicians' professional reputations. These reforms unfolded within a broader framework of themes that will be familiar to historians of American medicine and drugs, such as professionalization, specialization, regulation, and medicalization. Some doctors tried to redefine the opium "habit" as a disease called "inebriety" that ought to be treated by addiction experts in specialized clinics, akin to modern drug addiction rehabilitation facilities. Leading physicians also devalued opiates in the materia medica and self-regulated their prescribing to avoid causing iatrogenic addiction, a profound rejection of foundational therapeutic practices dating back decades. Exploring these medical responses to addiction helps situate Civil War veterans in the dynamic world of nineteenth-century American medicine and underscores the war's transformative effects on medical practice. Finally, the epilogue explores the memory of the postwar addiction epidemic in the twentieth-century United States, particularly how the example of opiate-addicted Civil War veterans was used to argue in favor of harsh drug policies throughout the War on Drugs.

Terminology

The use of terms like "opium slavery," "addiction," and "epidemic" warrants careful explanation. Many of the harms associated with substance use and addiction have historically been derived not from the inherent act of consumption but from perceptions ascribed to drug users by other people. To avoid perpetuating stigma, in recent years there has been a shift in medicine and the media away from harmful labels like "addict" and drug "abuse." *Opium Slavery* adopts this approach. For several reasons, I have chosen to employ nineteenth-century terminology instead. "Opium slavery" and similar contemporary terms appear throughout the book, especially when quoting or paraphrasing primary sources, but not without caution. Like "addict," older nineteenth-century labels such as "opium slaves," "opium eaters," and "opium habit" are problematic in their own right. If used without qualification, this language risks perpetuating the historical stigmatization of drug users. Describing addiction as "slavery" without qualification also falsely equates it to chattel slavery, an unrealistic and immoral juxtaposition. By using nineteenth-century labels, I do not seek to endorse the harmful characterizations of drug users that these labels were originally meant to convey. Rather, I employ these terms to reconstruct the medical and cultural context in which Civil War veterans used opiates. Omitting contemporary labels for addiction and addicted people would obscure veterans' experiences and shroud the cultural and medical construction of addiction that occurred during their lifetimes. It would also be impossible to write an accurate and complete history of the Civil War–era opiate addiction epidemic without quoting extensively from primary source material. I have taken care to add quotation marks around the term "opium slave" when discussing individuals to foster a critical distance from harsh nineteenth-century views of drug users.

I use the label "addiction" throughout the book, partly because nineteenth-century Americans themselves used the word to describe dependency to opiates, albeit far less frequently than other contemporary labels.[28] Of course, addiction has a malleable definition, meaning different things to different people in different times and places.[29] Recognizing that historical conceptions of addiction cannot be understood devoid of context and that historical diagnoses rarely map neatly onto their modern counterparts, I have taken care to avoid retrospective diagnosis. I only ascribe addiction to veterans when they, or close contemporary observers such as family, friends, or physicians, made such diagnoses. Nineteenth-century opiate users commonly switched back and forth between various preparations and modes of use. Reflecting contemporary language, I use such catchall terms as "opium addiction," "opium eating," and "opium slavery" when referring to various opiates in common use, including morphine and laudanum, except in cases where substances are specified in the relevant primary sources.

I approach the concept of addiction with a dose of medical realism. Drug historian Nancy D. Campbell has persuasively argued that to do justice to the history of narcotics, we must take the biology of addiction seriously—we must "think pharmacologically."[30] This approach allows historians to understand the changes that occurred in the bodies of Civil War veterans, ultimately leading to a more authentic reconstruction of the addiction epidemic and individual experiences within it. Considering modern knowledge about opiate pharmacology also offers a legible counterpoint against which we can contrast historical theories of addiction. Comparing earlier theories of addiction to present-day understandings makes it easier to clearly articulate otherwise murky historical ideas that do not always translate across time and cultures. It is delicate work to navigate the tension between explanations of addiction that prioritize biology and explanations that recognize addiction as being a socially constructed "problem."[31] Yet as historians Diane Miller Sommerville, Sarah Handley-Cousins, and Kidada E. Williams have noted, the tools of modern medicine *can* help us better understand the Civil War era. Indeed, it is impossible to fully comprehend the often-traumatic experiences of war survivors without such knowledge.[32]

The label "epidemic" is useful for characterizing the opiate crisis that plagued the United States during the late nineteenth century. The term was sometimes used by contemporary observers to describe a surge in opiate use and addiction. The phenomenon of mass addiction in the late nineteenth century also fits with historian Charles E. Rosenberg's classic definition of an epidemic as "elicit[ing] immediate and widespread response." Epidemics are characterized by the observers' perception that a crisis is afoot, which garners fear, soul-searching, scapegoating, and sometimes reforms—all of which characterized opiate addiction after the Civil War.[33] Several drug historians, including David T. Courtwright, Timothy A. Hickman, David Herzberg, Nancy D. Campbell, and Elizabeth Kelly Gray, have likewise characterized the Gilded Age as witnessing America's first opioid addiction crisis. These scholars rightfully observe that Civil War veterans represented only one demographic within a broader epidemic. No one counted how many veterans became addicted to opiates, and by no means was addiction exclusively the consequence of the Civil War or the domain of ex-soldiers. Unfettered capitalism, the unregulated and democratized state of medicine and health care, Gilded Age social changes, and myriad other forces created a sweeping addiction crisis. Although we cannot know with certainty how many veterans became addicted to opiates because of primary source limitations, it is clear that Civil War veterans comprised a minority among the hundreds of thousands of Americans who regularly used opiates.[34] Adopting the framework of an epidemic better situates addicted veterans within the broader opiate crisis that rippled throughout American society in the late nineteenth century.

PART I

Origins

Chapter 1

The Magnum Dei Donum of the Materia Medica

The Rise of Opiates in Antebellum American Medicine

By the time the Civil War erupted in 1861, American doctors viewed opiates as the most important drugs in their arsenal. They called opium the "magnum Dei donum," or God's great gift, and used opiates to treat hundreds of ailments. Opium and its many derivatives were so popular that it is tempting to assume their widespread use during the war was predestined. Yet their ubiquity during and after the conflict was not inevitable. A unique set of factors emerged in the antebellum era to catalyze the widespread use of opiates, setting the stage for an addiction crisis later in the nineteenth century. Charting the rise of opiates in antebellum America, including their medicinal uses and contemporary medical knowledge about their risks, is crucial to understanding the complex tragedy that unfolded during the war and postwar decades.

Opium from Origins to the Early Republic

Opium is among humankind's most storied drugs. Likely originating in Neolithic Europe, where farmers first cultivated poppies, opium has been a staple of Western medicine for thousands of years.[1] From ancient Greece and Rome through the Middle Ages and the Scientific Revolution, Western medical authorities wielded opium against a wide spectrum of maladies, although the drug was not yet the "magnum Dei donum" of medicine as it would later become during the Civil War era.[2] Eighteenth- and nineteenth-century Americans cited the medical authorities of antiquity and the Enlightenment as precedent for prescribing opium. Well-read doctors recalled how titanic figures such as Hippocrates, the ancient Greek "father of medicine," and influential Roman physician Galen extolled the virtues of opium. European medical luminaries from Paracelsus in the sixteenth century to Thomas Sydenham, John Brown, and William Cullen in the eighteenth century likewise embraced opiates and drilled their utility into American students who ventured abroad for top-notch medical educations, which were not readily available in the United States.[3]

American doctors of the early republic inherited an old opium tradition and embraced the drug with gusto. When John Jones, a Philadelphia physician who personally attended Benjamin Franklin and George Washington, published the republic's first surgical treatise in 1775, the landmark book zealously endorsed "the sovereign and almost divine power of opium." As if emulating Hippocrates and Galen were not reason enough to prescribe opium, the drug's pain-killing properties, to which Jones alluded, offered pragmatic justification.[4] Unsurprisingly, considering Jones's effusive praise for opium, some historians suggest that Benjamin Franklin became addicted late in life. As with many suspected addiction cases, it is difficult to know with certainty, but not implausible.[5] Opiates were among the only effective pain-relieving drugs available before the mid-to-late nineteenth-century introduction of aspirin, acetaminophen, the bromides, and chloral hydrate.[6] Opium made life in a harsh world bearable, a key reason why it outlived other ancient remedies and became a staple of American medicine.

The trouble with opium, however, was its addictiveness. The longer one took an opiate to treat pain or other ailments, the more accustomed to the drug the body became. After swallowing opium consistently for a few weeks or longer, it often became hard to quit, an outcome that was obvious to many doctors and laypeople long before the Civil War. If opiate use has deep roots in American history, so too does the recognition of opiate dependency and its framing as a problem. Observant travelers touring the fledgling republic occasionally noted cases of dependence. Passing through Nantucket in 1782, J. Hector St. John de Crèvecœur reported how some Quaker women practiced the "Asiatic custom of taking a dose of opium every morning; and so deeply rooted is it, that they would be at a loss how to live without this indulgence." They "would rather be deprived of any necessity than forgo their favorite luxury."[7] Even without the modern label of "addiction," Crèvecœur's language hinted at nascent understandings of opiate abuse. Within a generation, Americans would come to define opiate dependence as sinful, a gendered phenomenon mostly afflicting women, and an exotic custom of the racial other.

Doctors played an early and crucial role in defining opiate addiction as a concern. Benjamin Rush, the so-called father of American medicine, observed opium's dangers firsthand. As a student at Edinburgh Medical School, Rush learned from the influential William Cullen how to treat tetanus, colic, and fevers with opium.[8] Throughout his medical career, Rush routinely prescribed or recommended opium and laudanum, even to his patient Thomas Jefferson, who had opium poppies cultivated by enslaved people at Monticello.[9] Rush's letters describe multiple encounters with people whom the doctor perceived as addicted to opium. In 1795, he treated a twenty-five-year-old man who took "50 to 90 grains in a day," leaving him "in great distress of mind, and much debilitated in body." Rush advised the man to "leave off the use of opium gradually" and substitute it with "strong coffee," fern tea, garlic, ether, and zinc, among other medicines. Following this advice, the man endured weeks of diarrhea and other withdrawal symptoms.[10] In May 1812, Rush received a desperate plea for help from Bushrod Washington, Supreme Court justice and nephew of George Washington. The younger Washington's wife, Julia Ann Blackburn Washington, was severely dependent on laudanum. Washington sought Rush's advice on how to "conquer" his wife's addiction, hinting that her dependence was perceived as problematic. Rush's grave reply confirmed that "the habitual use of opium is often attended with the most serious and distressing consequences." Chronic opium use "weakens and disorders" the body, culminating in "idiotism and madness." To escape this harrowing fate, Rush urged Bushrod to taper down Julia's daily laudanum dose slowly over several weeks until she no longer craved the drug. Recognizing that this regimen of forced withdrawal would be physically agonizing and emotionally distressing, Rush advised that Julia should also be dosed with wine, porter, and assorted stimulants during the ordeal.[11] Considering Rush's well-documented obsession with alcohol and intemperance, it is unsurprising that he possessed a sophisticated awareness of the physical characteristics of opiate addiction and had a well-thought-out plan to treat it.[12] Indeed, the complexity of Rush's gradual withdrawal method suggests that, like alcohol dependence, opiate addiction as a consequence of long-term opiate use was known to educated, elite physicians, who recognized what to do for patients like Julia Washington because they had encountered such cases before.

Well-documented cases like that of Julia Washington notwithstanding, there is little evidence indicating that opiate addiction was a widespread problem in the United States before the 1820s. The conditions needed to facilitate widespread addiction had not yet materialized. Most important, opiates were not widely available. Most opium consumed in the nineteenth-century United States was imported from Asia and, until mid-century, was usually funneled through northeastern port cities. Although no statistics are available to gauge opium imports prior to 1827, the bustling Asia trade did not develop until the 1820s, which means opiates were most likely relatively scarce commodities prior to that decade.[13] Americans living near seaports, like the women of Nantucket and wealthy elites with well-stocked medicine cabinets, such as Benjamin Franklin, Thomas Jefferson, and Julia Washington, could readily obtain opium. But ordinary Americans probably had less access. An early nineteenth-century recipe book, compiled between 1800 and 1831 by a well-heeled New York City family, included scores of carefully scribed medicinal formulas for such maladies as "the bite of a mad dog," "putrid sore throat," dysentery, coughs, aches, and pains. Yet despite the family's financial means and location, opiates appeared in only 10 percent of the pre-1826 recipes, compared with 38 percent of the antebellum entries. The infrequent appearance of opium in the earliest recipes suggests that even wealthy families used opiates relatively sparingly before the 1820s.[14]

Opiates in Antebellum Medicine

The situation changed beginning in the 1820s, when geopolitical, commercial, and social trends converged to make opiates widely available to middling white Americans. Opium imports surged with the growth of the Asia trade. Most of the global opium supply in the nineteenth century originated in the sun-drenched poppy fields of Turkey and India. To produce opium, laborers (often unfree) cut small incisions into the bulb of an opium poppy, the *Papaver somniferum*. A milky white, viscous fluid oozed out and dripped into collection trays. As the latex oxidized and dried, it turned brown. Harvesters collected the raw opium and kneaded it into "lumps, varying in size from half a pound to three pounds of globular shape."[15] Balls of opium were loaded into crates, often stored in the vast warehouses of the British East India Company. From 1797, it monopolized the production of Indian opium for export to China. Wanting Chinese tea but with little to trade for it, the British turned to the sale of addictive opium to correct an unfavorable trade balance and underwrite their empire.

The British-dominated traffic in opium roughly doubled in volume with each decade between 1811 and 1839. Yet John Bull craved more and more profit and power. So, in 1839–42 and again in 1856–58, British naval guns forcibly opened Canton (present-day Guangzhou) and other Chinese ports to the opium trade against the wishes of the Qing imperial government, which despised the drug and repeatedly tried to ban it. The Opium Wars facilitated an unprecedented surge in the global opium supply. By 1839, the volume of opium flowing from India to China stood at 36,000 chests annually (about 6 million pounds), mushrooming to about 77,000 chests by 1870.[16] American newspapers derisively quipped that the opium trade was a kind of "slavery" imposed by Britain on China. Yet some Americans jumped at the chance to siphon opium from Chinese ports or to purchase it directly from Turkish suppliers.[17] Merchant firms imported the valuable commodity through New York City, Boston, San Francisco, and other ports. These firms—including Boston's Perkins & Company and the Canton trading house Russell & Company, founded by Warren Delano Jr., the grandfather of President Franklin Delano Roosevelt—enriched some of the nation's earliest millionaires.[18] Sporadic efforts made to cultivate opium domestically were dwarfed by opium imports.[19]

The transportation revolution that began in earnest during the 1820s facilitated the distribution of imported opium throughout bustling domestic markets. From coastal ports, a tentacle-like network of canals, turnpikes, and railroads carried opium to regional markets on the cheap. Like whiskey, coffee, and countless other commodities, the availability of opium skyrocketed while prices plummeted.[20] For the first time, ordinary Americans living far inland could consistently access a variety of inexpensive opiates. Pharmacies, general stores, and doctors sold raw "gum" opium to be taken orally. One South Carolina doctor sold a patient a piece of gum opium in August 1856 for a mere twenty-five cents.[21] However, opium has a bitter taste, which some consumers found nauseating. To appease sensitive stomachs, one could also purchase opium pills, neatly manufactured in humming apothecary shops or by individual doctors by combining raw opium with soap, gooey mucilage, powdered ginger, or cinnamon. The pills looked like a pea and were sold by the dozen.[22] Opium could also be combined with alcohol to create laudanum and paregoric, weaker but more palatable tinctures measured out in drops and fluid ounces. Laudanum was perhaps the most used opiate preparation in the first half of the century.[23] Some families prepared it at home with cinnamon and cloves.[24] Doctors, apothecaries, and home-healers also compounded powdered opium with various ingredients to make innumerable concoctions. Dover's powder, a standard formulation containing opium and ipecac, was popular until the Gilded Age.[25] Opium could also be synthesized into morphine, an alkaloid that was ten times more powerful and more palatable than gum opium. Yet "morphia," the Latin name, was scarce before the Civil War. The powerful drug required sophisticated chemistry to manufacture, unlike home-brewed laudanum or opium pills.[26] Hypodermic morphine injections were practically unheard of in the prewar years because American physicians had not yet adopted the hypodermic syringe. More often, morphine (and sometimes opium) was administered in salt form. Morphine sulfate could be swallowed or applied topically by rubbing the drug on the skin near a troublesome body part.[27]

Medical revolutions collided with wars and international trade to dramatically accelerate opiate use after 1820. In the early republic, opium had been merely one of many drugs that doctors could call on to treat illness. Physicians considered cinchona bark, ipecac, foxglove, camphor, and sassafras root, among many other drugs, to be just as useful for various fevers and maladies. But during the antebellum decades, opium emerged as a mainstay of the "heroic medicine" that became popular among American physicians, thanks in part to the influential Benjamin Rush and his acolytes. Rush believed in aggressive interventions, so the heroic physicians who emulated him prized therapies that yielded quick, visible, and dramatic effects. Heroics bled, purged, puked, and drugged their sick patients nearly—or occasionally—to death.[28] Extreme measures were appealing because heroics believed that sickness was primarily caused by imbalances in the body's humors and fluids, triggered by complex interactions between a person's constitution, habits, and environment.[29] Facial redness or a hot-to-the-touch forehead signaled a brain "congested" by too much hot blood. The obvious solution was to slice open a vein with a lancet and drain the excess fluid until the patient's temperature dropped.

Twenty-first-century Americans often find heroic therapies jarring. But to many antebellum Americans—blissfully unaware of the invisible microbes recognized later in the nineteenth century as the cause of many sicknesses—bleeding and other heroic measures made perfect sense.[30]

Like bleeding, opiates visibly *did something* to the body, and many sick people felt that opium's something was better than nothing at all, making opium and laudanum extremely attractive in the era of heroic medicine. At the bedside, medicine involved negotiation between doctors and health care consumers, and the latter had considerable leverage over what their doctors prescribed—after all, most "patients" were simply paying customers. As one doctor observed, "The public expect something more of physicians than the power of distinguishing diseases" and fatalistically relaying prognoses. Instead, the ill "look to them for the relief of their sufferings, and the cure or removal of their complaints."[31] For their part, doctors were equally enthusiastic about prescribing opiates, and not just because they believed in the drugs' clinical efficacy. Medicine was an intensely competitive and low-profit-margin business for most antebellum practitioners. To make a living, they had to provide remedies that literally *appeared* to work. Opium fit the bill nicely, quickly and visibly warding off the symptoms of everyday ailments like painful "Pointed articles, sticking in the Body."[32] Opiates induced sleep, a convenient way to calm frustrated patients with "agitated" brains.[33] Doctors and patients prized opium as an antidiarrheal, "a nervous stimulant, a pain-killer, a sedative, and a narcotic," discordant roles that the drug managed to fulfill simultaneously depending on bedside deliberations. The consumer's unique constitution and the variety and amount of opiate administered also influenced which of these seemingly contradictory effects might result from taking the drugs.[34]

Opium's antidiarrheal properties made the drug especially valuable. Twenty-first-century Americans tend to think of opioids as painkillers, but in the nineteenth century, opium, laudanum, and Dover's powder were commonly used to treat diarrhea. Opiates reduce intestinal motility, preventing stools from moving through the bowels. A hefty dose of opium or laudanum might trigger stubborn constipation, a useful effect for counteracting diarrhea, a major health problem in unsanitary nineteenth-century America.[35] Eating poorly cooked food contaminated by unseen bacteria from unwashed hands or drinking feces-laden water from a nearby stream often led to diarrhea a few hours or days later. Everyday nineteenth-century maladies like ague (malaria), gastroenteritis, and hookworm often involved severe diarrhea too. No mere nuisance, such cases could lead to deadly dehydration. Thus unchecked diarrhea had to be stopped to rebalance the constitution and restore health. Elisha Bartlett, a Kentucky physician and professor at Transylvania University, one of the nation's oldest and westernmost medical schools, described treating a patient suffering from severe diarrhea. Worried about the the man, Bartlett urgently consulted with a colleague steeped in knowledge about such health problems. Only one remedy would save the patient's life, the colleague insisted. Bartlett must "cork him up; plug him up. Give him opium. Give him opium."[36]

The momentum of westward migration intensified Americans' diarrheal distress and their appetite for opium. Between the 1820s and the 1850s, the United States grew voraciously, doubling in size with the Louisiana Purchase in 1803 and expanding again with annexation of Texas in 1845 and the Mexican Cession three years later. Having violently dispossessed Native Americans and Mexicans, enthusiastic settlers and the people they enslaved poured into newly opened territories and states. Yet these unfamiliar, unsettling landscapes boded ill for health. Settlers' letters reveal deep-seated anxieties about how slow, snaking rivers and low-lying swamps might affect their well-being. They were right to worry. Malaria was endemic in the South and West, punctuated by frequent epidemics of yellow fever. Unaware of the mosquito-borne microbes behind these diseases, settlers attributed them to miasmas, or unhealthy smells, that wafted from rivers and swamps.[37] To defend against malaria and yellow fever, which caused diarrhea, nausea, and malaise, settlers turned to opium. A dose or two, often coupled with some quinine, allowed settlers to go about the cruel business of manifest destiny. During the Civil War, when Union and Confederate armies surged back and forth across the sickly South, opiates would again defend armies against miasmatic fevers.

Antebellum cholera epidemics also accelerated the use of opiates. Cholera was relatively unknown to American doctors before the 1830s. They scrambled to find effective remedies when the terrifying disease appeared on American shores, arriving by steamships and spreading throughout the nation by riverboat.[38] Cholera struck with terrifying speed. Its hallmark rice-water diarrhea could kill within hours, although most people recovered. Cholera's penchant for striking in public places was also terribly embarrassing, unraveling the Victorian obsession with privacy and self-control. Opium seemed a godsend. Rhode Island physician David B. Slack explained in 1830 how opium could be used to check the "forceful discharge of fluids" that "often carries off" cholera patients. Because opium can "cut short the discharge," he argued, "I think we are bound to give it at the earliest intermission."[39] Another doctor warned in 1832 that "we shall unquestionably have occasion for its [opium's] boldest employment, in case our country should be visited with epidemic cholera."[40]

These insights were prescient. During the cholera epidemics that ravaged the nation over and over in the 1830s and 1840s, American doctors took Slack's advice, widely employing opiates to treat cholera patients.[41] Clinicians across the country experimented with various protocols and shared their findings. One doctor explained in the *Boston Medical and Surgical Journal* (*BMSJ*) that he treated cholera with three grains of oral opium, followed by an additional grain every hour until "discharges" ceased.[42] In an Indiana newspaper, another practitioner recommended a "pretty full dose" of opium for cholera.[43] Suddenly, opium was on everyone's minds. Newspapers circulated opium-based "specific" remedies for cholera. As ordinary folks desperately searched for anything that could ward off the terrifying traveling scourge, opiate remedies made their way into family recipe books.[44] The more severe the case, the stronger the dose warranted. Sometimes fatal overdoses resulted. "Opiates [were] of the first importance" during the antebellum cholera outbreaks, an elderly practitioner recalled in 1870, when cases of addiction found increasing newspaper coverage. But "no doubt they have been greatly abused. In the epidemic of 1849 especially their use was carried to great excess. I saw patients in a state of profound narcotism, who seemed to me to be dying from the effects of the medicine rather than the disease; and it was the remark of one of the best practitioners in Louisville at that day, Dr. Coleman Rogers, that 'opium was killing more people than cholera.'"[45] While hindsight likely swayed this impression, cholera doubtless helped popularize opium in the United States.[46]

As the example of cholera illustrates, opiates were especially useful when physicians needed to compensate for gaps in medical knowledge, many of which emerged in the antebellum decades. Although they practiced medicine decades before the development of germ theory, observant mid-century doctors recognized their inability to identify the root causes of many sicknesses that modern medicine ascribes to germs. The uncomfortable realization that unknowable forces might be behind diseases like cholera left antebellum physicians less confident in their abilities to cure sickness than the doctors of Rush's generation. This lack of confidence made opiates even more valuable at the bedside. Opium papered over creeping voids in medical knowledge by reliably relieving the symptoms of mysterious sicknesses that doctors struggled to understand with the diagnostic tools at their disposal.

Increasingly fatalistic about their ability to cure illness, many antebellum physicians embraced palliative medicine during the 1840s and 1850s. Opiates were already medicine's best-known painkillers, so this palliative turn only accelerated their use.[47] James Thacher of Plymouth, Massachusetts, spoke for many of his peers when he observed that if "the patient is tormented with intolerable pain, recourse must be had to opium as the only solace."[48] Extremely utilitarian substances, opium and morphine pills and salts, laudanum, and their milder cousins, paregoric and Dover's powder, could be swallowed, swigged, applied as a poultice, dusted into open wounds, or even inserted into the anus or vagina as suppositories. Nor did pain have to be intolerable to warrant a dose of opium. Minor aches also warranted relief. "A few drops of the tincture of opium mixed with warm oil" could be poured into the ear canal to relieve earache, coupled with "a proper dose of tincture of opium taken internally" for good measure. Opium offered comfort and a good night's rest for parent and child.[49]

Between the 1820s and the Civil War, the increased global and domestic trade in opium, westward expansion, burgeoning epidemics, and medical trends coalesced to make opiate use increasingly commonplace. Indeed, by the time that South Carolina guns fired on Fort Sumter in April 1861, American physicians were fully convinced that opiates were the most utilitarian drugs, so valuable that their use outweighed the long-understood risk of addiction. It was as if God himself wanted doctors to prescribe opium. A South Carolina medical student explained in 1857 that opium was "the 'Magnum Dei Donum' of the Materia Medica."[50] The young man, armed with a bottle of opium, entered his new practice confident that he could tackle the symptoms of any ailment under the sun, even if he did not understand its causes. Samuel DuBois, another soon-to-be physician, illustrated his faith in opium on the cover page of his 1855 University of Michigan medical thesis. In careful, sentimental quill and pencil strokes, DuBois sketched an angel descending from heaven, carrying an opium poppy down to earth for mankind's benefit. "Opium," DuBois wrote, "is a divine gift from heaven." (See fig. 1.1.) This rhetoric was more than artful flourish. Nineteenth-century America was a cruel world, full of sickness, starvation, and violence. Yet if God allowed Americans to suffer such hardships, physicians like DuBois—who identified overwhelmingly as Christian amid a backdrop of the Second Great Awakening's evangelical revivals and reform movements—took solace in their faith that the Heavenly Father provided opium for his children to ease their corporeal misery. "Thank God for opium!" added another doctor in 1854. "It is an undoubted blessing that the Creator should have permitted such an antidote to the sufferings of mankind."[51] Eleven years later, President Abraham Lincoln would remind Americans that God's wrath over slavery had brought on the Civil War. The 750,000 deaths "drawn with the sword," Lincoln explained, were payment for centuries of "blood drawn with the lash."[52] Yet if the war was indeed divine punishment, at least the Civil War generation could again turn to opium, God's gift, to assuage his wrath.

Armed with the conviction that opiates were a gift from God, antebellum doctors prescribed them for more ailments than ever. "The diseases in which opium is applicable . . . are almost as numerous as the list of diseases which human flesh is heir to," a medical student observed in 1856.[53] Antebellum medical textbooks, materia medica commentaries, medical guidebooks and dictionaries, prescription books, and home health guides named approximately 150 medical conditions that physicians believed could be remedied or alleviated by opiates. These maladies ranged from the most familiar afflictions of nineteenth-century life—the "common Griping of Children," consumption,

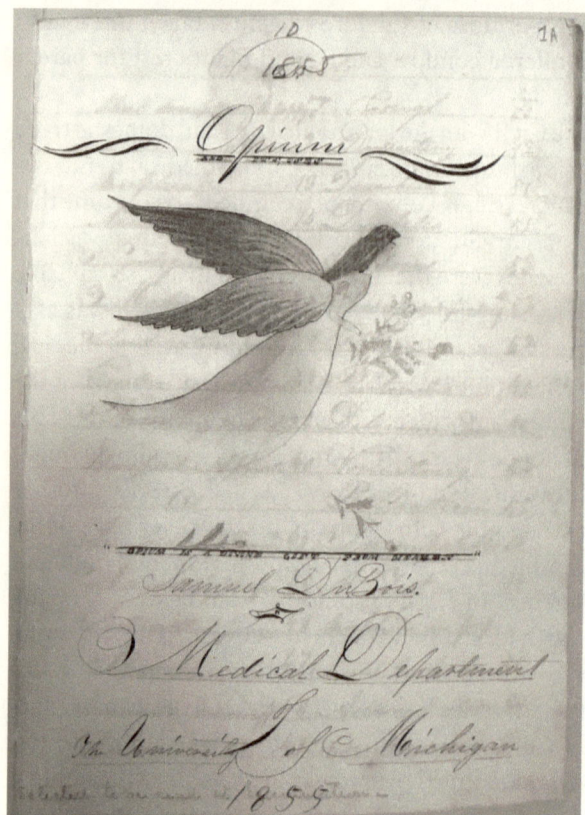

Figure 1.1 This drawing depicts an angel descending from heaven with an opium poppy. The caption reads: "opium is a divine gift from heaven." Frontispiece, Samuel DuBois medical thesis, 1855, Bentley Historical Library, University of Michigan, Ann Arbor.

coughing fits, diabetes, fatigue, various fevers, hangover, hiccups, muscle spasms, nausea, syphilis, and toothaches—to the odd and idiosyncratic, even by antebellum standards, such as arsenic and mercury poisoning, the "bite of a mad dog," "sloughing ulcer," and "St. Vitus's Dance."[54] A South Carolina doctor prescribed an opium and zinc ointment to a nursing mother who suffered from sore nipples in May 1858.[55] Another doctor considered opium and laudanum "the sovereign remedy[s]" for painful snake bites.[56] A budding practitioner recommended injecting laudanum into the urethra to treat urinary incontinence.[57] Whereas previous generations of physicians might have given any number of alternative drugs for these ailments, antebellum doctors' first impulse was often to prescribe opium. In fact, in the mid-1840s, when Connecticut physician Allyn Merriam Hungerford compiled a personal compendium of prescriptions for various ailments, he included opiates in about half of the formulas.[58]

Utilitarian opiates thus became among the most widely prescribed drugs in the United States by the time of the Civil War. Rare mid-nineteenth-century prescription records left behind by doctors, pharmacies, and hospitals illuminate the prescribing practices of "regular" allopathic physicians, confirming that doctors prescribed opiates heavily. Three New Jersey physicians trained in Philadelphia—the epicenter of American medicine for much of the nineteenth century—who shared a prescription book in 1853 and 1854 included opiates in about 36 percent of their prescriptions, mostly in combination with other drugs. Overall, opium was their second most prescribed ingredient, second only to mercury.[59] Not only were opiate prescriptions ubiquitous, but their use also became increasingly common as the antebellum decades progressed. John Harley Warner's analysis of the casebooks kept at Massachusetts General Hospital indicates that opiates were present in roughly 45 percent of prescriptions written during the 1820s and 1830s. This rate skyrocketed to an astonishing 62 percent in the decade preceding the Civil War.[60]

Naturally, the opiate prescribing rate varied by region and individual practitioner. Choices were influenced by proximity to well-stocked marketplaces and the ailments peculiar to any given locale. Individual training, skill, temperament, and one's professional networks also mattered. University training and access to the bustling marketplaces of Philadelphia, Boston, and New York City meant that elite Northeastern physicians had numerous alternatives to opium, potentially reducing reliance on it. This was certainly true of calomel, another drug prized by heroic physicians, but one that elite doctors at Massachusetts General Hospital prescribed less frequently and in lower doses than did their western colleagues.[61] Yet even accounting for training and region, evidence suggests that by mid-century the opiate prescribing rate was high across the board. In the South, where diarrheal fevers and dangerous miasmas seemed especially common and well-trained physicians were fewer in number, doctors relied more heavily on opiates. Orders filled at Charleston's Pankin Drug Store were heavily laden with opium, present in about 43 percent of prescriptions filled between November 1853 and June 1855, considerably higher than in previous decades.[62] In 1834, opium was present in only 19.1 percent of prescriptions filled at a Baltimore pharmacy.[63] Farther west, where the land was even more insalubrious and well-educated physicians fewest in number, the opiate prescribing rate was even higher. At Cincinnati's Commercial Hospital, a facility catering to sick riverboat workers and poor migrants, opiates were present in a staggering 78 percent of prescriptions in the 1830s. Bucking national trends, the hospital's opiate prescription rate declined to 59 percent in the 1840s and 53 percent in the following decade. Even still, the Commercial Hospital's high opiate prescribing rate remained on par with national averages.[64]

Doctors' daybooks and account books provide a close-up view of prescribing patterns at the ground level, underscoring the zeal for opiates. These invaluable but underutilized sources recorded information such as doctors' comings and goings, daily appointments, medical visits, and fees. The practice of medicine sometimes contrasted sharply with the lofty ideals expressed in medical commentaries. Yet concerning opiates, most doctors seem to have practiced what the textbooks preached. The young Philadelphia physician Henry Hartshorne recorded in his daybook how he treated a Mrs. Rogers for an attack of severe abdominal pain and bloody diarrhea in October 1848. For six days, Hartshorne administered opium pills, laudanum "injections" (possibly enemas), and paregoric, which did the trick and suppressed the diarrhea. Despite earning a measly seven dollars for his efforts—"poor pay for hard work!" he complained—Hartshorne was proud of himself, gleefully reporting on the final day that Rogers had "no pain since the injection! Pulse elegant!!!" "How delightful it is to find all my patients doing so well as they are today! Thank God!" he added. Opiates rarely failed young Hartshorne, it seems. He even used them on himself, treating his own painfully "diseased teeth" with morphia. A mastery of opiates was foundational for Hartshorne's long, successful career. He battled cholera epidemics in Philadelphia during the 1840s before working in Civil War hospitals there and at Gettysburg. Hartshorne went on to cofound the American Public Health Association in 1872. Yet in the Gilded Age, he changed his tune on opium. In 1893, Hartshorne moved to Japan and became an advocate against the international opium trade, a cause célèbre among American missionaries.[65] Hartshorne's evolving views mirrored the shifting American medical and cultural discourse on opiates throughout the nineteenth century.

As antebellum physicians such as Hartshorne became increasingly reliant on opiates and enamored with their therapeutic benefits, dosages grew precipitously, even dangerously. At the Commercial Hospital of Cincinnati, the average initial dose of opium administered to patients swelled by 27.3 percent between 1830 and 1840. It dipped by about the same figure in the 1840s but rebounded with a 45.5 percent increase in the 1850s. By the time the Civil War broke out, the mean opium dose at the hospital was 3.2 grains—about 207 milligrams—enough to poison uninitiated patients, potentially fatally.[66] Unsurprisingly, skyrocketing dosages sparked a fierce backlash. The 1830s and 1840s witnessed a rejection of heroic medicine by healers who were not allopathic and by health care consumers in some quarters. This was especially true in the West, where physicians relied most heavily on opium. Against the backdrop of the growth of white-man democracy, one can read the anti-opium backlash as a democratic rejection of elitist physicians and their claims of special medical knowledge. But opium's critics also had pragmatic concerns about the drug's very real dangers.

The over-prescribing of opium was a major inflection point for critics who accused heavy-handed heroic physicians of doing more harm than good. One homeopath fumed that the use of opium "is always [the] production of evil" because it "frenzies the brain, stupefies the mental faculties, blunts the senses, vitiates the moral emotions and social affections and thus degrad[es] the whole man." This was especially true of "the class of people, who are naturally fond of artificial stimulants."[67] Among the most outspoken opium critics was Samuel Thomson, an herb doctor who believed that the cure for any and all ailments was a hearty dose of *Lobelia inflata*, or pukeweed. Thomson soured on opium after his mother was fatally poisoned by a heroic practitioner. Understandably enraged, Thomson thereafter characterized opium as the "whip" used by doctors to drive unfortunate patients to their deaths. In the context of the expanding domestic slave trade, Thomson's juxtaposition of doctors, who endeavored to remedy pain, with slave drivers, who inflicted suffering, was a shot across the bow of regular medicine. Thomson urged Americans to reject heroic physicians and their deadly drugs and instead take up his own brand of herbal medicine. He amassed legions of followers before the Thomsonian movement collapsed in the late 1830s. Pukeweed, it turned out, was not as effective as opium for most sicknesses. Ironically, Thomson's penchant for gigantic doses of the weed also seemed not so different from physicians' use of opium and mercury.[68]

Opium weathered the Thomsonian storm. Despite the success of democratic health movements in challenging physicians' authority, most antebellum doctors continued prescribing opiates, and most ordinary Americans kept on taking the drugs enthusiastically. Some heroic physicians actually doubled down on opiates, calomel, and bleeding to deflect the sectarian backlash and distinguish themselves from the competition.[69] Even some homeopaths and sectarian practitioners prescribed opiates.[70] Across the board, opiates remained among the nation's most widely prescribed medications until the 1870s. But Thomsonianism left a lasting mark on the medical marketplace. In the Civil War's wake, proprietors of patent medicine addiction remedies would revive the spirit of Thomson's critiques, reaping huge fortunes from pharmaceutical sales while undermining physicians' reputations and authority.

Opiates were immensely popular home remedies, which helped insulate them against the antebellum backlash against heroic medicine. Physicians were few and far between in many rural areas, where three-fifths of Americans lived. Few rural health care consumers—or poor city dwellers for that matter—could access or afford doctors' services. Yet because opiates were abundant and unregulated, many people doctored themselves with opium and laudanum. Ordinary folks relied heavily on didactic home health guides for medical advice. Before and after the Civil War, enterprising physicians published dozens of titles that matched the signs and symptoms of diseases with appropriate remedies for readers to thumb through in times of need.[71] More often than not, home health guides simply advised sick readers to take opiates. *Gunn's Domestic Medicine*, an especially popular title, referenced opiates nearly 250 times, far more than any other drugs. According to author John C. Gunn, "the inexpressible delight produced by opium, when the poor sufferer is prostrated, can scarcely be described. It always soothes the irritations of the cough, and mitigates all those symptoms which cannot be removed. The influence it exercises over the mind and imagination of the patient no human language can describe."[72] Lydia Maria Child, the influential women's suffrage activist, abolitionist, and author of *The Family Nurse*, likewise praised opium, laudanum, and paregoric. She even included instructions on how to grow poppies, harvest the opium, and formulate homemade laudanum and paregoric.[73] Ordinary Americans put great stock in the advice conveyed by home health guides, so it is unsurprising that opium comprised the active ingredient of many homemade medicines recorded in family recipe books.[74] In fact, doctors frequently complained that mothers, wives, and nurses relied too much on opiates.

According to physicians, the unsupervised use of opiates in the home was particularly dangerous because opiates were so powerful, "capable, in certain doses, of destroying brute animals."[75] Medical men believed that they alone possessed the training and insight to safely administer the "'Sampsons' of the materia medica."[76] Male practitioners leveled their fiercest denouncements toward women, who bore the primary responsibility for health care in antebellum America. The physician Calvin Cutter barked that "mother[s] should never give one iota of medicine, without knowing the cause of the disease, the state of the system, and the definite effects of such medicine," wisdom that could only be learned through an allopathic medical education.[77] Another physician accused "parents and nurses . . . disturbed by the crying of a child, and its wakefulness at night" of indiscriminately sedating their charges with opiates "because they read in the '[*Gunn's*] *Domestic Medicine*,' that laudanum soothes pain and procures sleep."[78] Certainly, accidents occurred. A two-year-old in Baltimore died in April 1849 from "a spoonful of laudanum, administered to it by its mother in mistake, supposing it to be paregoric."[79] Yet much of the ire directed at laudanum-wielding mothers and nurses reflected the gender bias of male doctors against female healers, as well as physicians' apprehensions about being squeezed out of the increasingly democratic antebellum medical marketplace.

Opiates were easy for consumers to get when instructed by a doctor, home health guide, or knowledgeable family member: one did not need a prescription. There were few legal restrictions on the sale of narcotics until the late nineteenth century, although regulations on poisons sometimes included opium in the interest of consumer protection or to keep narcotics out of the hands of the enslaved.[80] Most Americans could freely purchase opiates at local stores or pharmacies. Druggists, merchants, and wholesalers saturated newspapers with advertisements for the drugs.[81] In Louisiana, where oral opium was a common remedy for miasmatic fevers, rural stores sold opium on demand for fifty cents to a dollar per ounce.[82] In Chicago, then a frontier town, travelers could stop by druggists Brinckerhoff & Penton on Lake Street to have an opium-laced prescription compounded.[83] Itinerant doctors also peddled opiates. In March 1825, one man bought an opium prescription "for a neighbor" from Daniel Swinney, an Ohio physician trained by Benjamin Rush.[84] Laudanum was even cheaper. In April 1857, another Ohio doctor charged a mere twenty-five cents for two ounces of laudanum, an enormous quantity of the drug considering that dosages were often measured in drops or drachms instead of ounces.[85] A year later and across the country, Dr. William M. Parsons of Bennington, New Hampshire, charged Isaac Pratt the same price for a supply of laudanum to use at home, likely for pain following a tooth extraction.[86] The price of opiates stayed consistently low throughout the antebellum era in most places, a testament to the transformative effects of the China trade and the Transportation Revolution. In November 1852, South Carolina doctor John W. Ogilvie charged a mere $2.25 for two dozen calomel and opium pills, enough to last a typical yeoman family for months.[87]

Opiate Addiction and Antebellum Medicine

Widespread prescribing and relatively unfettered access to opiates meant that cases of opiate poisoning and addiction became increasingly commonplace and visible as the Civil War lurched closer. Although most American doctors continued to view opium as the "magnum Dei donum" of the materia medica, some physicians could not help but fixate on opium's dangers. These doctors believed that intoxication, overdose, and addiction mostly occurred when people misused opiates by taking the medicines outside of physicians' direct or indirect guidance or by continuing a prescription for too long. To a vocal minority of doctors, these perceived "abuses" made opium seem more like a Faustian bargain than God's gift to medicine. Yale medical student Moses Clarke White warned in an 1854 medical thesis that "none of the bounties of Providence when abused, are capable of producing greater evil to the human family." "The habitual and excessive use of opium" left users liable to a host of dangers ranging from the unsettling—upset stomach, loss of appetite, apoplectic fits, premature aging, and a "yellow complexion"—to the downright dangerous, including stupor, "wasting of the body," derangement of the nervous system and mind, delirium, early death, and, most alarming of all, an insatiable "craving" for opiates. Indeed, White claimed, "the torments of the opium eater when deprived of his stimulant are as dreadful as his bliss is complete when he has taken it." In the early 1800s, only a few doctors, most notably Benjamin Rush, had expressed such concerns. But by 1854, White was just one of many voices sounding the alarm about opiate addiction.[88]

Numerous observers echoed White's warning about addiction. One popular medical textbook praised the use of opium in fevers but warned about the dangers of prescribing the drug too often or for chronic conditions. Opium should "be resorted to on urgent occasions only, lest the patient become addicted to a practice which can never be relinquished."[89] Home health guides also cautioned laypeople that "opium, to the physician, is a most valuable remedy." But "the practice of opium eating cannot be too strongly condemned . . . like the baneful habit of drinking spirituous liquors, the quantity must be from time to time increased, until at length the constitution becomes so undermined that life becomes a burden."[90] Warnings about the addictiveness of opiates appeared over and over in antebellum medical literature, to the point that by the 1850s, one could hardly read about the virtues of the "magnum Dei donum" without accompanying warnings about its risks.

Such warnings reflected the reality that opium eating was far more widespread in antebellum America than it had been in the early republic, although its frequency paled when compared with alcoholic intemperance. Statistical evidence documenting the extent of opiate addiction in the nineteenth century is hard to come by. Few states, counties, or municipalities recorded vital statistics until after the Civil War. Countless Americans were born, got sick, and died without leaving behind even a scrap of paper, beyond barebones census entries, for future historians to find.[91] An accurate estimate of opiate overdose deaths—a yardstick for addiction, albeit an imperfect one—is thus impossible to determine for most regions. Nevertheless, certain strands of evidence strongly suggest that opiate addiction had become endemic in antebellum America, although it was still a more limited phenomenon than during the post–Civil War decades. Tariff records provide a bird's-eye view of opium eating. Weighing the volume of opium imports against estimates of the amount needed to sustain an addicted person, David T. Courtwright suggests that the national opiate addiction rate stood at no more than 0.72 per thousand Americans in 1842, which translates to roughly 11,000 people. Courtwright adds that tariff records from this era were haphazardly kept and by nature do not account for smuggled opium, so in all likelihood, this estimate is an undercount.[92] William J. Rorabaugh suggests the booze-saturated "alcoholic republic" counted perhaps a thousand drunkards for every opium eater.[93] Although these imperfect figures suggest a rate of opiate addiction that was much lower than the contemporary rate of alcoholism, they nonetheless underscore how, by the 1840s, opium eating was prevalent enough to alarm doctors.

Coroners' inquests provide a more textured, close-up view of opiate addiction in certain locales, where death investigators were tasked with uncovering and interpreting the circumstances surrounding unusual, sudden, or suspicious deaths. Coroners' inquests are far from perfect sources, as most deaths went uninvestigated. White, middle- and upper-class corpses largely avoided the stigma of an inquest, whereas xenophobic New York City authorities went out of their way in the 1830s and 1840s to document Irish deaths, pathologizing Irish immigrants in the process.[94] But even with such limitations, inquests go a long way toward illuminating nineteenth-century mortality patterns.

New York City coroners kept particularly robust records, providing a macabre window into the grisly deaths befalling the denizens of America's biggest, busiest metropolis. Coroners' inquests suggest that opiate use, overdoses, and likely addiction were endemic in antebellum New York City. At least 413 New Yorkers died from opiate overdoses, often recorded as "poisonings," between 1823 and 1849 out of some 9,700 inquests. Opiate overdoses were responsible for just over 4 percent of deaths investigated by coroners during the twenty-six year period. Overdose deaths were much more common among adults than children, a surprising pattern considering the volume of medical commentary framing laudanum as a mother's helper. Only thirty-nine overdose deaths were recorded among children ten years of age or less, compared with 373 deaths among people ten or older; 98 percent of the latter were aged eighteen years and over.[95] In general, urban child mortality was so high that infant overdose deaths were perhaps deemed unremarkable and went unrecorded. Among adults, addicted individuals were not necessarily the most likely to fatally overdose. Although nineteenth-century observers believed that tolerance could lead to the consumption of dangerously high doses, culminating in overdose, it is plausible that inexperienced users without tolerance were more likely to do so fatally. Antebellum New York City's opiate overdose mortality suggests that drug use in the city was widespread enough for accidental overdoses to have been fairly common occurrences and that the city perhaps boasted a moderately sized population of addicted users. It is unsurprising that opiate use in the city also generated sporadic media attention in the 1850s. New York City's opiate outlook was perhaps higher than other locations but likely not very exceptional. Rural Americans also used opiates and died from overdoses, although their deaths were less meticulously documented than deaths in New York City.[96]

Coroners' inquests also reveal that opiates served as an accessible means of suicide in antebellum America, in and outside of New York City, underscoring the dangers of opiate "abuse" in the minds of physicians. As one doctor lamented in 1836, the "tincture of opium is not infrequently resorted to, for the destruction of life."[97] Inquests, newspapers, and medical journals are replete with reports of attempted and completed suicides by laudanum or opium overdose.[98] In New York City, apparent suicides represented about 75 percent of the overdose deaths investigated by the coroner's office, but this figure demands scrutiny. Nineteenth-century Americans rarely left suicide notes to explain their motives or even if they intended to die, so the line between accidental overdose deaths and suicides was opaque. For example, Sarah Barker "took a quantity of laudanum," according to the coroner's report, and died on June 6, 1843.[99] But did Barker mean to die, or did she simply take too much laudanum, perhaps to overcome tolerance that inevitably developed after years of use? The coroner could not conclusively determine the answer to this thorny question. Separating suicides from accidental overdoses is further complicated by the reality that suicide sometimes overlapped with opiate addiction. The hardships of life as an opium eater often drove people to suicide. In 1850, an elderly man, an "opium eater for many years," became "tired of such a wretched life," so "he decided to cut it short" by poisoning himself with a half dram of morphine, an amount far exceeding his usual dose.[100] Moreover, the use of opiates for suicide served to amplify antebellum doctors' unease about them. Like addiction, death by suicide was deeply stigmatized because most Americans deemed "self-murder," a common contemporary label for suicide, to be un-Christian.

The mounting number of overdose deaths in and outside cities convinced doctors that opiate "abuse" was a growing problem, not the least because they were often summoned to attempt to reverse overdoses. Physicians strove to develop methods to counteract opium poisoning, some of them dubious whereas others were ingenious.[101] One medical textbook included a list of botanical remedies that might help when patients took "too large quantities" of opium "for the horrid purpose of self destruction."[102] A vice president of the American Medical Association (AMA) advocated for caffeine as the best antidote for the "poisonous narcotism of opium."[103] *The Physician's Visiting List*, a popular appointment book used by doctors, included a guide for reversing opium overdoses.[104] The use of a stomach pump to evacuate poisonous opiates was a common method—the only one with much chance of success.[105] But sometimes it failed, as in the case of a twenty-five-year-old man named Davis who in 1825 bought a bottle of laudanum from a New York City druggist and promptly drank the entire contents. Doctors were summoned, and "a considerable quantity of laudanum was got up" by a stomach pump, but "after an agony of more than an hour he died."[106] For such scenarios, an 1852 medical dictionary included timetables spelling out exactly how long it would take for poisoned patients to succumb.[107] These early harm-reduction techniques hint at an undercurrent of sympathy for opiate users on the part of doctors, who often wanted to help their patients survive overdoses even as they viewed dependence with contempt.[108] Such medical innovations also serve as clear evidence that addiction had become prevalent enough to warrant sustained medical attention.

By the 1840s and 1850s, opiate addiction was so worrisome that the faculties of fifty-odd US medical schools took it upon themselves to educate soon-to-be doctors about the phenomenon. Students at the Medical College of the State of South Carolina learned to use a stomach pump on overdosing patients, as did

Moses Clarke White at Yale.[109] With increasing frequency, students wrote about opiate use and "abuse" in their medical theses, capstone essays that represented the final hurdle before obtaining a coveted medical degree. Students at the South Carolina college wrote at least twelve theses on opiates during the 1840s and 1850s. Nine theses were produced between 1852 and 1860 alone, underscoring the growing perception of opiate abuse in the decade before the Civil War.[110]

Medical theses also provide a frank, clear-eyed view of doctors' clinical understandings of addiction on the eve of the Civil War. Eight South Carolina thesis writers described addiction, warning that patients who took opiates for too long or outside a doctor's supervision were liable to intoxication, overdose, and addiction. As one student explained, "the continued use of opium" to relieve pain "does more harm finally than good, for the sufferer becomes habituated to its use."[111] A second student elaborated at length about opium's evils, admitting that "without it [opium] the Materia Medica would be wholly inefficient to combat with many symptoms of diseases that with it can be subdued as they arise."[112] But no one could mention opium's benefits without warning about its dangers in the next breath. As the student cautioned, "the adage 'that the greater the benefits which naturally result from anything the more pernicious are its effects when diverted from its proper course' applies to opium[;] this is daily seen in the extensive opium eating which many persons are daily and hourly in the habit of and the greater though less frequent evil that of poisoning by opium."[113] Another thesis writer described an acquaintance who took opium "extravagantly." The man "became accustomed to taking it for a calculous affection, which it apparently cured." But "like all bad or dissipating habits," opium eating "cannot be eradicated."[114]

Frequent and stirring warnings by medical students illustrate how, with ample opportunity to read about or observe cases of opium eating, doctors developed a much more sophisticated understanding of addiction than had doctors of Benjamin Rush's generation. Antebellum doctors recognized that people who took opiates for months and years eventually lost sensitivity to some of the drugs' beneficial effects, such as pain relief and euphoria. As one physician explained in 1832, "one grain" of opium, a small dose, "will produce upon an adult, unaccustomed to its use, all the effects of a narcotic; whereas ten grains will not do so . . . in the same individual, when long accustomed to its use."[115] Some, but not all, of this variability could be attributed to individuals' distinct constitutions. Yet doctors realized that tolerance was an eventuality for *any* patient who took opiates for too long, regardless of their constitution. Tolerance meant that "to produce the desired effect" of opium, "the dose must constantly be augmented."[116]

Physicians also believed that escalating consumption was dangerous because this process could result in fatal overdoses when the dosage required to sustain an addicted person reached poisonous levels. Doctors feared that even the bodies of chronic opium eaters, habituated to huge doses, could only take so much "abuse." Snowballing dosages eventually "brings on debility and premature decay" and death.[117] Long-term opium use was thus framed as "extremely injurious" to the body of "the opium eaters themselves—they lost their appetites—become feeble and tremulous—the necks wry, and their fingers contracted." Physicians also recognized that missed doses would lead to painful withdrawal symptoms. When a dose was delayed, "they are perfectly miserable until the hour arrives for the gratification of their indulgence."[118] In 1835, a physician described the case of a frail elderly woman with a "nervous temperament," who had been addicted to opium for nineteen years before her death. She was originally "advised to take tinc. opii. [laudanum]" and, after contracting the opium habit, built up extreme tolerance to the drug's effects, requiring at least thirty grains every night before she felt the drug's soothing effects. She "could not sleep without it, but would scream till she had" laudanum. Opium use might have hastened the woman's death after a five-week period in which she did not defecate.[119]

Although physicians had discovered certain clinical hallmarks of addiction, such as physical dependency, tolerance, and the risk of fatal overdose, the state of medical knowledge in the mid-nineteenth century prevented doctors from understanding a fuller picture of addiction. Even the best-educated physicians, like Yale's Moses Clarke White, puzzled over why opium eaters could not simply quit using the drug through willpower. Doctors also wondered why some individuals became "slaves" to opium, whereas other people were able to take opiates without developing a compulsion to use them.

Modern medicine answers these questions by pointing to the brain and nervous system. Unknown to antebellum doctors, the human body has a network of opioid receptors in the brain, spinal cord, and even the intestines. Opiate agonists (including opium and morphine) bind to opioid receptors, releasing neurotransmitters that cause euphoria, analgesia, drowsiness, and depressed breathing. Opiates thus trigger powerful physiological responses when swallowed, smoked, injected, or applied to the skin. If one has not developed tolerance through long-term use, or even if one consumes opiates outside their usual environment, the resulting overdose can prove fatal. But if a person uses opiates over and over, their body usually develops tolerance. Regularly consuming opiates over long durations means that eventually the body cannot feel or function well in their absence. Some recent studies have also suggested that long-term opiate users may even experience an increased sensitivity to pain.[120]

Yet antebellum doctors could not readily understand this complex phenomenon with the medical tools or biological knowledge at their disposal. Instead, nineteenth-century Americans had to content themselves with cultural explanations for the mysteries of opium eating. Observers ultimately decided that perceived racial, moral, mental, and physical inferiorities made certain people more prone to opium eating. This explanation reflected the racism, misogyny, classism, and ableism that pervaded nineteenth-century American medicine as well as the influence of the missionary and temperance movements, which reached a fever pitch around the time when antebellum doctors began firming up their ideas about addiction. Chapter 2 reconstructs these formative antebellum cultural understandings of opiate addiction, which would ultimately persist beyond the Civil War and animate the experiences of addicted veterans.

Chapter 2

So Dreadful an Evil

The Cultural Construction of Addiction in Antebellum America

Decades before opium "enslaved" any Civil War veterans, opium eating emerged in the antebellum American consciousness as a malady that mostly afflicted women, weak-willed men or those with disabilities, or Chinese immigrants. The editor of the influential *BMSJ* encountered a woman in his practice who fit the bill of an archetypal opium eater in 1833, narrating her heart-wrenching story in a widely circulated article. Framed as an appeal for help on behalf of a sympathetic, but very sick, young white wife and mother "of the most touching character," the doctor painstakingly described the woman's troubling "addiction" to opium. Suffering from "some slight degree of nervous irritation" a few years before, a well-intentioned practitioner had prescribed opium. Realizing the drug's remarkable capacity to soothe nerves and make life more bearable, she kept on taking it. Days of taking opium stretched into weeks, then months and years.

Opium began as a godsend but soon became "so dreadful an evil," transmogrifying the woman from a paragon of domesticity into "a bound and servile slave." The daily rhythm of her once happy life now revolved around doses of opium. Believing herself to be hopelessly dependent on opium and afraid of being judged as intemperate, the woman kept her drug use secret, even from her husband. She might have been content to carry on that way forever, but as the years passed her body developed a stubborn tolerance to opium's palliative effects. To ward off agonizing withdrawal pains, she was forced to swallow more and more opium every day and eventually became afraid that a fatal overdose might kill her. Unable to quit the addictive drug at will, she approached the journal's editor and confessed her darkest secret. Considering the woman's identity and station in life, the doctor was sympathetic. But the complicated case stubbornly defied his best therapeutic know-how. So he took the case public, appealing to the journal's national audience of esteemed physicians in hopes that some kindhearted, knowledgeable doctor would reply with a "sure and safe method of curing a person of the habit of opium eating." The stakes were high, for "still young and with a family of children, what must become of her a few years hence, when already an ounce [of opium] a day scarcely sufficed" to stave off withdrawal?[1] If the woman fatally overdosed, her children would be left motherless and her husband wifeless. Slavery to opium thus appeared to threaten the woman's life, ruin her reputation, humble her doctor, and separate her family.

This chapter illuminates cultural perceptions of opium eaters, such as the woman profiled in the *BMSJ*, who embodied so many antebellum ideas about opium users and opiate addiction. Understanding how Americans viewed opium eaters before the Civil War is crucial to fully grapple with the experiences of addiction for veterans. The antebellum era was formative in the development of American cultural ideas about drug addiction and drug users, although until recently historians have largely overlooked the period's significance.[2] Opiates were among the era's most ubiquitous and utilitarian drugs, used by doctors and ordinary folks to treat pain, diarrhea, and anything and everything in between. Addiction was a natural consequence of widespread opiate use. Consequently, between the Missouri Compromise of 1820 and the outbreak of the Civil War in 1861, opium eating became increasingly visible. It never reached crisis levels or generated much hand-wringing outside medical circles until after the Civil War, however, because it was seen as mainly affecting women and, to a lesser extent, Chinese immigrants or white men deemed to be effeminate or disabled. The phenomenon thus appeared to pose little risk to most white men or American society at large. Yet even with lower levels of addiction than the postwar decades, plenty of cases still occurred for doctors and other observers to develop sophisticated medical understandings of addiction and to form concrete opinions about the sort of people who "abused" opium. After the Civil War, antebellum perceptions of opium eaters carried over to veterans who contracted the "habit."

Antebellum views about gender and the era's social reform movements informed how doctors and other Americans came to view addicted people. Medical and popular accounts of opium eaters convinced readers that the archetypal American opium eater was a white, frail, weak-willed, "nervous" wife and mother who began using opiates medicinally but whose life and reputation were endangered by out-of-control use. Opium eaters who fit this mold usually elicited sympathy, whereas other opium users warranted condemnation. These narratives linked characteristics of bourgeois white womanhood, especially dependency and physical infirmity, to opium eating. Even though white male opium eaters were relatively rare before the Civil War, the fusion of femininity and opium eating ultimately seemed to feminize the few white men who became addicted. The temperance and missionary movements also shaped how antebellum Americans viewed opium eaters. Temperance rhetoric that framed intoxication as sinful and missionaries' descriptions of opium smoking among the allegedly racially inferior Chinese people became increasingly salient by the 1850s. These strands congealed into a gendered, racialized, ableist understanding of opiate addiction as "slavery" by the eve of the Civil War. During the

1860s—the first time a large cohort of white American men became addicted to opiates—observers judged them through antebellum cultural sensibilities, which the war buffeted but did not always overturn. Ultimately, the antebellum cultural construction of opium slavery would directly inform veterans' experiences with opiate addiction in the postwar decades.

Gendering Addiction

By the outbreak of the Civil War in 1861, American doctors had already probed deeply into various facets of opiate addiction, developing robust, sophisticated clinical understandings of the phenomenon. Elements of addiction such as tolerance, overdoses, and even the gradual withdrawal method of treatment were widely known in American medical circles. But opium's mysteries still abounded. The most perplexing questions revolved around the profile and behaviors of opium eaters. Why were some people able to use opiates medicinally without becoming dependent, whereas others became addicted? And why were opium eaters unable to quit the drug, despite usually being desperate to rid themselves of it? Medicine could not provide satisfying answers to these vexing questions. Instead, deeply rooted cultural ideas gave contemporary observers a useful frame of reference for puzzling out answers to these confounding questions.

During the 1830s and 1840s, physicians increasingly relied on gendered rhetoric to understand and describe opiate addiction and the kind of people who doctors believed "abused" opiates. Medical literature portrayed the typical opium eater as a white woman of marriageable age, with frail constitution, who initially began taking opium on medical advice. The description of the "lady" opium eater that appeared in 1833 in the *BMSJ*, for example, emphasized her domestic background and her delicate, sickly constitution. She seemed physically weak and infirm, a "useless thing, lolling about in idleness and pain" and left unable to attend to her children. It was to "quiet some slight degree of nervous irritation" that her family doctor had originally prescribed opium, and only after "many years" of opium use had she become "a bound and servile slave" to the drug. This gendered description of opium eating reflects the era's prevailing belief that white women were inherently more prone to pain, nervousness, and infirmity than were white men. Most Americans also believed that white women were naturally dependent. These ideas about womanhood mapped neatly onto opiate addiction, which became associated with inherent physical infirmity, weakness, and dependency. Gender constructs thus helped doctors explain why some people seemed more prone to becoming addicted to opium than others. Indeed, such women "illustrate the kind of opium eating that we apprehend is most common with us, and that which calls most loudly for the sympathy and aid of the humane physician," according to the *BMSJ* editor.[3]

Did doctors' firm belief that most opium eaters were bourgeois white women match reality? It is difficult to know for sure if most antebellum opium eaters were women, chiefly because the scarcity of contemporary vital records makes it impossible for historians to quantify overdose deaths, a rough proxy for gauging the demographics of opiate use and addiction. Most overdose deaths went unrecorded because most deaths in general went unrecorded. Addicted people also tended to hide their condition to avoid the stigma associated with drug dependence. "The unhappy victims of this habit labor" to "conceal the fact from notice," a physician condescendingly observed in 1832. Family doctors were often "entirely ignorant" of their patients' daily "indulgence" in opium.[4] Indeed, the woman profiled by the *BMSJ* managed to keep her husband and family oblivious to her opium use for years. Her case is known to historians only because she had the social and financial capital to seek medical help from a well-connected physician who created a paper trail.[5]

Yet fragmentary sources allow historians to overcome gaps of secrecy and anonymity in the historical record. Coroners' inquests indicate that women and girls comprised about 55 percent of the 413 overdose deaths investigated by the New York City coroner's office between 1823 and 1849, which suggests that women outnumbered other demographics among the overall addicted population.[6] Antebellum mental asylum records likewise illuminate demographics, suggesting that women were more likely than others to be institutionalized for opium eating. Nineteenth-century psychiatry posited that long-term opium use could overexcite and disorder a person's mind and body, resulting in insanity that sometimes warranted institutionalization. Between 1843 and 1866, twenty individuals were committed to New York State Lunatic Asylum at Utica for insanity that the asylum doctors—among the foremost psychiatrists in the nation—attributed to long-term opiate use. Seventeen of these individuals were white women.[7] Prewar asylums were relatively small facilities usually sporting a few dozen beds, a handful of staff, and one or two doctors to treat patients. With such limited capacity, asylums treated only a fraction of the nation's addicted population.[8] Women were often overrepresented in asylums, stemming in part from the widespread belief that women were uniquely liable to insanity.[9] But even accounting for these caveats, gendered institutionalization patterns, coupled with coroners' inquests, suggest that women probably comprised a majority among antebellum American opium eaters.

Responding to demographics and cultural ideas about womanhood, the antebellum medical and popular media became convinced that the typical American opium eater was a white woman. The influential *BMSJ* published at least 121 articles describing various facets of opiate addiction and overdose in the three decades preceding the Civil War.[10] White women were featured most prominently in these articles. In an 1832 case, a physician described a woman who was "addicted to the habit of using laudanum in considerable quantity," which she developed accidentally by using the tincture to treat "uneasy sensations connected with a dyspectic [sic] state of stomach." She was the first case of opiate addiction the doctor had treated, and he found the encounter particularly illuminating, considering that his previous knowledge about opium eating had been gleaned from Thomas De Quincey's 1821 *Confessions of an English Opium-Eater*. In the wildly popular book, the British romantic author had framed opium eating as a euphoric pursuit that inspired literary genius, even if one that was ultimately destructive. The book was widely read in Britain and the United States from the 1820s until well beyond the Civil War. Scholars have noted De Quincey's sway over antebellum American readers, who were deeply influenced by his romantic, if harrowing, portrayal of opium eating. Some Americans, trying to emulate De Quincey, even claimed to have experimented with opium to induce "fantasies." Exposure to *Confessions* had given young American doctors the impression that most opium eaters were literati or intellectuals like De Quincey. Yet his version of opium eating did not match the reality experienced by most American opium eaters. In fact, having studied a case of addiction firsthand, the newly enlightened doctor rejected De Quincey's portrayal as "fanciful and exaggerated." *Confessions* was "interesting and highly wrought[,] considered as a literary work," but it romanticized the agony of addiction and misleadingly framed opium eating as a pastime instead of a compulsion. De Quincey himself, an Englishman, also contrasted sharply with the identity and characteristics of the white, female American opium eater under the physician's care.[11]

Case narratives provided doctors a venue in which to hash out gendered notions of opium eating and to probe why more women became addicted to opiates than men. First and foremost, doctors began to recognize their own role in facilitating women's addiction. Physicians often remarked how their patients became addicted after initially taking opium or laudanum under medical advice for gendered conditions such as "nervousness." As the psychiatrist Edward Jarvis explained, white women were "more frequently nervous" and "more under the influence of the feelings and emotions" than were men.[12] Hence doctors prescribed opiates to women suffering from "some slight degree of nervous irritation" far more than they did to men.[13]

After discovering the utility of opiates, many women understandably kept on taking the drugs, only to find they were unable to quit. Case narratives and coroners' inquests informed doctors that women often ate opium or swigged laudanum to relieve painful menstruation or venereal disease, conditions that women were often reluctant to discuss with male clinicians. One woman took an opium and belladonna concoction to medicate "a w [*sic*] eruption on the vulva" that had "tormented [her] for some months." One day in 1830, the woman's husband discovered her in a catatonic state. Surprised and dismayed to find that his wife had been taking opium, he summoned doctors, who promptly intervened with leeches, bleeding, and purgatives to rebalance the woman's constitution.[14] Prostitutes in New York City often used laudanum to self-medicate for venereal diseases contracted on the job and to cope with the stresses and physical demands of dangerous sex work. Eliza Middleton, "a common prostitute," died from "taking laudanum" in August 1840.[15] Although the coroner did not speculate as to why she had been using laudanum, this description implied a connection between sex work and opiate use. Stories like Middleton's thus played into a broader cultural panic about prostitution and the "fallen women" who haunted the alleyways and tenements of American cities. The association of opiate abuse with prostitution thus served as potential justification for regulating vices, while also contributing to the stigmatization of opiates when used outside the bounds of medicine.[16]

Doctors of course recognized that even "respectable" women took opiates to self-medicate for various maladies. Corinna Brown Aldrich married Edward Aldrich, an ambitious but frenetic and financially unsuccessful country doctor, in 1837. During the California Gold Rush (1848–55) he moved to the booming town of San Francisco to set up a fledgling medical practice, leaving Corinna and their young daughter in New York City with relatives. Isolated and impoverished, Corinna began taking morphine twice daily to cope with her stressful living situation. Yet the drug seemed to worsen her emotional and mental state, her family reported. Ashamed of his wife's morphine addiction but recognizing that the drug "ha[d] become necessary to her very existence," Edward was at a loss about how to "reform and save" Corinna. Eventually he resorted to having Corinna institutionalized at New York City's Bloomingdale Asylum, where she died in November 1854.[17] Corinna was not alone in using opiates to cope with stress or separation from loved ones. In the South, where plantations were often spaced miles apart with neighbors few and far between, "plantation mistresses" frequently remarked in their diaries about boredom and isolation. Euphoric laudanum may have offered these lonely women a tempting solution. It is also likely that some women used laudanum as a substitute for alcohol, as some men did.[18] For women to imbibe in spirits was deeply taboo, especially in such regions with strong temperance roots as upstate New York. Because laudanum was consumed in private, it also offered a discreet alternative for whiskey consumed at rowdy, male-dominated taverns and workplaces.[19]

Whether through a doctor's prescription for gendered maladies or the understandable impulse to dull the senses, many American women became opium eaters in the decades before the Civil War, although we can never know precisely how many. What *is* clear is that Black women were much less likely to become opium eaters because of limited access and exposure to the drugs. Enslaved people's use of opiates was curtailed by several factors, including laws in Southern states designed to prevent their access to poisons that might be turned against slaveholders. In 1748, for example, Virginia made it a felony for slaves to "prepare, exhibit, or administer any medicine whatsoever" under penalty of "death without benefit of clergy."[20] Although anti-poison laws largely curbed enslaved people's access to opiates, these laws were not foolproof. Confederate diarist Mary Chesnut discovered as much in March 1865 when she instructed Ellen, a woman whom she enslaved, to retrieve a packet of Dover's powder from a physician. Perhaps sensing the war's end at hand, Ellen burned the directions about how much to administer the medicine and then gave Chesnut the whole packet at once. Chesnut's doctor later described the act as a "murder" attempt. This act was not so different from burning down a plantation house or fleeing to Union army lines, forms of resistance to slavery that crippled the institution during the Civil War.[21]

The nineteenth-century medical belief that Black bodies possessed extraordinary physical strength and an imperviousness to pain was also paramount in shaping the demographics of addiction. Historian Deirdre Cooper Owens has described this idea as the "Black superbody."[22] Under attack from abolitionists, white proslavery doctors developed elaborate medical theories to defend slavery by defanging torture. Samuel A. Cartwright—a Mississippi doctor who infamously espoused the notion that slaves who ran away from their masters must be suffering from insanity, or "drapetomania"—claimed in *De Bow's Review* in 1851 that a "natural disposition to idleness and sloth" meant that Black people's blood became "unfit to stimulate the nerves of sensation distributed to the body." Black bodies thus lost "feeling in so great a degree, that he [the slave] burns his skin by the fire he hovers over without knowing it."[23] If enslaved people could not even feel burns, Cartwright implied, then they must not mind being whipped to shreds by the overseer's lash. A Georgia physician concurred, adding that "the nervous system" of Black bodies "with reference to sensation is less developed than in the white" body. Thus "the lash is not very painful" for slaves. Further still, he alleged that "the negro" even "suffers less pain from dental extraction" than do whites. Cartwright's inclusion of this mundane procedure illustrated the broad applicability of the racist medical belief in Black imperviousness to pain.[24] Black and white abolitionists loudly disagreed, insisting that Black people could, and did, feel every flesh-splitting stroke of the lash, emblematic of slavery's many cruelties. Frederick Douglass recalled how Edward Covey, an infamous Maryland "slave breaker," once set upon Douglass "with the fierceness of a tiger, tore off my clothes, and lashed me till he had worn out his switches, cutting me so savagely as to leave the marks visible for a long time after." "I was seldom free from a sore back," Douglass pointedly remarked.[25] Yet abolitionist counterarguments failed to convince slaveholders or the doctors at their beck and call.

Proslavery medicine purported that Black bodies did not require painkillers, so white doctors rarely gave opiates to enslaved people. This absence of basic medical care was deeply hypocritical considering slaveholders' paternalistic claims that they took good care of their slaves.[26] John W. Ogilvie, a South Carolina planter and doctor, routinely prescribed and sold opiates during the 1840s and 1850s. Yet his detailed account books suggest that he prescribed opiates much less frequently to enslaved Black people than to his white customers. Despite practicing plantation medicine in a majority-Black region, between 1845 and 1859, Ogilvie only recorded prescribing opiates to five Black patients compared with about eighty white patients.[27] Some overseers withheld medical care from slaves, recognizing that plantation owners despised large medical bills.[28] Slaveholders also devalued enslaved people with disabilities and subjected them to medical neglect.[29] Perhaps these factors help explain Ogilvie's prescribing patterns. But he was also probably influenced by the widespread belief among white doctors that Black bodies were impervious to pain. Moreover, white planters and physicians were inherently skeptical when Black voices expressed physical pain. Slaveholders often grumbled that enslaved people feigned pain to avoid backbreaking work in cotton fields, allegations that left them less likely to receive opiates than whites, whose pain was taken more seriously.[30] For their part, many enslaved and free Black people were skeptical of opium and the white doctors who peddled it, for good reasons. Black healers played crucial roles in delivering health care, administering remedies derived from African medical traditions and local plants. "Root doctors" and conjurers used herbs and roots as balm, rejecting the "magnum Dei donum" of white doctors. Most enslaved people preferred the techniques and medicines offered by these Black healers.[31]

African Americans also had to overcome barriers in pharmacies if they wanted to procure opiates. Although a web of commercial exchanges linked enslaved and free Black and white communities in the South, a relative lack of freedom of movement worked against Black Southerners who might have had the financial means to purchase the drugs, even if they could find a white doctor or druggist willing to do business.[32] Such access barriers reduced the potential for self-medication that often fostered addiction among whites, which translated to a racial gulf in opiate overdose mortality. Free and enslaved Black people were far less likely to die from opiate overdoses. Out of 1,066 inquests of Black Virginians sampled between 1757 and 1900, coroners did not record even a single overdose death.[33] Coroners in antebellum New York City recorded only 22 overdose deaths among the city's Black residents between 1823 and 1849, compared to 391 overdoses among whites.[34] Medical racism linked to slavery caused an enduring disparity that persisted for decades and eventually translated to a lower rate of addiction among Black Civil War veterans.

Contrasting the experiences of white and Black women who endured painful gynecological surgeries under the knife of James Marion Sims puts the racial disparities of opiate use into sharp relief. Between 1845 and 1849, the influential Alabama gynecologist conducted experimental surgeries without anesthesia on coerced enslaved women while developing surgical solutions for vesicovaginal fistula. Sims subjected one enslaved woman, Anarcha, to at least thirty surgeries without anesthesia. Like most antebellum doctors, Sims sang the praises of opium and he regularly administered it to his enslaved subjects—but *not* as a painkiller. Hyperfocused on surgical success, Sims was willfully ignorant when it came to Black women's pain. To Sims, it was unthinkable to administer ether during surgery or opium afterward to mitigate the agony his enslaved subjects' must have felt. Rather than pain relief, Sims administered opium to cause constipation. He feared that if his unwilling subjects, fresh out of surgery, strained their abdominal muscles during bowel movements, the motion might inadvertently rip out their sutures. Sims's solution was paralyzing the bowels with opium. After announcing his pioneering surgery in 1853, Sims gained an international following and relocated to New York City, where he founded a women's hospital and performed gynecological surgeries on wealthy white women. In those cases, Sims routinely administered opiates for pain relief, not merely to induce constipation. Sims's cross-purposes—the compassionate use of opium to ease white women's pain versus the use of opium to paralyze Black women's bodies for personal gain—powerfully illustrates the medical racism that fostered white women's overrepresentation among American opium eaters and Black women's underrepresentation.[35]

If whiteness was a key factor in determining women's likelihood of becoming addicted, then it also shielded many women from being held personally responsible for their conditions. Opiates were complicated, Janus-faced substances that affected users differently depending on one's identity and the context of use. On the one hand, many doctors celebrated opium as an essential medicine that, when used properly, enabled the performance of gender-prescribed domestic roles. A dose of laudanum prescribed to quell the nerves enabled white women to do the hard work of cooking, cleaning, and raising children. Consumed in this context, opiates buttressed the patriarchal order of antebellum American society. Consequently, white women who became addicted under these circumstances seemed to warrant a degree of sympathy. The editor of the *BMSJ* explained as much in his 1833 appeal on behalf of the nervous wife and mother. "When we allude to opium eaters," he explained, "we mean only those who took it originally as a medicine for some nervous affection, and continue it from necessity . . . who take it, not to intoxicate, but to strengthen and balance the nervous system and enable them to attend to business, and to appear like other people." C. L. Seeger, a Massachusetts doctor, echoed this sentiment in a reply published the next month in the journal. Seeger was motivated to write by his "feeling of pity for the poor lady."[36] Opium eaters who "had no hand in bringing it upon themselves" but had been exposed to the drugs by doctors or friends "while on the bed of affliction . . . of course should be entitled to our sympathy," added a New York City doctor in 1859.[37]

On the other hand, opium abuse by individuals who did not live up to the prevailing gendered, racial, and class-based ideals of antebellum American society or who used opiates outside of medical advice warranted condemnation. The *New-York Daily Tribune* reported one such unsympathetic case in 1843. "On Saturday last a Mrs. Lovejoy committed suicide . . . by taking opium." Little wonder she died from opiate overdose, the paper reasoned, for "she appears to have been of intemperate habits" and was a reported opium eater. So was Lovejoy's husband, "who, from a state of comparative independence, has been reduced to deep reverses by [the] indulgence" of opium eating. Intemperate opium users like the Lovejoys represented the kind of users who "need less of our sympathy," the editor of the *BMSJ* sneered.[38]

The antebellum era saw the emergence of a wide gulf between two kinds of opium eaters, contingent on identity and circumstances of use. Doctors saw bourgeois white women addicted to medicinal opiates as the "right" kind of opium eater, worthy of sympathy and assistance. By contrast, physicians branded opium eaters who were not white or not women or who consumed opiates outside medical advice as the "wrong" sort of opium eater, deserving of castigation, not kindness. Historians have traditionally periodized this categorization of drug users later in the nineteenth century. David T. Courtwright, Joseph F. Spillane, Timothy A. Hickman, David Herzberg, and Elizabeth Kelly Gray have illuminated how Gilded Age doctors viewed middle-class women who used morphine and laudanum with much more understanding and sympathy than Chinese immigrants who smoked opium. Federal legislation enacted in the early twentieth century to regulate the sale of opiates formalized the cultural bifurcation of drug users. Heavy-handed laws such as the Harrison Narcotics Act of 1914 and its enforcement measures cemented race- and class-based "white markets" and "black markets" for drugs that segregated users who lacked a doctor's stamp of approval from users who could obtain legal prescriptions.[39] Yet the division between the socially acceptable drug use among middle-class white women and unacceptable drug abuse by other, less sympathetic groups had even deeper roots than historians have realized, dating back to the antebellum era.

The early nineteenth-century delineation of "right" and "wrong" opium users becomes especially apparent in descriptions of white men who "abused" opiates.

Although fewer in number than women opium eaters, men who depended on opiates were deemed particularly notorious and unworthy of sympathy or medical aid because they violated ideals of manhood. Naturally, these ideals varied by race, class, individual, region, and age, with some white men embracing "restrained manhood" while others gravitated toward "martial manhood." Some men proved their manliness by adventuring in the West; others idealized the role of family man and provider.[40] Proponents of restrained manhood espoused self-control, abhorred violence, and prided themselves on temperance and reliability. In contrast, men who embodied martial manhood derived their self-worth in part from the ability to dominate others. Losing oneself in flashes of aggression or short bouts of violence was not immoral but rather an expression of how masterful men were supposed to behave. Despite these clear differences, however, opium eating defied all the prevailing models of white manhood. Restrained men gravitated toward the temperance movement and denigrated those who imbibed intoxicating substances like alcohol or opium. Martial men strove to assert their dominance, yet opium intoxication seemingly rendered men docile and unable to control their own bodies and behavior, let alone command women or enslaved people.[41] In an era of white male social, political, and economic dominance, white manhood above all stressed independence. White men were not supposed to be beholden to the dictates of another master, human or chemical.[42] Yet dependency, the ultimate hallmark of opium eating, defied this ideal, branding addicted men as less than manly in the eyes of doctors, families, and communities.

Opium eating seemed to emasculate men, making their cases particularly shocking and unsettling in a society ordered around gender conventions. If addicted white women often garnered sympathy, male opium eaters were met with disgust. Describing such men, a doctor seethed that "nothing makes one more *miserably* dependent than the use of opium."[43] Addiction left men "ready to sell wife and children, body and soul for the continuance of his wretched and transient delight," added another observer.[44] These descriptions conveyed the unthinkable: that white men had lost their independence and self-mastery and instead had become abjectly reliant on opium, which controlled their bodies and actions. This state of dependency to opium was not necessarily alarming when ascribed to women, who were widely considered to be inherently dependent and "servile." But it seemed unnatural and deeply troubling when embodied by white men. Gendered understandings of dependency help explain how doctors could call for "charity" for sympathetic female opium eaters while in the next breath condemning male opium users.[45]

Not only did male opium users seem odiously dependent, but their bodies also violated the widely held conviction that white men should be strong, whole, and able-bodied.[46] Opium eating seemed to "destroy" one's "mental and bodily powers." In the cases of white women opium eaters, sickly, nervous constitutions were not terribly alarming to observers, who believed that white women's bodies were inherently frail. The same could not be said of male opium eaters. Observers remarked that opium "abuse" debilitated and deformed the male body, transforming it into a twisted mockery of the idealized masculine form. Moses Clarke White noted with horror his belief that opium eating led to "total attenuation" of the body, "bending of the spine," "lame gait," and "withered yellow countenance[s]."[47] Similar accounts of emasculated male opium eaters circulated in antebellum magazines and newspapers, painting a decidedly unsympathetic portrait predicated on dependency, weakness, and debility. In a sensational 1833 story in *New England Magazine*, a purported male opium eater decried how laudanum left him "as weak as a child—weak alike in mind and body."[48]

If unmanly bodies were a consequence of addiction, observers also pointed to weak, frail bodies to explain why some men became opium eaters, whereas other individuals used opiates without negative consequences. An 1856 story in *Flag of Our Union* reported the case of a young man from Elmira, New York, whose "yellow and haggard visage gives fearful evidence of the presence of the coiled serpent" of opium eating. The unfortunate "laudanum drinker" was "a dwarf, about fifteen years of age, quite small and delicately formed." Disability explained why the teenager "ha[d] been a victim of the habit for years, and all attempts to prevent his indulgence in the stupefying drug have been in vain." Repeated efforts by family and friends to help the young man failed, so the community gave up. Instead, a local drugstore negotiated a contract to supply the young man with laudanum at a discount rate. Yet this arrangement, which the people of Elmira saw as a pragmatic solution, horrified outsiders because addiction seemed to rob the boy of all claims to manliness. "The only object for which this strange creature seems to live," the author lamented, "is this deadly narcotic, and his only care and ambition is centered in producing the little means required to buy the two-ounce draught." His relationship with laudanum was that of "the destroyer and the destroyed." Already seen as wanting in manliness and prone to addiction because of his size, the young man was further emasculated by laudanum, which sapped his independence as well. The moral of this account was unambiguous. Dependency and physical infirmity meant that male opium users could not embody manhood and did not warrant the same degree of sympathy as women opium eaters.[49]

Male opium eaters were met with condemnation even when their condition could be traced back to medical care. "I know of one case of a gentleman," wrote an observer in the *New York Daily News* in 1852, who "was afflicted for several years with Neuralgia. His sufferings were intense and his physician prescribed Morphine. The doses increased until they became enormously large." Soon, "the poor sufferer had contracted what was far worse" than neuralgia, "a nervous condition which demanded the continuance of the Opium." Recognizing that addiction violated his manhood, the gentleman "deeply lamented his bondage and made desperate efforts to free himself, but in vain." Physician B. W. M. McCready encountered a male opium eater in 1835 whose "health was ruined" by overstudy. Resorting to opium, he developed the "wretched habit." Opium eating left him even more "languished, nervous, and dejected" with "a very pale and unhealthy look." Considering himself a charitable fellow, McCready attempted to treat the opium eater using the withdrawal method. But soon the doctor caught his patient forging prescriptions to obtain extra doses. Before long, the man made off with McCready's pocketbook, leaving the good doctor with nothing but contempt for his former patient and the "vicious and degrading" addiction.[50] Considering this antebellum groundwork of hostility toward men who used opium regularly, it is not surprising that addicted Civil War veterans would be met with antipathy, and even outright hostility, in the coming decades.

The notion that opium eating was an effeminate and emasculating condition deeply affected men's emotional and psychological well-being. Male opium eaters despaired at their apparent inability to live up to standards of manhood. A rare letter from an opium-addicted man, Sylvanus Cobb Jr., captured this haunting feeling of self-loathing. Cobb was a temperance activist who publicly denounced drinking, despite being secretly addicted to opium. Originally prescribed by a physician in 1848 for rheumatism, Cobb often took "a small pill of gum opium . . . for the purpose of aiding me at work, never once dreaming there was to be formed a habit that could not be easily broken off." After "using it daily for about six months," he began experiencing "weakened . . . virile power" and the loss of "carnal desire," convincing Cobb to quit the drug. But from the first pill he skipped, "one little set of nerves began to dance a jig, then another." Withdrawal brought on the "sensation of electric shocks . . . through every avenue of my system." Overpowered by cravings that "*would not* be quiet," Cobb "got up and went to my opium drawer" and swallowed a pill. Eventually he was taking a hundred grains of opium a day. Multiple attempts to quit during the 1840s and 1850s failed, forcing Cobb to confess his condition to his wife. Depressed, hopeless, and emasculated by his lack of willpower, Cobb described himself as "the living epitome of mental and nervous unrest" and "a bound victim" to opium for life.[51] Such powerful emotions illustrate how addicted men took society's views of their manhood seriously, to the detriment of their emotional and mental health. After the Civil War, addicted veterans likewise internalized the idea that opium slavery was emasculating and disgraceful, leading to a profound sense of despair, emotional turmoil, and in some cases even suicide.[52]

Lacking a medicalized vocabulary for drug addiction, antebellum doctors and other observers frequently adopted the metaphor of "slavery" to describe the dependency and infirmity characteristic of opium "abuse." "There is no slavery so complete as that of the opium-taker," one commentator brooded in 1849.[53] This metaphor reflected a broad cultural reliance on slavery to explain dependency. Opium was merely one of many things that might "enslave" white antebellum Americans. Southern planters loudly decried the Yankees who economically "enslaved" the South. "Financially we are more enslaved to the North than our negroes," an Alabama judge told John C. Calhoun in 1847.[54] For their part, Northern and Midwestern antislavery Republicans fumed about the "slave power" that dominated the federal government. From countless church pulpits and convention stages, temperance speakers railed against "slavery" to drink. These metaphorical slaveries conveyed broadly recognized fears about the loss of white male independence in a society that was profoundly in flux politically, economically, socially, technologically, and even spiritually. Against a backdrop of dizzying change, the metaphor of opium slavery caught on because it made sense to antebellum observers who were already worried about anything that might endanger white male independence. Little wonder one doctor quipped that opiate addiction was "worse than African slavery."[55] Such fears were ironic and misguided, considering that white men by their own design possessed far greater rights than other Americans. Even if the opium slavery metaphor made sense to many antebellum Americans, the comparison of addiction to chattel slavery was also deeply flawed and unrealistic. Opium "slaves" were not bought and sold or subjected to the brutal, systematic violence endured by the roughly 4 million African Americans held in bondage in 1861. If the clumsy opium slavery metaphor provided a convenient vocabulary for antebellum Americans to express their uneasiness about drug use and users, by falsely equating addiction and physical bondage, the label also mocked the experiences of Americans who endured literal slavery.

Antebellum Social Reform Movements and Addiction

The opium slavery metaphor also drew on the racial and moral discourse of the temperance and missionary movements. The antebellum missionary movement supplied a racial counterpoint to white opium eaters through widely circulated descriptions of Chinese opium smokers. As the US maritime trade with China bloomed during the early nineteenth century, white American missionaries flocked to China, taking up the Great Commission in Hong Kong and other Chinese ports. Once there, missionaries were shocked to witness the practice of opium smoking, a common social activity among Chinese men, much like drinking among white American men. Missionaries became vocal critics of opium smoking among the Chinese whom they hoped to "save," even as American merchants carried boatloads of opium back home to US ports and enjoyed handsome profits. One missionary warned in 1841 that "the use of opium" was among the "greatest stumbling block[s]" to bringing "the light of the Gospel" to China. He urged devout Americans to pray for Chinese deliverance from opium.[56] Some missionaries desperately tried to cure Chinese opium smokers by giving them laudanum, a seemingly less exotic form of consumption that might allow for tapering off.[57] Americans also loudly denounced the British for "enslaving" the Chinese to opium against the Qing government's wishes, even as some observers pointed out American complicity in opium trafficking.[58] With Chinese immigration to the United States increasing in earnest during the 1840s, it did not take long for American politicians to latch on to missionaries' warnings about opium smoking and smokers.[59] During a January 1855 hearing on a would-be Pacific railroad in the House of Representatives, Milton Latham, a Democrat from California, cautioned that "opium eating and smoking are now rapidly on the increase in every part of China." Decades of opium trafficking had been "carried on by armed vessels" that "distribute both chests of opium and the Scriptures." Yet "the eagerness of the [Chinese] people to buy the poison" far outweighed their enthusiasm for the Bible. Opium, the congressman warned, "ruins the country."[60]

Like doctors who linked opium eating to unmanliness and disability, missionaries linked opium "abuse" to the supposed Chinese racial inferiority, with disturbing implications for white opium users. Moses Clarke White, the Yale medical student who wrote an 1854 thesis about opiate abuse, was a missionary in China before taking up his studies in New Haven. Firsthand observation of Chinese opium smokers indelibly shaped White's views about opiate use among white Americans. Although the opium smoking practiced in China and the opium eating that occurred in the antebellum United States were very different—smoking was a recreational social practice, like the saloon culture of American men, whereas opium eating occurred primarily in an individual medical context—White lumped these distinctive forms of consumption together under the label of "slavery." "The habit of opium smoking (like that of opium eating)," he explained, "is exceedingly enslaving." The Chinese opium smoker and the white American opium eater alike ended up in the same dismal fate, with "mental and moral powers enfeebled" by opium and without "energy or resolution to break away from the chains which bind him."[61] White went so far as to equate the bodies of white opium eaters with those of Chinese opium smokers. Ordinarily, nineteenth-century Americans focused on racial differences embodied by white and Chinese men, represented by skin color, facial features, hair, and dress. To xenophobic Americans, these visual markers served as evidence of white racial superiority.[62] Troublingly, White suspected that chronic opium intoxication diminished racial differences between Chinese and white men. He claimed that opium turned the skin of white opium eaters "yellow."[63] Opium abuse, White reasoned, chipped away at whiteness, thus branding American opium eaters with the stigma of racial inferiority. In nineteenth-century American society, organized along racial lines, few allegations could be more unsettling than to challenge the whiteness of a white person. Yet according to the young missionary-turned-medical student, this disturbing racial transformation was the certain outcome of opium eating.

White's racialized understanding of opium eating seemed particularly alarming in the context of Chinese immigration to the West Coast beginning in the late 1840s.[64] In the wake of the California Gold Rush, which triggered mass migration from China followed by a violent white backlash, lurid stories about alleged Chinese racial inferiority circulated widely in the popular and medical media. These racist stories often explicitly linked opium abuse to supposed Chinese racial, moral, and national decline, heightening public concern about the dangers of opium in the United States.[65] In the 1860s, amid the racial upheaval of the Civil War and Reconstruction, when white fears about "miscegenation" and the erosion of white supremacy were front and center in American society and politics, the gravity of these stories only increased as nativists and Republicans grappled with the "Chinese question."[66] Soon, the menace of opium smoking fueled a burgeoning movement to restrict Chinese immigration and to heavily circumscribe the lives of Chinese migrants already living in the West. In 1862, a California doctor predicted the imminent collapse of American civilization, not because of Confederate victories at the Seven Days Battles, the Second Battle of Bull Run, or Fredericksburg but because of immigration from China, a nation that was itself "poisoned with opium." The immediate exclusion of Chinese immigrants and a ban on opium imports to the United States were the only true means of saving the Union.[67]

Racist and hyperbolic newspaper stories notwithstanding, there is little tangible evidence to indicate that a large population of opium smokers actually existed in antebellum America. Even in 1881, a year before Congress passed the Chinese Exclusion Act banning immigration from China, the *New-York Times* estimated there were only 10,000 Chinese and 4,000 "native American" opium smokers in the United States.[68] Yet nativists throughout the Civil War era nonetheless floated the specter of rampant opium smoking among Chinese immigrants because it helped justify racial discrimination and immigration restrictions. Linking opium slavery to racial decline was the other side of the coin.

The missionary movement and anti-Chinese xenophobia thus profoundly affected Americans' perceptions of opium slavery. For decades, opium eating had been primarily seen as afflicting white women or effeminate white men with disabilities. But in the 1850s, race became an increasingly salient factor in the cultural constitution of opiate addiction. The racialized discourse around Chinese opium smokers raised disturbing questions about white opium users.[69] If white Americans were racially superior to the Chinese, then why did some white men become "enslaved" to opium, a vice of the racial other? Did abusing opium somehow degrade one's whiteness, or worse still, did white men's addictions signal a broader decline of the white race? After all, if opium smoking played a key role in the collapse of Chinese civilization, as American missionaries alleged, would a large population of white opium eaters threaten the future of the United States as well?[70] After the Civil War, with addiction alarmingly on the rise among veterans and other white Americans, Gilded Age race scientists would take up these questions with renewed urgency.

In the short term, however, the antebellum temperance movement helped distract doctors and other Americans from these complex racial questions by providing a palatable explanation for opium eating among whites that was rooted in contemporary notions of morality. As Moses Clarke White explained, opium eaters' "moral powers are enfeebled."[71] Addicted white men, he implied, must be inherently sinful and thus more liable to opium dependency. White's rationalization reflected not only his experiences as a missionary but also the influence of the antebellum temperance crusade, a cultural juggernaut closely linked to evangelical Christianity. Temperance was a mass movement that boasted more adherents and influence than any other contemporary reform movement.[72] Since the days of Benjamin Rush, temperance activists and doctors (not always mutually exclusive groups) had classified opium intoxication as one of many branches on the tree of intemperance, alongside drinking, tobacco use, gambling, and other vices.[73] Lyman Beecher, the influential cofounder of the American Temperance Society, once lectured that "opium," like whiskey, "is only another mode of producing inebriation." Opium could act as a kind of gateway drug, Beecher warned. Opium "not infrequently unites its own forces with those of ardent spirits to impair health, and destroy life."[74] According to the Sons of Temperance, the "consumption of opium" was an immoral form of "self-destruction." When the "opium-eater" invariably "increases his dose grain by grain," it "terminate[s] in uncontrollable and beastly excess."[75] Like liquor, opium threatened to overshadow all other physical, emotional, and spiritual desires, from the "love of women" to "the peacefulness of religion" and "even sleep . . . that chief nourisher in life's feast."[76] Not all temperance advocates considered opium to be as dangerous as alcohol, but most agreed that opium and alcohol shared many dangerous parallels.[77] Both substances were intoxicants moonlighting as medicines. When used outside medical advice, opium and alcohol "enslaved" users and degraded their moral character. As *Gunn's Domestic Medicine* warned, opium, "when it is used as a stimulant or luxury, and not as medicine, produces the same sufferings as those which arise from intoxicating liquors. . . . Therefore use not this drug, but as intended by the Great Father of the universe."[78] "Who has not experienced the soothing restorative operation of opium, that divine medicine . . . [and] 'magnum Dei donum[,]' the great gift of God," added another home health guide, "and who has not known its demoniacal influence when imprudently employed?"[79]

Temperance advocates considered the moral and spiritual fruits of opium eating to be especially problematic, with dark implications for one's soul. For starters, opium intoxication seemed to cause an alarming loss of self-control.[80] Like whiskey, opium "induces a suspension of the will" that "make[s] men beat their wives or starve their children."[81] This loss of self-control not only inverted proscribed gender roles and physically endangered families but also seemed to directly clash with the Bible, the foundational text for the temperance movement. As Lyman Beecher warned, opium eaters were simply acting out "a temptation to intemperance." Opium eating was merely a "sensual and criminal indulgence" in the desires of the flesh, added a Boston newspaper.[82] For these reasons, temperance activists urged "young men" to "totally abstain" from opium.[83]

Detractors of opium often used familiar biblical language and allegories to convey the apparent sinfulness of opium eating. "When used for no necessitous purpose, and taken habitually," one writer warned, opium "acts as a horrible demon." "In no other way does" a man "so much demonize his manhood and brutify his mind, as in the habitual indulgence of such a drug."[84] Alluding to the devil and the fall of man in the Garden of Eden, another writer cautioned that opium "coils itself, like a deadly snake, round the victim . . . until escape is impossible."[85] For the opium eater, "heaven is converted into the gloom of hell."[86] The spiritual imagery of temptation, abstinence, demons, and serpents would have resonated deeply with American Christians. Most Americans were familiar with such biblical motifs as well as Bible verses condemning drunkenness as a sin, while praising self-control as one of the "fruits of the spirit."[87] Ultimately, by equating alcohol and opium addiction, antebellum temperance rhetoric defined opium eating as a sin. This classification persisted throughout the nineteenth century, eventually resulting in profoundly negative repercussions for addicted Civil War veterans. In 1877, as addiction surged, Henry Ward Beecher echoed the anti-opium religious convictions of his father Lyman. "Opium eating and dram drinking are acts of vicious self-indulgence" that warranted condemnation, the younger Beecher explained.[88]

Endemic, Not Epidemic

Long before the Civil War erupted in 1861, opiate addiction had become a well-documented and widely recognized phenomenon in American society. With physicians, missionaries, and temperance activists leading the way,

Americans had developed distinct understandings of opium slavery rooted in contemporary medicine, culture, and social reform movements. However, despite a constant stream of commentary about opium eating in antebellum medical literature, addiction failed to generate sustained attention in the popular media. If lurid stories about opium "slaves" were titillating, popular depictions of opium eating in newspapers and magazines were also sporadic. This limited media coverage reflected the reality that cases of addiction were relatively few in number compared to the postwar decades. Opium eating was endemic. It had not yet flared into an epidemic. As the *BMSJ* observed in 1833, "There are not many in this country addicted to the free and constant use of opium."[89] An equally important factor in limiting antebellum media coverage was the identity of opium eaters themselves. Doctors, writers in newspapers, and other observers were convinced that addiction was relegated to white women, the archetypal American opium eater, or to "other" men with predisposing factors, such as those who were intemperate or disabled or Chinese. These beliefs about the identity of opium eaters meant that the phenomenon appeared contained to the margins of society and did not necessarily pose a broad threat. Thus in the antebellum era, the phenomenon of opium eating rarely generated sustained public alarm or coverage in the popular media, relative to the postbellum decades.

Even in New York City, few observers outside the coroner's office and a handful of doctors seemed to care much about opiate addiction or overdoses before the Civil War. In 1852, John S. Schofield, a physician familiar with local mortality patterns, tried to raise the alarm in the *New-York Times*. He observed that New York's 500 pharmacies collectively sold 1,000 pounds of opium per week, enough to support many opium eaters. The drug was so cheap and abundant that "recruits from the alcoholic ranks" might be tempted to switch from whiskey to opium. "Something should be done at once to meet and arrest the evil" before it "bringeth forth tears, disease, and death," Schofield urged. But aside from a few concerned physicians, these warnings failed to catch on.[90] As the coroner could attest, most opiate overdose deaths occurred among women, especially the poor and immoral women whose deaths typically garnered little sympathy or notice.

It would ultimately take the nation's worst health crisis, the Civil War, to spark enough cases of opiate addiction among white men to attract sustained media attention. Doubling down on therapeutic patterns established in the antebellum decades, Civil War surgeons and soldiers relied heavily on opiates to cope with the war's carnage. Predictably, white veterans became addicted by the thousands. Observers in medicine, the media, and government agonized about the numbers and identity of these new American opium eaters. Consequently, opiate addiction among Civil War veterans sparked a national panic that eclipsed the antebellum era's compartmentalized coverage of women opium eaters and Chinese opium smokers. Foreshadowing this looming postwar addiction epidemic, Moses Clarke White concluded his 1854 Yale medical thesis with the prescient warning that "we . . . as a people may soon be deeply interested in the means of curing patients addicted to the abuse of opium."[91] Within a decade, the Civil War proved White's prediction all too accurate.

Chapter 3

The Drs. Put Me on Morphine

Civil War Medicine and Addiction

Alpheus M. Chappell never got "entirely over" the wounds he received at Gettysburg, as he explained in a tragic 1886 letter. The Confederate captain was shot while storming Union lines alongside Gen. George Pickett's ill-fated Virginia division on the sweltering afternoon of July 3, 1863. The other officers above Chappell had apparently been shot, so it fell to him to lead the 14th Virginia Infantry as the men charged through clouds of smoke toward Union lines. But a white-hot lead minié ball stopped Chappell in his tracks, smashing into his left kneecap at full force and pancaking on impact with the bone. The ball angrily ripped through cartilage and soft tissue at the joint, tearing a huge exit hole in the leg. Chappell dropped to the tall, dry grass in unspeakable pain. His unit struggled on under withering rifle and cannon fire, even briefly breaching the infamous Angle before being routed by its stalwart defenders. As the adrenaline of the Civil War's only named charge faded to shock and loss, retreating Confederate soldiers collected their maimed captain and dragged him behind the lines to a field hospital. When the Army of Northern Virginia and its seventeen-mile-long wagon train retreated from Gettysburg, Chappell bounced along with them on the bumpy wagon ride through Pennsylvania and Maryland. Every rut and rock in the road added to his misery.[1]

The Civil War produced thousands of war stories like Chappell's, which too often ended in grisly deaths from infection or exposure. Yet judging by outward appearances, surgeons would have considered Chappell to be one of the lucky ones. Arriving back home in Virginia, Confederate surgeons reset Chappell's bones, stitched up his wound, and tried to help however they could as the wounded man's body battled infection. But the surgeons could only give food, water, and morphine. Large and repeated doses of the drug seemed to help. Miraculously, Chappell's wound healed, and infection subsided. Somehow, he had managed to survive one of the Civil War's most notorious, suicidal frontal assaults. But the pain lingered, so the captain kept taking morphine. Ultimately, the medical care that Chappell received for his wound would haunt him, inhibiting a true recovery in the fullest sense of the word as contemporaries understood it. Twenty-three years after Gettysburg, the wound's unexpected consequences still dominated the older soldier's life. As Chappell explained in the 1886 letter, the "Drs. put me on Morphine and I can't stop that." He had become addicted to the painkillers that surgeons administered after Gettysburg. Although the gunshot wound had long since healed, the drug refused to release Chappell from its chains.[2]

Nor was he alone. Thousands of veterans became addicted to opiates because of medical care during the Civil War, when opium and morphine were among the most widely used remedies for pain and sickness. In this chapter I investigate how the war triggered an epidemic of addiction among veterans, illuminating the events that led wounded and sick soldiers like Chappell from the surgeon's tent down the path of addiction in their postwar lives. The Civil War created a health crisis on a scale unprecedented in American history, leaving millions of soldiers sick and in pain. To cope with this unparalleled influx of suffering, military doctors fell back on time-honored medicines even as they innovated new therapeutic techniques and organizational forms. Opiates, already the "magnum Dei donum" of the materia medica, were drafted into wartime service. American physicians were well aware that addiction was a potential outcome of the medicinal use of opiates, a phenomenon that had been noted in medical journals for decades. Yet the immediacy of the Civil War's health crisis was front of mind, outweighing the potential risk of addiction in the future. Union and Confederate surgeons administered opiates widely to treat soldiers' painful injuries and debilitating sicknesses. In the war's sickly swamps, sun-bleached cornfields, and dirty camps, soldiers also self-medicated with opiates for sickness, pain, boredom, and anxiety. Predictably, these medical practices often resulted in addiction, sometimes beginning during the war years and in other cases much later.

When weary, lean-faced veterans like Chappell finally straggled home from war, limping on wooden crutches or ill-fitting prosthetics and with "empty sleeves" pinned to their waistcoats, many kept taking opiates as they had done during the Civil War. Just as the drugs helped armies stay in the field, they also helped ailing veterans cope with the lingering effects of wartime wounds and sicknesses, which often lasted a lifetime. Military officials during and after the war, families, doctors, public health officials, journalists, and even some veterans themselves were horrified to witness a nascent addiction crisis grow into a full-blown epidemic among war survivors. Panicked observers sounded alarm bells in medical journals, public health investigations, newspapers, and even novels. The Civil War was not the only cause of addiction, nor were veterans the only Americans who used drugs during this era. Yet a firm cultural association between veterans and opium slavery solidified in the public's consciousness as the stereotype of the morphine-addicted old soldier, an oft-referenced character in histories of the Civil War.

Opiates in Civil War Medicine

As war loomed during the secession crisis of 1860–61, well-read American doctors recognized—in the back of their minds, at least—that injured and sick soldiers ran the risk of becoming addicted to medicinal opiates. Since the days of Benjamin Rush, addiction cases had been reported in medical journals and sometimes in newspapers, even if such cases were mostly women or "unmanly" men. Scattered reports of addicted veterans of the antebellum Indian Wars and the Mexican-American War circulated as well, reminding doctors that the brutality of nineteenth-century warfare could foster addiction.[3] Prominent medical journals during the 1850s provided reports of opium eating after painful amputations, raising awareness of the perceived risks attendant to the procedure and foreshadowing the coming addiction epidemic.[4]

Although addiction was a known risk of extended opiate use, Civil War doctors ("surgeons," in military parlance) relied heavily on the drugs given their antebellum training and because there were few alternatives. When the war broke out, opiates were the most dependable and widely used drugs in the medical arsenal. They were natural tools for surgeons tasked with the impossible: waging a defensive war against relentless, poorly understood sicknesses, pain, and suffering. Unlike generals, who could rest their minds and refit their armies in the downtime between battles and campaigns, surgeons' work rarely stopped. Armies in winter quarters might be crippled by camp diseases, struck down by pestilence on the march, or overwhelmed and immobilized by injuries after battle.[5] To complete their herculean tasks, surgeons needed opiates. Not using them in many cases was unthinkable. As a Confederate medical handbook explained, "Opium is the one indispensable drug on the battlefield—important to the surgeon, as gunpowder to the ordnance."[6] No soldier could have misunderstood this martial metaphor.

Opiates were so important because they were utilitarian. Surgeons and stewards could administer opium, morphine, laudanum, and Dover's powder effectively against hundreds of ailments, as civilian doctors had done before the war. Doctors recognized that opiates could not cure sicknesses or heal wounds outright but could reliably mitigate symptoms such as pain, diarrhea, and coughing. Joseph Woodward, Union army surgeon and wartime apostle of the sanitary movement, reminded Union surgeons that "opiates are not to be regarded as specific or curative agents." But because opiates "control the frequency of the stools," they were immensely useful for camp fevers, even if they did not cure the underlying disease. He advised the use of opium, morphine, Dover's powder, paregoric, laudanum enemas, and even a compound of strychnine and opium for "simple diarrhea," dysentery, chronic diarrhea, enteritis, typhoid, malaria, measles, catarrh, pneumonia, and rheumatism.

Opium or morphine should also be given "in large doses" to comfort dying soldiers.[7] The Confederate medical handbook that described opium as "one indispensable drug on the battlefield" told surgeons to employ opiates not only to mitigate pain but also to arrest vomiting, diarrhea, and internal bleeding; relieve the muscle spasms of amputees' stumps; and sedate shrieking patients who arrived at hospitals overnight until surgeons could attend to them in the morning. "Large and repeated doses" of morphine could numb soldiers, easing their passing.[8] To medical staff, opiates seemed like a godsend. With the drugs' remarkable utility in mind, Union Army of Kentucky's medical director reminded his surgeons on the march that "a pill of opium . . . will be found exceedingly convenient . . . if carried in the pocket of the Surgeon."[9]

Opiates were also important because they enabled the military to fulfill its obligation to provide for soldiers' health needs. When soldiers enlisted, they surrendered their basic freedoms to their respective governments. They lost the power to decide for themselves where to go, when to sleep, and what to wear. In return, the military agreed to provide wages, clothing, shelter, and medical care to keep men healthy.[10] Considered within these negotiations between the military and soldiers, opiates functioned like rations, uniforms, and pay stubs. Without painkilling, diarrhea-suppressing, sleep-inducing opium and morphine, the military would have failed to hold up the medical end of the enlistment contract.

Surgeons took guidelines to dispense "large and repeated" doses literally. Civil War armies swigged, swallowed, and injected opiates in mind-boggling quantities. They were among the most widely used medicines of the Civil War, eclipsed only by diet and alcohol. Union military forces requisitioned 9,875,808 opium pills, 448,864 ounces of powdered opium, 492,706 ounces of Dover's powder (opium and ipecac), 901,467 ounces of laudanum, 998,599 ounces of paregoric, and 29,828 ounces of morphine. These figures dwarfed the 3,044,437 ounces of ether and 1,588,066 ounces of chloroform used to anesthetize wounded soldiers during surgery, or the 1,273,505 ounces of quinine and cinchona used as a malaria prophylactic. Opiate requisitions were surpassed only by alcohol, including 77,785,120 ounces of whiskey, 17,991,072 ounces of brandy, and 29,239,168 ounces of sherry, drinks that doubled as medicines and a way to appease rowdy soldiers. Enumerating the vast quantity of opiates requisitioned by the Union army underscores the drugs' centrality to Civil War medicine. Sizing up this huge stockpile is also a roundabout way to measure the carnage unleashed by the Civil War. It took millions upon millions of opium pills and morphine injections to help soldiers cope with the suffering they endured in America's bloodiest war.[11]

Tallying the sicknesses and injuries that plagued Civil War armies puts the need for such giant quantities of medicines in stark relief. More than 6.5

million cases of sickness, wounds, and injuries were reported during the war, spread among some 3.2 million soldiers. Only about 500,000 of these reports were battle wounds or accidental injuries, including 235,585 gunshot wounds among Union troops alone.[12] Disease accounted for the vast majority of the Civil War's medical emergencies and was responsible for about two-thirds of the war's roughly 750,000 deaths.[13] Millions of soldiers took opiate painkillers and antidiarrheal medicines during the war. Dysentery and diarrheal sicknesses were prolific, afflicting more than 70 percent of Union troops. "Fevers" abounded too, and nearly six in ten soldiers in blue contracted malaria.[14] All things considered, the average Civil War soldier was sick enough to report to the surgeon twice a year, not to mention the countless times that soldiers treated their own ailments in camp without reporting ill at sick call.[15] No soldier's diary or letters home were complete without referencing his health, usually to grumble about malaise. When soldiers needed medical care for any one of hundreds of maladies, they could expect to be given a dose or two (or more) of opium or morphine. Indeed, *The Medical and Surgical History of the War of the Rebellion*—the US government's official medical record of the Civil War, spanning thousands of pages in six volumes published between 1870 and 1888—is replete with medical case histories describing the ubiquitous use of opium, morphine, laudanum, paregoric, and Dover's powder for all manner of sicknesses and injuries.[16]

Opiate use increased throughout the war, mirroring the quickening pace of slaughter. Early on, medical supplies were notoriously understocked. After the First Battle of Bull Run in July 1861, swarms of wounded soldiers ended up in Richmond hospitals. According to the *Richmond Dispatch*, "a vast amount of physic"—or, medicines—would be needed to help them, but supplies were already short. The war had barely begun, so armies had not yet stockpiled enough of any supply, let alone opium.[17] But surgeons and quartermasters caught on quickly. When casualties mounted during the bloody battles of 1862, armies began to stockpile opiates near field hospitals before the shooting began. In the lead-up to the Battle of Fredericksburg in December 1862, Jonathan Letterman, the pioneering medical director of the Union Army of the Potomac, stockpiled 200 drams of morphine, 400 dozen opium pills, 50 dozen pills of opium and camphor, and 25 pounds of powdered opium. These "extra" opiates merely supplemented medicines already supplied to surgeons.[18]

Between the butchery of the battlefield and the pestilence of camp, government contractors struggled to keep up with the vastly increased demand for opiates in the United States. So much opium flowed into the country that Congress implemented an aggressive tariff of $2.50 per pound for opium and ounce of morphine. Opium could help armies remain in the field while the revenue raised on imports could help fund the war effort.[19] Yet the unpredictability of campaigns and leaks in medical purveyors' offices meant that surgeons faced localized shortages of drugs. The US Sanitary Commission—a civilian relief organization that partnered with the military to provide medical supplies, hospital workers, and sanitary expertise—supplemented the Union army's opiate stockpile with shipments of opium and morphine and encouraged hospital staff to administer the drugs in earnest. One Sanitary Commission doctor boasted how opium "has always been used more freely by surgeons in this country than in Europe," seeing little downside to dosing surgical patients with opiates. Another doctor writing under the aegis of the commission reminded military surgeons to "carry in his pocket a phial containing pills of opium" so the medicines would always be within reach.[20] Accordingly, the Sanitary Commission tried to make sure opiates were always on hand in Union hospitals. In the aftermath of the May 1864 Battle of the Wilderness, which saw many soldiers burned and killed in an inferno, the commission issued 6,000 pills of opium, 2,000 pills of camphor and opium, and 17 ounces of morphine to Union forces near Richmond.[21]

Yet even the Sanitary Commission's relief efforts were not enough. As the war dragged on longer than most Americans had initially feared, the military's appetite for opiates outpaced the nation's capacity to manufacture and supply them. In well-equipped army hospitals, stewards—soldiers responsible for compounding and dispensing prescriptions—used apothecary tools to make opium pills in small batches by mixing raw opium with gum arabic, soap, ipecac, or camphor.[22] But regimental surgeons and those working at field hospitals lacked pill-making machines and rarely had time to spare for making opium pills by hand. An opium supply crunch prompted Union surgeon general William A. Hammond to take unprecedented measures. Over the opposition of private sector pharmaceutical wholesalers, which had traditionally supplied bulk medicines to American doctors and pharmacists, in 1863 Hammond created the first federally funded pharmacies to manufacture medicines for the military on an industrial scale. In government pharmaceutical labs in Philadelphia and Astoria, New York, women and men worked shoulder to shoulder to fill the military's insatiable hunger for drugs (fig. 3.1). Hammond's scheme marked a turning point for the Union war machine's ability to provide medical supplies to military hospitals in the North and the occupied South. Thereafter, Union medical purveyors directed a steady flow of medicines to Northern troops, helping to sustain the war effort in the bloodiest years of 1864 and 1865.[23] These government pharmaceutical labs also saw the entry of a large number of American women into the pharmacy sector, a male domain before the war. Women's crucial wartime medical work, like their efforts in government offices, farms, and weapons factories, later provided ammunition for the postwar women's movement.[24] The crushing medical demand sparked by the Civil War proved

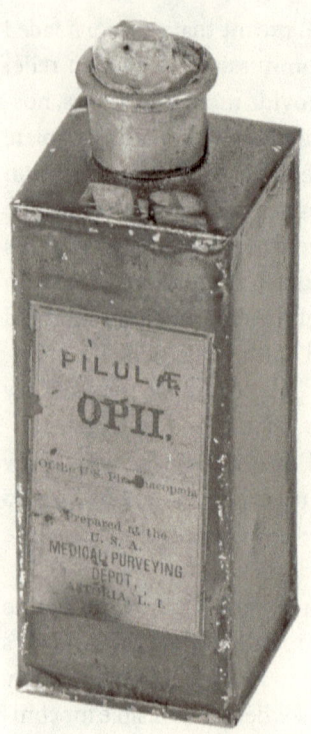

Figure 3.1 Tin of opium pills produced at the government pharmaceutical laboratory at Astoria, New York. Courtesy Wood Library-Museum of Anesthesiology, Schaumburg, IL.

a boon for the American pharmaceutical sector as well, launching the industry into decades of unprecedented growth and reorganization.[25]

Like the Union military juggernaut, the Confederate military also consumed enormous quantities of opiates.[26] But considering the severe shortages afflicting the Confederacy, many Southerners had to make do without opiates.[27] One Confederate soldier was forced to substitute lettuce juice for opium, although the leafy green perhaps did little good.[28] Like other manufactures, most medicines had to be imported to the South. Blockaded by the Union navy's "anaconda," the Confederacy resorted to plundering and smuggling opium. Union supply trains and depots were the easiest sources of drugs, and opportunistic Confederates looted medicines whenever they could. When Union general Nathaniel Banks and his army fled Winchester, Virginia in May 1862, "Stonewall" Jackson's Confederate soldiers seized 500 pounds of opium from "Commissary Banks."[29] A few weeks later, after the Confederate defeat at Gettysburg in July 1863, Lee's retreating army plundered drugstores as it passed through Chambersburg, Pennsylvania.[30]

The Confederacy's opium supplies dwindled in 1862 and 1863, even as demand skyrocketed. "There is great want of opium in the Confederate States," the *Richmond Christian Advocate* complained in November 1862, while Lee's army recuperated from the bloody Battle of Antietam two months prior. Desperate Confederates looked inward for solutions, seeking domestic substitutes for imported drugs.[31] Surgeon General Samuel Preston Moore commissioned physician Francis Peyre Porcher to identify indigenous plants that might serve as decent substitutes. Porcher's resulting *Resources of Southern Fields and Forests* (1863) noted that *Papaver somniferum*, the opium poppy, might be cultivated on Southern farms but that horse chestnut, onion, red poppy, and prickly poppy could perhaps serve as alternatives.[32] From Richmond to Houston, Confederate newspapers echoed Porcher's suggestion that civilians take up poppy cultivation instead of cotton or tobacco. Southern opium could be profitable for planters and good for the war effort. The harvest could even be "carried on by children" or "small negroes" in regions where most farmers had left to join the army.[33] Twenty-nine enslaved people were forced to work on a farm in Louisiana, where the governor tried to emulate the success of the Union's pharmaceutical labs using white prickly poppy, a native species, instead of *Papaver somniferum*.[34] Calls to use children and enslaved people to grow poppies underscores the Confederacy's desperation for medical supplies as the war dragged on. Finally, in March 1863, Surgeon General Samuel Preston Moore ordered military medical purveyors to furnish women with opium poppy seeds. Women could "render the Confederacy [an] essential service" by delivering their opium harvests to the military.[35] Unrealistic at best, Moore's scheme reflects the Confederate government's delusional faith in white women's undying zeal for the Confederate cause. Yet with husbands, sons, fathers, and brothers absent, enslaved people to control, hungry mouths to feed, and Yankee "bummers" to ward off, opium cultivation was the last thing on most Confederate women's minds. Just a few months later, poor white women all over the Confederacy revolted, demanding "bread or blood."[36]

Little ever came of efforts to grow Confederate poppies. Instead, smugglers and blockade-runners supplied most of the Confederacy's opium. The *Bermuda*, a blockade-runner out of Liverpool, England, slipped past Union warships and landed at Savannah, Georgia, in October 1861 carrying a load of Enfield rifles, cannons, and morphine.[37] How many blockade-runners managed to slip through Union ships is difficult to gauge. During the early war years, they appear to have kept Southern ports well supplied with opiates. About 40 percent of prescriptions sold at Charleston's Pankin Drug Store between January 1860 and August 1862 contained opiates, a slight rate increase compared with the previous decade that suggests a consistent supply of opiates made it to the South before the Union blockade became effective later in the war.[38] Wholesalers in Atlanta, Richmond, and Charlotte advertised opiates "from John Bull" throughout the war, evidence that the drugs also remained available in Southern cities.[39] As the Union naval blockade of the Confederacy became increasingly effective from 1863 onward, it seems likely that the volume of sea-smuggled opiates diminished. A more reliable option was to smuggle opiates through the relatively porous overland border between North and South. One clever smuggler loaded morphine, quinine, ether, and whiskey into a wagon with "SMALL-POX" emblazoned on the side to scare away border guards.[40] Confederate sympathizers in the North and militant Confederate women in Union-occupied regions engaged in smuggling to support the war effort. In November 1862, a secesh woman crossed through Union lines into Chambersburg, Pennsylvania, with a pass issued by Union general Banks himself. Suspicious residents notified Union soldiers, who arrested the woman after finding hundreds of dollars' worth of opium and quinine "for the use of Uncle Sam's enemies in the land of Dixie ... concealed in secret recesses of her dress."[41]

With demand for opiates surging and supplies growing scarcer, prices skyrocketed and a black market developed, perhaps for the first time in American history, considering that opiates were largely unrestricted before the war. In June 1864, a Richmond man tried to sell a few ounces of morphine and a quart of quinine to a pharmacist for $100. The suspicious apothecary turned the man over to the police, who traced the illicit medicines back to a drug smuggling ring operating within Richmond's Chimborazo hospital.[42] This illicit opium economy foreshadowed the cultural association of opium with criminality that would emerge in the coming decades. The boldness of soldiers who engaged in the opium black market also underscores the dire medical needs of civilians in the Confederate capital, where tens of thousands of sick and injured soldiers took precedence over the health care needs of noncombatants. Yet the fact that hospital staff at Chimborazo still possessed any opiates to steal also reveals that opiates remained on hand in at least some Confederate general hospitals, even late in the war. Certainly, medicines were in short supply in the South, especially in isolated regions.[43] But overall, opiates seem to have been accessible to Confederates in certain places for much of the war.

Surgeons North and South thus prescribed opiates liberally whenever and wherever they could. Naturally, there were variations by individual surgeon and in areas where supplies were scarce, but military clinicians generally relied heavily on opiates. Extant Civil War prescription records are rare, meaning no comprehensive data on opioid prescribing exists as it does in the twenty-first-century United States. However, a sampling of rare regimental and hospital prescription books reveals that military surgeons prescribed opiates on par with antebellum American doctors and often more frequently. Run-of-the-mill camp fevers and minor complaints were usually treated by regimental surgeons, who doled out doses of opium, quinine, or calomel. Twenty-six percent of the prescriptions recorded by the 210th Pennsylvania Infantry's regimental surgeon, W. Stockton Wilson, over a ten-day period in October 1864 contained opiates, mainly for diarrhea and fevers contracted in muddy trenches that ringed Petersburg, Virginia.[44]

At field hospitals, surgeons triaged the wounded men dragged off the field by messmates, carried to the rear by ambulances, or who stumbled in on their two legs in the nighttime hours. Hospital volunteers and surgeons assessed these patients, determining who needed urgent care, who could wait, and which cases were hopeless. This system of triage, developed by Jonathan Letterman in 1862, revolutionized military medicine.[45] Rudimentary surgeries like amputations and bullet extractions tended to occur at the field hospital level. Men whose cases were not too serious often recovered and returned to their units. Cases needed to be processed quickly, and drugs kept the workflow running smoothly in field hospitals. Contrary to enduring myths, there was little bullet biting. Men who needed surgeries were almost always given anesthetics like chloroform and ether before going under the knife. After surgery, opium and morphine dulled the pain. At Petersburg, across the lines from W. Stockton Wilson and his 210th Pennsylvania Infantry, surgeons at the 2nd North Carolina Infantry's field hospital included opiates in 40 percent of prescriptions.[46] The drugs kept patients stable while they slowly recovered or wasted away and died from infections.

As armies jockeyed for position after battle, bumpy wagon trains carried wounded men off to regional medical hubs away from the front lines, such as the Confederate hospital at Camp Stokes, near Greensboro, North Carolina. At these facilities, men were often drugged heavily with opiates. The prescription and diet book of the Camp Stokes hospital describes in detail the medical care administered to 149 soldiers transferred to the facility in August 1864. Surgeons gave opiates to sixty-six of these men, or about 44 percent.[47] Regional medical hubs were notoriously cramped and starved for resources, however. To make do, surgeons often furloughed any soldier who could travel, outsourcing their recovery to civilians, who had to feed, clothe, and medicate their wounded loved ones. Even these furloughed men got opiates, from families or local civilian doctors. William Rutherford, a prominent physician in Harrisburg, Pennsylvania, treated at least fifty-nine Union soldiers on furlough, suffering from a nightmarish array of war wounds and disease. Rutherford prescribed opiates, often repeatedly, to thirty-one of these patients, about 53 percent. On October 12, 1864, Rutherford visited a soldier, John Black, who had been bayoneted. Rutherford examined and dressed the sloughing wound, leaving Black with eight opium pills to manage the pain.[48] No matter where soldiers turned, to military or civilian doctors, the odds were high that wounded men would receive opiate painkillers.

The most severely wounded soldiers, including men with botched amputations, mangled nerve injuries, or minié balls hiding in the torso, were usually sent behind the lines by rail to large general hospitals such as Chimborazo in Richmond, Armory Square Hospital in Washington, DC, and Philadelphia's Satterlee General Hospital. These large-scale facilities had little precedent in the United States, as most antebellum hospitals had been small affairs. But the war demanded a scaling up of the nation's health care system. Before long, the Union and Confederate medical corps ballooned into vast, intricate health care networks, with thousands of hospitals staffed by tens of thousands of surgeons and hospital workers. General hospitals practically ran on opium and morphine. Surgeons dosed soldiers with anesthetics and morphine while they corrected hasty field amputations or performed experimental procedures. Opiate painkillers flowed freely as legions of nurses, orderlies, and stewards attended to convalescing soldiers for months on end before they returned to the ranks, received discharges, or finally succumbed to their wounds.

Diarrhea and Opiate Addiction

Diarrhea was by far the most common malady prompting the use of opiates during the Civil War. Like boredom and homesickness, it was a soldier's constant companion. "Diarrhea runs me hard," a Union soldier artfully wrote in his diary.[49] Indeed, "divers miseries in the bowels" stalked the men wherever they went, echoed a Confederate surgeon.[50] Whenever soldiers congregated for a few weeks, "camp fevers" like dysentery, typhus, and malaria erupted, bringing on mass outbreaks of the runs. "I have bin in bad health for ten days with my bowels," reported Robert C. Caldwell of the 10th North Carolina Heavy Artillery in October 1863. The diarrhea "has worried me bad," so "I am taking Spirits of terpin" and one "ons lodnum all the time."[51] Caldwell was right to worry. Diarrhea could easily prove lethal for dehydrated, hungry, vitamin-deficient soldiers subsisting on just a few hundred calories a day.[52]

Since diarrhea could kill through dehydration, surgeons praised the constipation-inducing properties of opium. "Opium is the most valuable medicine in diarrhea," a doctor explained, "for it keeps the sphincter in a state of permanent contraction."[53] At a Union hospital on Hilton Head Island, South Carolina, surgeons gave oral doses of Dover's powder, morphine, and opium to "quiet the stomach."[54] At the Staunton, Virginia, general hospital, experience taught Confederate surgeons that a pulverized opium mixture was the most successful treatment for "Soldier's Diarrhea."[55] Most men appreciated the relief that opium provided. Ferdinand Sophus Winslow, an Iowa quartermaster, contracted dysentery in January 1862, shortly after enlisting. His attack of "diarrhea lasted eight days," Winslow recounted to his wife, so "the Doctor gave me powders (opium and camphor) to stop it—it did so most effectually."

In fact, the opium "closed me up too much," eventually necessitating a dose of castor oil to reverse the constipation.[56]

Ordinary diarrhea was bad enough. But when diarrhea turned chronic, it could result in decades of debilitating gastrointestinal distress that often called for long-term opiate regimens. Among the most common disabilities that affected Civil War soldiers, chronic diarrhea sometimes became severe enough to warrant a discharge from the army, often enough that Union army surgeons conducted major medical studies to identify the etiology and pathology of the disease, hoping to stop the hemorrhaging of troops from the ranks. The mere passage of time rarely resolved the condition, and many chronic diarrhea sufferers never improved after the war.[57] As one observer explained in the *National Tribune* in 1877, "Wounds do not grow less grievous by lapse of time. Arms and legs lost in service do not sprout from the stump. Disabilities from disease are likely to grow worse as time rolls on . . . [and] never grow better, but generally proceed from one stage of decay to another."[58] No mere nuisance, chronic diarrhea was a deathly serious, long-term condition that could wreck veterans' bodies and health through malnutrition. When Benjamin F. Fairbanks, formerly of the 19th Maine Infantry, appeared before Maine doctor Thaddeus Hildreth for a pension examination in June 1870, the doctor noted that the soldier had lost twenty pounds since contracting chronic diarrhea during the war. Fairbanks was unable to digest solid foods without an attack, so for years he had been reduced to a milk diet. Hildreth examined another veteran who suffered from such severe chronic gastrointestinal disease that he "bleeds half a cup when he evacuates the bowels."[59] Chronic diarrhea left veterans miserable and seriously impeded their ability to function in their day-to-day lives. As one older soldier recounted in 1917, "chronic diarrhea was one of the inheritances from army life that a great many Civil War soldiers carried home with them at the end of the great four-years struggle." He explained that "not one of them could tell what moment nature would sound an urgent call to evacuate the bowels. One might be pleading at the bar, another might be ministering to the wants of a suffering patient, and yet another might be in the pulpit invoking the blessing of the Father of us all, when nature, insistent nature, gave a call that had to be heeded . . . and the victim's linen would be soiled." Some humiliated veterans were even "compelled to wear diapers" just "like babes."[60]

Mystery shrouds the etiology of such cases. Nineteenth-century diagnostic labels do not always translate clearly into the modern medical lexicon, and even in the 1860s, the chronic diarrhea label was a flexible one. Unsanitary Civil War camps, hospitals, and prisons were brimming with plausible suspects behind the mysterious ailment. Because soldiers and surgeons lacked awareness of microbes, they were not fully cognizant of the destructive effects that poor

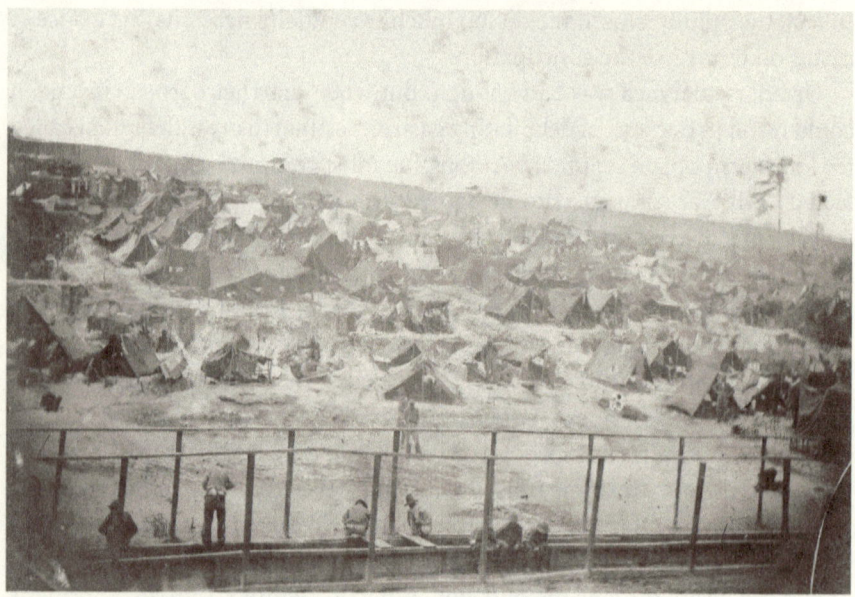

Figure 3.2 A. J. Riddle, *Andersonville Prison, Georgia. South End View of the Stockade Showing the Sentry Stands in the Distance,* August 17, 1864. The prison's latrine (*foreground*) was located mere feet from the tents that housed prisoners and the stream that supplied water, just out of sight opposite the latrine. Unsanitary conditions sparked rampant sickness and many deaths. Courtesy Library of Congress, Washington, DC.

sanitation could have on their lifelong health. Even the herculean efforts of the US Sanitary Commission to educate soldiers about the dangers of filth and miasma did not fully drive home the point. Oblivious to bacteria and viruses lurking around every latrine, soldiers often failed to wash their hands after defecating or dug latrines too close to tent rows, contaminating water supplies. At Andersonville prison in Georgia, the prison latrine immediately abutted the makeshift tents where prisoners ate and slept (fig. 3.2). To make matters worse, the festering creek that supplied water to the camp was also contaminated with feces from a Confederate camp upstream. Thousands of Union prisoners died of diarrhea, and conditions were so grim that the prison's superintendent, Henry Wirz, was later hanged for war crimes.[61]

Nineteenth-century gender roles also contributed to soldiers' intestinal malaise. Before the war, the skilled labor of cooking most often fell to women. Male soldiers now forced to cook for themselves, perhaps for the first time, tended to be quite bad at food preparation. Tired, hungry soldiers on the march also loathed cooking food slowly. Meat often went undercooked and vegetables unwashed. Daniel Holt, surgeon to the 121st New York Infantry, explained to his wife how this perfect microbial storm of camp life once gave him a nasty case of diarrhea. "A few head of cattle had been driven in and butchered," Holt recounted, and "I obtained a small piece which I ate almost raw, so hungry was I." Predictably, the "next day . . . cramps in my stomach and bowels took place to such an extent that I verily thought my last day had come." Stumbling over to his medical chest, Holt tried opium and ether for the diarrhea, but he could "not find relief . . . until every part and parcel of the offending substance was ejected from the system."[62] The Civil War's unsanitary living, eating, and drinking conditions could introduce any number of unhealthy bacteria like *E. coli*, *Salmonella*, and *Shigella* or parasites like *Trichinella* into soldiers' delicate gastrointestinal systems, with disastrous results.[63]

One or two doses of opium taken in an army hospital to squelch a bad case of diarrhea was often beneficial and usually did not culminate in addiction. But when camp diarrhea morphed into the chronic form, it called for a more dangerous therapeutic regimen. Veterans who were given opiates in the army often kept taking the medicines at home, mimicking the care provided by surgeons during the war. It did not take long to become dependent or addicted to opiates under these circumstances. Jansen Beemer Mattison, a Gilded Age expert on opiate addiction, observed patients who became addicted to opiates after using the medicines daily for as little as a month. A second doctor recounted how he became addicted to morphine after just two weeks of self-medicating with the drug. Certainly, every veteran's physical constitution was distinct, and not everyone who treated themselves with opiates became addicted. Yet modern addiction research corroborates these Gilded Age accounts, suggesting that it takes some individuals as little as two weeks of consistent morphine use to develop tolerance—a key indicator of physical dependence.[64]

Taking opium or laudanum over an extended duration to manage chronic diarrhea ultimately caused many veterans to develop opiate addictions. As the Massachusetts Board of Health reported in 1872, "Chronic affections, especially of the bowels, [are] perhaps the more common" cause of opiate addiction.[65] In 1889, Massachusetts doctor and former Union surgeon James F. A. Adams likewise observed that "among the veterans of the war, a very large number are still suffering from this disease [chronic diarrhea]. . . . As might be expected, some have become opium-eaters."[66] A New York veteran returned home from the war with a severe case of chronic diarrhea in 1867. A doctor prescribed opium and "after the diarrhea was controlled," the veteran "continued taking opium, gradually increasing the amount until he was taking one drachm of morphine a week."[67] Frank E. Pray, an Ohio veteran who fought with several infantry outfits and did a stint as a hospital steward, likewise contracted chronic diarrhea during the war. In 1880, Pray was admitted to a soldiers' home in Dayton. Upon medical inspection, the facility's doctors discovered that Pray had developed an "opium habit" after decades of taking the drug, originally prescribed by army doctors for diarrhea.[68] A Connecticut soldier contracted chronic diarrhea during the war and upon returning home "had recourse to laudanum." He quickly became addicted, and as tolerance to the drug's effects mounted, his daily dose increased so much that the veteran decided to quit. He entered the care of the Boston physician Albert Day in the late 1860s, hoping the doctor could set him free from the "horrible nightmare" of opiate addiction. In 1871, Day noted that he had recently seen "perhaps forty cases of analogous character" to the soldier he treated for laudanum addiction.[69]

Day's findings were echoed by many doctors in the postwar decades, who often remarked on the link between chronic diarrhea and opiate addiction. Thomas Davison "T. D." Crothers, once a Civil War surgical cadet, explained this connection at the AMA's annual meeting by telling the story of a Union veteran who checked himself into Crothers's private Walnut Lodge Hospital in Hartford, Connecticut, in the early 1880s. Crothers "found that opium had been used twenty years before for a chronic diarrhea following a term of service in the Civil War. He was given opium pills daily for nearly two months; then recovered." However, the veteran continued to use opium off and on for two decades after the war, because, as Crothers explained, "the use of opium for the chronic diarrhea impressed the organism, creating a diathesis which called for its use from the slightest exciting causes." In other words, Crothers believed the man's exposure to opium during the Civil War generated a disposition for using and abusing opiates. Thus, when the veteran suffered from "slightest exciting causes" later in life, he resorted to opium, leading him down the path of addiction. At first, the veteran kept his drug use secret, but eventually "he threw off all restraint and used it boldly and in large quantities," which led Crothers to the discovery of his case.[70]

Crothers was on to something. Opiate prescriptions and general knowledge about the drugs flowed freely in Civil War hospitals and camps, leading to soldiers becoming acculturated to medicinal opiate use. Wartime experiences taught men to reach for the opium, morphine, or laudanum bottle when battling sickness, pain, or stress. Once they learned this lesson, soldiers shared their wisdom with sick messmates. Scribbled inside the cover of Reverend Andrew Jackson Hartsock's diary was a recipe for a malaria remedy comprised of ten grains of opium mixed with tartarized antimony and divided into ten pills. This "infallible remedy for ague" had been shared with Hartsock by another Union army chaplain.[71] Once soldiers learned the benefits of opium, they rarely forgot. As the case treated by Crothers at Walnut Lodge underscores, veterans remembered the efficacy of opiate remedies when faced with injury and sickness in their postwar lives. Acculturation to opiates in Civil War hospitals and camps thus facilitated the likelihood of opiate addiction later in life.

Pain, Morphine, and Addiction

The same pattern held true for opiate painkillers, which took on new importance during the Civil War when more Americans than ever before needed such drugs. Like diarrhea, pain was never far from Civil War soldiers. At any moment, soldiers could be shot or stabbed on the battlefield, accidentally burned by fires or boiling water in camp, or crushed by wagons or trains while on the march. High-caliber minié balls fired with accuracy from rifled muskets could shred a man's body to pieces, leaving behind the tattered remains of limbs and nerves. One soldier in the 77th Pennsylvania Infantry was shot in the right thigh. The ball went cleanly through uniform and flesh, exiting the back of the leg and luckily missing an artery. The wound healed nicely at first, and surgeons were optimistic about the soldier's recovery. But after two months, just as the scar began forming, the wound turned inexplicably painful—an intense "shooting and darting" kind of nerve pain that never relented, and one that surgeons did not yet understand how to fix. All they could do was to keep the man under "constant hypodermics of morphia."[72] Most American doctors had never encountered such traumatic wounds before. As one Union surgeon explained in 1862 to his civilian counterparts back home, "The expression, 'only a flesh wound,' used to imply" before the war "that the wound was of little consequence. . . . But experience has shown that even a flesh wound, inflicted by a Minié ball, is by no means to be despised."[73] Mason Smith, a young Confederate lieutenant, was struck by a bullet that pierced the abdomen and lodged itself against a nerve, too deep for surgeons to extract. The case was hopeless, and as Smith slowly lay dying, the pain became unbearable. Hearing word of her son's case, Smith's mother somehow managed to navigate the war's maelstrom and arrived to comfort her son on his deathbed, like thousands of other family members who doubled as impromptu nurses for the army. But even a mother's word was not enough to soothe the dying Smith, who "begged me to stop, saying 'Mamma it hurts me to think.'" Unable to go on in agony, he begged "to be shot through the head." In this impossible situation, morphine offered the only practical measure of solace for Smith, his horrified mother, and beleaguered hospital workers. So, surgeons dosed the dying soldier to ease his passing.[74]

Opiate painkillers were popular during the Civil War because they met not only the medical needs of soldiers but also the logistical needs of overworked surgeons. Morphine allowed surgeons to do the frantic work of triage, sorting dozens or hundreds of wounded men, screaming, bloody, and in shock, during smoke-filled loud battles or the immediate aftermath of combat. Surgeons had to allocate scarce human and medical resources to the most critical (but still survivable) cases. Men whom the surgeons passed over might receive a dose of morphine to keep them calm and quiet while they waited their turn for proper care. S. G. Bremen of the 26th Ohio Infantry was shot through the shoulder at the Wilderness in May 1864. Because the ball had gone through and through, Bremen's case could be safely put on the back burner. He was "kept under morphine" until surgeons finally cleaned and dressed the injury three days later.[75] Exhausted medical staff also leaned on morphine to placate soldiers whom they could not, or simply did not want to, spend much time on. A Confederate from the 3rd Maryland Infantry was shot twice at Chancellorsville in May 1863, first in the chest while advancing on Union lines and again in the back while retreating. After the second wound, he dropped to the ground and was swiftly overtaken by Yankees. For two months, the prisoner received scant medical attention from his captors, save for hypodermic morphine injections. The shots took mere seconds to administer, keeping the man subdued while enabling Union surgeons to focus on their own wounded men. Finally, on July 5, 1863, two months after his wound, the Confederate received a full medical exam from Union surgeons at Philadelphia's Turner's Lane Hospital.[76]

Hypodermic morphine also provided a tempting way to ease the passing of mortally wounded soldiers. Union surgeon John G. F. Holston never forgot a Confederate prisoner brought to a field hospital hours after the Second Battle of Corinth in October 1862. A Union shell had smashed the man's head in, leaving him missing "both eyes and the upper part of the nose." All that remained of his head was "begrimed with blood and dirt and already containing . . . some maggots." The dying man clung to life for 48 hours, but during his final hours, he "could not be restrained from pulling the bandage down and delving with his fingers in the brain, to stop the itching." Holston's staff could not bear to look any longer. "So distressing was his state, not to himself, but to his surgical and nursing attendants," Holston wrote, "that by several parties I was importuned to have a ten-grain dose of morphia administered to end the distress." Euthanizing the soldier presented an unthinkable ethical dilemma. In the end, Holston could not bring himself to do it. The soldier died a few hours later.[77]

Every day, disheartened surgeons and horrified nurses fell back on opiates to care for their injured patients and manage an impossible workload. Yet faced with an endless deluge of patients in pain as the war's cadence quickened, surgeons realized the need to develop better management protocols. Before the Civil War, opium, laudanum, and, less often, morphine salts had been administered orally, topically, or by suppository. These methods could bring pain relief, but only slowly. The damage that minié balls, grapeshot, and heavy artillery shells could do to the body required something speedier. Responding to the crush of wounded patients needing immediate relief from pain, Union surgeons turned to the hypodermic syringe, which they began using to inject liquid morphine directly into gunshot arms and severed leg stumps. This clinical practice revolutionized how Americans took painkillers, while laying the groundwork for the postwar addiction epidemic.

Few American physicians had heard about hypodermic syringes in the 1850s, but most doctors remained unaware of the device until the Civil War. Elite European physicians invented the first such syringes and pioneered a method of localized "hypodermic" morphine injections directly into injured body parts to bring immediate pain relief. Anglophone medical journals published reports on the procedure, and these articles quietly circulated among well-read American physicians, some of whom launched small-scale clinical experiments beginning in 1856. But few ordinary practitioners recognized the promise of hypodermic medicine until prompted by the Civil War's carnage.[78] Some well-heeled Union surgeons arrived at their posts with self-purchased hypodermic syringes early in the war. Assistant surgeon John Shaw Billings began duty in Washington, DC, in July 1861 with his personal syringe in hand.[79] Surgeons marveled at the efficacy of injectable morphine to bring near-instantaneous pain relief, even for men with "crushed and torn off" limbs.[80] Morphine was ten times more powerful than opium, and injections administered directly to the tissue or veins of the injured appendage allowed the drug to metabolize faster than through the oral route, bringing a rush of pain relief and euphoria. Soon, the morphine made men sleepy and pliable, a godsend for soldiers in agony and the stressed hospital workers who cared for them. Billings's hypodermic syringe was "constantly in requisition" by his colleagues, as a grassroots hypodermic movement emerged in the Union medical corps.[81] From there, the practice spread to civilian doctors in Philadelphia, New York City, and elsewhere.[82] Eventually, the Union army requisitioned 2,093 hypodermic syringes to share between 12,000 surgeons.[83] These early devices varied in form. Some models had glass tubes equipped with screw pistons that pushed morphine through a blunt needle into the skin. Other models used leather plungers to pass the drug through pointed needles (fig. 3.3). But with too few syringes in circulation to meet demand, some army surgeons improvised. With a scalpel, they sometimes sliced open wounded limbs and used their fingertips to insert a few grains of morphine salts. While this method might have brought relief, it unknowingly spread dangerous germs.[84]

The experimental use of hypodermic morphine was part of a broader scientific movement in the Union medical corps. The war presented surgeons with an urgent glut of mangled and diseased bodies that needed novel cures. In a hierarchical military context, soldiers could not easily resist surgeons' poking and prodding. Young practitioners could hardly help but take advantage of the unprecedented opportunity to conduct scientific research involving not only hypodermic syringes but microscopes, rudimentary disinfectants,

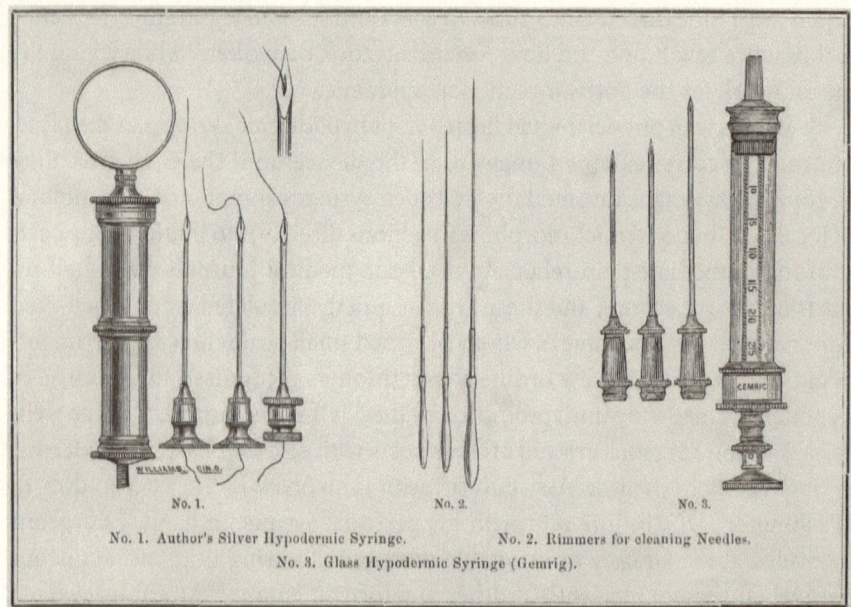

Figure 3.3 Civil War–era hypodermic syringe kit, owned by the Union army surgeon Roberts Bartholow, a pioneer of hypodermic medicine. Union army surgeons used such devices widely, helping to popularize them in the US. From Roberts Bartholow, *Manual of Hypodermic Medicine* (Philadelphia: J. B. Lippincott, 1869), frontispiece.

surgical photography, and epidemiological techniques. After the war, the US government would publish much of this research in *The Medical and Surgical History of the War of the Rebellion*, one of the earliest peer-reviewed medical publications in the United States. Physical specimens gathered during the war went on to be housed at the Army Medical Museum, a major postwar center of scientific medicine.[85] Many scientifically minded Union surgeons later went on to become the most elite physicians in the nation, spreading the gospel of hypodermic medicine through published accounts and high-profile clinical practices. Billings ultimately became a towering figure in American medicine during the Gilded Age, establishing the National Library of Medicine and laying the groundwork for the Johns Hopkins University medical school and hospital.

Silas Weir Mitchell, a Union contract surgeon, was likewise at the cutting edge of hypodermic medicine. Later in life, he achieved great notoriety for his pioneering neurological research, including the first description of phantom limb syndrome, as well as his infamous "rest cure," the subject of Charlotte Perkins Gilman's 1892 novel *The Yellow Wallpaper*, a brilliant and biting critique of women's oppression by a male-dominated medical profession. Before the fame, Mitchell was an overworked young clinician at Turner's Lane Hospital in Civil

War Philadelphia—lauded as the birthplace of American neurology—where he learned to practice "hypodermic medication—at that time somewhat novel."[86] Mitchell and his colleagues specialized in treating the most severe wounds, especially nerve injuries, which involved managing long-term pain over the course of multiple surgeries and extended convalescence. Naturally, injectable morphine aided in this work. Together with surgeons William W. Keen and George R. Morehouse, Mitchell administered twenty to thirty injections of hypodermic morphine a day to injured soldiers. The team was impressed with the results. "In one case," they gleefully reported, "half a grain to a grain of morphia was injected thrice a day, and the man finally recovered after having used nearly four hundred injections."[87] Morphine was such a smashing success that it "became a part of the everyday routine of practice" at Turner's Lane, according to Mitchell, who claimed that Turner's Lane administered some 40,000 morphine injections annually at the height of the war.[88]

Yet for all of the drug's wonders, Mitchell quickly learned that hypodermic morphine had a downside. In one case, Mitchell's colleagues treated a botched leg amputation that had left a Union soldier in "intolerable" pain. It took six amputations and resections performed over three years to repair the stump. The soldier spent most of the war hospitalized and drugged with morphine. When it came time for discharge, Mitchell observed that the soldier's "craving for opium caused him to malinger" in the hospital.[89] Mitchell had come to realize that hypodermic morphine, which he had helped pioneer, often resulted in addiction among amputees and other disabled veterans. Alarmed, Mitchell began investigating, and he was horrified by what he uncovered. A. F. Swann, a captain in the 16th Pennsylvania Cavalry, was shot at the battle of Cold Harbor in May 1864. Mitchell described Swann's case for his pioneering 1872 book, *Injuries of Nerves and Their Consequences*, one of the first longitudinal studies in American medical history. "From the moment he [Swann] was struck" by the bullet, "he suffered the most intense pain in the arm and hand." The pain in Swann's arms and hands was "constant and excruciating, as if grasping a ball of red-hot iron." Morphine was the only thing that dulled the "indescribable" sensation. Swann soon became addicted, consuming "a vast amount of morphine ... estimated by him to amount to from two hundred and fifty to three hundred drachms, requiring the use of the syringe from six to twenty times every day for six years and some days." When he tried to quit the morphine in the early 1870s, Swann told doctors that he "craved" the drug.[90] The cases of Swann and other addicted veterans deeply troubled Mitchell, who began questioning if morphine did more harm than good. After the war, Mitchell would take measures in his clinical practice to mitigate the problem of prescription opiate addiction and even advanced an anti-opium position in his influential medical writings. The apostle of morphine would ultimately become an apostate.

Numerous postwar medical and popular accounts linked the hypodermic syringe to the growing problem of addiction among veterans and others. "Of all forms of continued opiate-taking," J. B. Mattison insisted in 1884, "hypodermic taking is by far the most frequent."[91] The role of the syringe in spreading addiction made Roberts Bartholow regret ever writing his pioneering manual of hypodermic medicine. "The introduction of the hypodermic syringe," he despaired in 1879, "has placed in the hands of man a means of intoxication more seductive than any." Because of the precipitous spike in addiction, "it may well be questioned whether the world has been the gainer or the loser by the discovery of subcutaneous medication."[92] While many Civil War veterans did become addicted to hypodermic morphine, Bartholow's rhetoric was somewhat overblown. Most addicted veterans gravitated toward oral opium. This preference stemmed in part from the complexity of administering a morphine shot. Users had to be taught by their doctors how to properly mix morphine salts with a liquid, draw the solution up into the syringe, and safely inject it into the skin, a risky process without instruction. Additionally, most veterans had originally been prescribed oral opiates during the Civil War. Such surgeons as Mitchell and his colleagues at Turner's Lane, who pioneered the use of hypodermic morphine, were in the minority. Most Civil War surgeons probably lacked consistent access to hypodermic syringes, instead relying on tried-and-true oral opium. Postbellum prescription records also suggest that oral consumption remained the most popular method during the Gilded Age. The Massachusetts Board of Health reported in 1888 that only about 15 percent of opiates prescribed by doctors in that state were injected hypodermically.[93] An 1885 investigation on behalf of the Iowa Board of Health surveyed 225 opiate users for their drug of preference, finding that only 25 respondents took morphine hypodermically. The rest consumed morphine, gum opium, laudanum, and other opiates "by the mouth."[94] Although the hypodermic morphine pioneered during the Civil War cast a large shadow in modern medicine, most addicted veterans probably stuck to older, easier-to-use oral forms of opium.

Despite the perception that "veterans as a class" were addicted to opiates, most men who became addicted were white. The racist antebellum myth that Black bodies were impervious to pain animated clinical care during the Civil War, skewing the demographics of the postwar veterans' addiction epidemic.[95] According to one Union surgeon, the Black man "differs as widely from the white man physiologically and psychologically as does his skin or hair; hence the importance of understanding his peculiarities, in order to treat his diseases successfully." Whereas the white soldier could feel the sear of the minié ball when it pierced his flesh, the wounded Black soldier "complains but little of pain," even when shot. According to this line of thinking, opium and morphine were not meant to be administered to Black troops as frequently or in as strong doses as whites received.⁹⁶ The systematic undertreatment of Black individuals' pain left African American veterans far less likely to become addicted to opiates than their white counterparts.

Extant prescription records for Black regiments are exceptionally rare, but anecdotal evidence suggests that army surgeons, who were overwhelmingly white, avoided prescribing opiates to wounded Black soldiers because they believed that Black bodies could not feel pain. One white Union surgeon assigned to a Black regiment refused to give painkillers to a soldier whose foot was mangled by shrapnel because the man "was not suffering much pain."⁹⁷ Considering the gruesome nature of his wound, the man's supposed absence of pain was highly unlikely. A more realistic explanation is the surgeon's racial bias, which prevented him from recognizing Black people's pain. Under these circumstances, the standard of care for white soldiers was to give morphine early and often.

Surgeons also appear to have refrained from giving opiates to Black soldiers suffering from diarrhea. They knew that well-timed, liberal administration of opium saved dysentery-stricken men from death by dehydration, the risk of poisoning or addiction notwithstanding. The widespread use of opiates therapy kept the mortality rate for diarrheal sicknesses among white Union troops to a relatively low 17.3 percent. In contrast, mortality among Black troops was 33.9 percent, nearly double that of white soldiers.⁹⁸ These "excess deaths" along racial lines strongly suggest that surgeons did not prescribe opiate antidiarrheals equitably to Black soldiers. The paucity of extant medical records for Black units makes it difficult to know for sure, but medical records from Freedman's Bureau hospitals can help fill in the evidentiary gaps. In July 1865, surgeons at a Freedman's Bureau hospital in New Orleans treated ninety-four Black men, women, and children for dysentery, chronic diarrhea, and other maladies. Only nine of these patients received opiates, or 9.57 percent, far below the opiate prescribing rate for the antebellum and wartime hospitals that catered to white patients suffering from similar ailments. George Mansfield, a military-aged Black man, came to the hospital with a bad case of dysentery. Yet surgeons failed to give him opium, despite the drug being the standard of care for white soldiers with dysentery. Another freedman, Lafayette, came to the hospital on July 20, 1865, apparently seeking care for a recent leg amputation. The hospital record does not reveal the circumstances of the amputation, but perhaps Lafayette had been injured in a workplace accident or was a discharged veteran of the United States Colored Troops (USCT). In any case, the surgeons treated his painful injury not with morphine but with "cold dressing," ferric sulphate, "brandy 3 times a day," and half rations. Lafayette must have been in agony, yet Freedman's Bureau doctors seem blinded to his pain. On August 1, Lafayette finally got a dose of opium. Yet even then, the drug was not administered for pain management but "to control the bowels," much like Anarcha, the enslaved woman given opium as an intestinal paralytic by James Marion Sims in the 1840s.[99] Tragically, Black soldiers and freedpeople's inability to access opiate analgesics and antidiarrheals was not exceptional within the well-documented, pervasive racism in Civil War military and humanitarian medicine. The substandard medical care available to Black soldiers and refugees also resulted in tens of thousands of preventable deaths from smallpox, scurvy, and other maladies.[100]

Racial disparities in wartime medical care meant that Civil War veterans who became addicted to opiates were overwhelmingly white. Although nearly 200,000 Black soldiers and sailors comprised roughly 10 percent of Union military personnel, they were not proportionately represented among the cohort of addicted veterans. Not even one Black veteran appeared in the archival records that yielded 200 addicted white veterans identified for this book. There are several plausible explanations for the apparent racial gulf among addicted veterans. As scholars of slavery and Reconstruction have demonstrated in recent years, the white surgeons and clerks who generated the Civil War's medical archive were largely uninterested in documenting sickness or deaths among freedpeople and Black soldiers, which led to archival silences.[101] Hospital records and government reports rarely speak directly or in detail about the health of USCT veterans. Rather than uncritically accepting the premise that fewer Black Americans became addicted to opiates, it is possible to read along this "archival grain" by interrogating sources to illuminate the reasons behind Black opium eaters' absence from historical records that document opiate use among white veterans.[102]

Postwar physicians and psychiatrists observed a distinct racial gap in the demographics of opiate addiction and provided several racialized explanations. Just as antebellum doctors like Samuel Cartwright hoped to justify slavery, so too did the next generation of psychiatrists marshal medical theories to defend Jim Crow. In 1885, a doctor reported that the Eastern North Carolina Insane Asylum had admitted an exceedingly rare case of a "colored insane man" of whom "it was alleged that his insanity was caused from the opium habit." To the doctor, the patient's otherwise pedestrian case was worth writing about not because of his addiction but because "this was the *only* case of opium habit he [the doctor] had ever seen in the *negro*."[103] This apparent racial gap persisted for generations. Few Black patients appear in the records of the morphine maintenance clinics that dotted the nation during the 1910s and 1920s, which catered to white and Black people alike.[104]

Gilded Age doctors conveniently explained away this glaring racial disparity by doubling down on contemporary theories of racial difference. Nineteenth-century psychiatry posited that, among other causes, opiate addiction could result from mental overstimulation, which prompted substance use. This could only occur among intelligent, sensitive white Americans. In contrast, white medical authorities sneered that Black people were too "simpleminded" to experience the same degree of mental overstimulation as whites. Consequently, "the opium habit is rare" among freedmen, claimed a Selma, Alabama, doctor in 1886.[105] J. D. Roberts, a white North Carolina physician, elaborated that Black bodies lacked "the same delicate nervous organization" as white bodies and thus "d[id] not demand the form of stimulant conveyed in opium." Black people, Roberts claimed, also had a "general ignorance" of medicine, an assertion implying that Black veterans lacked the wherewithal to self-medicate with opiates as white veterans often did.[106] Like the belief in Black imperviousness to pain, this argument about Black simplemindedness stemmed from antebellum white Southerners' attempts to justify slavery and to ward off abolitionist critiques.[107] After the Civil War, apologists of Jim Crow simply fine-tuned this rhetoric and used it to explain why whites became addicted to opiates more often than did Black Americans.

Observing that more white Civil War veterans experienced addiction than Black veterans need not require historians to endorse racist theories but instead formulate better explanations for this disparity. In reality, the relative infrequency of opiate addiction among Black veterans and other African Americans stemmed from racist medical practices. One possible explanation is that Black veterans were more successful than white veterans at hiding their addictions, going unnoticed by white doctors and authorities who were already primed to neglect the health needs of Black people. Indeed, Black Americans, for good reasons, tended to mistrust white doctors and often avoided them. Many postwar medical facilities were also racially segregated, excluding Black veterans who might otherwise have received treatment for addiction. An even more compelling explanation is structural racism in medicine, which led to separate pain management protocols for white and Black soldiers during the Civil War and subpar medical care for Black troops overall that lessened exposure to opiates and perhaps reduced the prevalence of addiction among Black veterans. Jim Crow similarly informed racial patterns of cocaine use. Historian David Farber has argued that the underprescribing of opiates to Black Americans led to relative higher levels of cocaine use among African Americans in the late nineteenth century.[108] In any case, whether there actually were fewer Black veterans addicted to opiates than were whites, or whether white doctors simply did not notice (or care to notice) them, a distinct racial gap emerged among the cohort of addicted Civil War veterans. Yet this infrequency of opiate addiction among Black veterans should not be celebrated as a metaphorical silver lining or a protection from opium eating. Instead, this racial gap merely underscores the profound and disturbing ripple effects of medical racism during the Civil War era.

Surgeons might have been convinced that not all soldiers needed opiates, but clearly many men wanted the drugs. Mortally injured soldiers sometimes begged for morphine on their deathbeds, knowing that the drug numbed pain and might allow one to maintain manly self-control and Christian devotion to the bitter end. Dying soldiers felt the need to die a "good death," and they recognized morphine as an ally in this final struggle. Sergeant William K. McCoy of the Charlottesville Artillery Battalion was grievously wounded at Chancellorsville on May 3, 1863. Struggling under the physical weight of his wound and the spiritual weight of his impending death, McCoy fought to maintain his composure. Morphine helped bridge the gulf between the idealized death McCoy wanted and the reality of the painful, terrifying death at hand. Word soon reached McCoy's family that he was dying, and they rushed to the hospital. Knowing they must watch him die and hoping not to disappoint, McCoy "asked for a little morphine as he was afraid he would be too much excited" by his painful wound. As McCoy's death drew near, the wound "began to pain him very much and indeed he was in agony as he expressed it all over" his face. McCoy's sister, a hospital nurse, arrived first. Recognizing the cracks that had emerged in her brother's stoic facade, she "had to give him morphine more frequently which made him dream a great deal and talk in his sleep." McCoy awoke one last time to find that his mother had arrived. With the pain now at bay, the dying soldier restored his self-composure and sang a few hymns, a performance meant to prove that his manliness was beyond question and his soul was right with God.[109] Morphine made this good death possible for McCoy and countless other dying soldiers.

While dying men often welcomed morphine to help them maintain composure, some wounded soldiers worried that taking painkillers could make them seem weak and unmanly. They recognized an inherent tension between the pragmatic, physical need for pain relief and the prevailing cultural expectation, albeit unrealistic, that men simply grit their teeth and bear pain stoically, unaided by drugs. As boys in the 1840s and 1850s, Civil War soldiers had learned to celebrate pain through childhood games, violent pranks, and brawls.[110] They came to war indoctrinated into a cult of pain, which the war's brutality reinforced. Indeed, inflicting and receiving pain with bullet and bayonet were the central tasks of soldiering. Nor was pain compartmentalized to battlefields. Soldiers relished painful social activities like bare-knuckle prizefighting in their downtime. These rituals reinforced the manly cult of pain by lionizing men who could endure and overcome physical suffering.[111] Without doubt, many of the war's survivors returned home with serious emotional and psychological scars from the pain they inflicted, endured, and witnessed. Yet most American men continued to celebrate soldiers, especially disabled ones, who bore pain without complaint.

If pain was celebrated, then battle wounds and medical care presented a unique opportunity for men to stoically perform the rituals central to the cult of pain. Severely wounded men who refused to let a groan escape their lips or a grimace cross their face exhibited what the historian Gerald F. Linderman has called "hospital courage." While some men valued opiates' painkilling properties, other soldiers recognized that morphine's other side effects might prevent one from attaining said courage.[112] One green recruit witnessed a tough-as-nails veteran enduring an amputation at the elbow without painkillers in 1862. "He lay there like a *man*," the young soldier admired. The old soldier embodied hospital courage by refusing to flinch even when the first cut from the surgeon's knife sliced open his flesh. A weaker man might have screamed as the back-and-forth motion of the surgeon's bone saw gnawed into the mangled limb. But here was "a *soldier*, every inch of him," who refused to give in to the pain by expressing the discomfort he surely felt. Admiring this example, the younger recruit hoped that he too would be able to endure pain with such manly fortitude when his time came.[113]

"Stonewall" Jackson was likewise lionized for his hospital courage after being accidentally shot by Confederate pickets at Chancellorsville in the dark hours of May 2, 1863. Jackson's aides rushed their commander to the rear, where surgeon Hunter McGuire praised the general's stubborn refusal to give "an expression to his suffering" until carried out of sight and earshot of his soldiers. McGuire considered it to be a "remarkable" display of "iron will." After a few days, he amputated Jackson's arm successfully, but the weakened general caught a bad case of pneumonia. As he lay dying, a Confederate newspaper claimed that Jackson said that he "would not part with" his wounds "if I could," despite "suffering great pain." Jackson recognized that his painful injuries provided an opportunity to showcase manly hospital courage for a keen audience, and clearly the general's exhibition resonated during the Civil War and long after.[114] Jackson's deathbed performance helped launch the Lost Cause "cult of Jackson" that emerged shortly after his death.

Although wounded soldiers were expected to embody hospital courage, gunshot wounds, amputations, and other physical traumas were often simply too painful to bear without drugs. Men were often forced to juggle overwhelming physical pain against burdensome masculine norms. Recognizing the impossibility of this task, pragmatic soldiers often elected to take their chances with morphine and worry about their manly image later. One sufferer, Lt. Albert T. Shurtleff of the 49th Pennsylvania Infantry, was wounded twice at the Third Battle of Winchester in September 1864. Lying in a ditch awaiting attack orders, an exploding Rebel canister shell broke Shurtleff's right elbow, followed a split second later by a metal ball in the right leg that embedded in the hip. Surgeons told Shurtleff that both limbs would have to come off, but he "preferred death rather than lose both an arm and a leg," as such an injury would be debilitating and seemed emasculating. Faced with two unsatisfactory choices, morphine offered Shurtleff a compromise solution. He would let the surgeons take his arm, which they gingerly removed. But Shurtleff insisted on keeping his leg and being given morphine for the pain. The surgeons obliged, sending him home to convalesce for eleven months under "the severest pain conceivable." "Had it not been for morphine," Shurtleff wrote, "I could not have endured it."[115] Faced with disfigurement and pain, many soldiers opted for morphine, despite the risks of looking unmanly for taking painkillers.

Stress, Self-Care, and Addiction

Most Civil War soldiers enthusiastically embraced opiates, even outside hospitals. Although these grim facilities and their saw-wielding surgeons are emblematic of Civil War medicine, most day-to-day doctoring occurred in camp or on the march. In these settings, men took their health needs into their own hands, falling out of ranks to bathe or sleep when tired or sick.[116] Opiates played an important role in soldiers' self-care practices. Trekking through a humid Mississippi swamp in August 1862, Confederate soldier J. W. Henderson would have been stopped in his tracks by fever and diarrhea if not for his stash of opium. "I had to live on opium nearly the whole trip," Henderson told his sister.[117] Anticipating such a journey in the winter of 1863, a Union soldier told his sister that he "had been taking opium for some time to prepare for the shake."[118] Charles Brewster once had "a terrible attack of Cholic" and took twenty-five drops of laudanum and four opium pills during an eight-hour window, not without ill effect. "I was so weak the next day," he reported, "that I had to lie abed."[119] Soldiers knew that opium worked, but neophytes sometimes did not know how much to take. Predictably, mishaps occurred. In July 1864, O. C. Shelton of the 4th Iowa Infantry took opium, camphor, and blackberries to quiet his stomach. It helped, so when symptoms recurred a few days later, Shelton swallowed twice as much opium, expecting twice the relief. The overdose left him feeling "very dull" and intoxicated, with a "head [that] felt like a bullet."[120] Charles Francis Adams Jr., a Union colonel and great-grandson of President John Adams, buckled under a "smart attack of [his] friend the dysentery" in 1862. Adams tried swallowing some opium as a remedy, but he was displeased with the drug, which left him "cross and disgusted."[121] Opiate use in camp was ubiquitous, even if soldiers were not always satisfied by the effects.

Soldiers often went to great lengths to obtain opiates for self-medication during the Civil War. A Union officer hospitalized after the 1862 Battle of Fort Donelson felt that surgeons were not giving him enough morphine to take his mind off a badly broken femur, so he bribed his night nurse a dollar for an extra dose.¹²² Men also endeavored to get opiates for their messmates. One Confederate in Hood's Texas Brigade claimed to have walked a mile to obtain a dose of morphine for his wounded friend.¹²³ Other men sent letters requesting opiates by mail. Suffering from a cold at Fairfax Courthouse, Virginia, Lt. Col. Charles Cummings of the 16th Vermont Infantry asked his wife in Vermont to mail him opium, "my sheet anchor in such complaints."¹²⁴ Sick and starving at Andersonville prison, Union soldier George W. Nailer wrote home in August 1864 asking for a package with "2 or three boxes good pills" and "Laudinum [sic] Golden tincture" for himself, along with "painkiller" for a comrade on the verge of succumbing to the scorching Georgia sun.¹²⁵ Confederate soldiers also tried to get opiates from Northern relatives through the mail. In 1863, a rebel sympathizer in New York City mailed opium and quinine to his nephew in Richmond, although federals intercepted the contraband.¹²⁶ When the mail failed, soldiers could buy opiates from sutlers, who stocked morphine-laced patent medicines like Dr. King's New Discovery for Consumption, which retailed for a dollar per bottle.¹²⁷

Many soldiers found that simply approaching surgeons and asking was the easiest and cheapest way to obtain a dose of opium or morphine. New York surgeon Daniel Holt recounted in a letter to his wife how a Union soldier appeared one afternoon with "*such* a case of diarrhea," begging piteously for a dose of opium. "I'm almost dead," the man pleaded, "give me a camphor and opium pill, and mark me sick to-day."¹²⁸ Observing a fellow Confederate surgeon dispensing opiates to a long line of soldiers in June 1863, one North Carolina surgeon wryly described the men as "very willing" patients.¹²⁹ These occasions complicate the persistent myth that Civil War soldiers avoided surgeons like the plague. Certainly, some men feared "old sawbones" because of his harsh surgical interventions and steered a wide berth around the hospital tent.¹³⁰ But this sentiment was not universal.¹³¹ When it came to opium or morphine, the opposite was often true. Soldiers knew that sympathetic surgeons could be cajoled into supplying the drugs, and a surgeon's prescription might also legitimize one's complaints of sickness and score an excused absence from duty, a doubly attractive prospect for tired, overworked soldiers.

If sickness prompted soldiers to cope with opiates, so did emotional and psychological distress. Many Civil War soldiers found the experience of combat to be unspeakably traumatic, literally. Men often struggled to describe the emotional effects of the carnage they witnessed. It was "useless to attempt to describe" the slaughter, although some soldiers felt compelled to try.¹³² Lewis Sylvester Branscomb, a transitionally literate teenager in the 3rd Alabama Infantry, strained the limits of his vocabulary to recount the Seven Days Battles of June and July 1862. "I will try to describe the battle field to you," he wrote to his father," but I hardly know how[.] Just imagine yourself walking over a large field half leg deep in mud scattered all over with dead men and horses[,] wounded men lying all about groaning in the agonies [of] death begging you for assistines [sic] and you will have some idea of a battle field[.]" "Pa," Branscomb added, "I am Fairing very bad."¹³³ Ambrose Bierce, a Union soldier-turned-author whose rare gift with words made him a stand-in for less well-spoken veterans, spent the rest of his life after the war trying to do justice to the horrible scenes he and Branscomb had witnessed. Again and again for decades, Bierce's pen reenacted the combat that undid men's fragile bodies and minds. Bierce once recalled a dying man he saw at Shiloh, "a Federal sergeant . . . who had been a fine giant in his time." Lying on the ground, surrounded by dead horses and broken caissons, the man's shallow breaths came in "convulsive, rattling snorts" punctuated by "sputters of froth which crawled creamily down his cheeks." "A bullet had clipped a groove in his skull," Bierce explained, "and from this the brain protruded in bosses, dropping off in flakes and strings. I had not previously known one could get on . . . with so little brain." One of the men in Bierce's platoon, "a womanish fellow," proposed to put the sergeant out of his misery, but Bierce refused.¹³⁴ Bierce survived the war but never got over this scene. How could he? Branscomb became part of such a scene, dying in battle at Harpers Ferry on July 4, 1864. After the war, veteran surgeons compiled a meticulous medical archive documenting the Civil War's physical sicknesses and injuries. Counting up the dead and physically wounded was a way to intellectually cope with the war's carnage.¹³⁵ They left the difficult task of assessing the war's emotional and psychological injuries to historians, who in more recent years have reconstructed a harrowing portrait of the mental health crisis sparked by the war. Suicides, domestic violence, and alcohol dependence were rampant among the war's survivors, manifestations of emotional and psychological distress.¹³⁶ Opium eating fits into this broader pattern of suffering.

Unnerved by the emotions of war, some soldiers took opium and morphine to compose themselves. Homesick Union soldier George Phillips explained how war "is [a] hard place to be sick away from Home and friends." Lonely and in "great pain," he "took a dose of opium to make me sleep" and forget his troubles.¹³⁷ William Diamond of the 1st New Orleans Volunteer Infantry washed down twenty-six opium pills in twenty-four hours with beer and whiskey. During his October 1865 court-martial trial for resisting arrest with a loaded rifle, Diamond recalled that his "mind was so disordered" that he "did not know an officer from a civilian."¹³⁸ Although Diamond did not make his motivations clear, it is difficult to imagine that he did not expect to get high and drunk, a welcome release from the tedium and tension of occupation duty.

George House, a sergeant in the 9th Alabama Infantry, swallowed morphine before going into battle to ease his stress and fatigue. The drug made him feel "exhilarated and indifferent to all danger," House told a doctor after the war.¹³⁹

Under the influence of morphine, House became a model soldier—strong and brave enough to execute dangerous maneuvers under withering rifle fire but indifferent enough to carry out the emotionally taxing work of killing.[140] The 9th Alabama did plenty of this work. Boasting 550 men at the start of the Peninsula Campaign in spring 1862, the regiment suffered at least 260 casualties. The next year, 111 men fell at Chancellorsville and another 58 casualties followed at Gettysburg a few weeks later. By the time the regiment surrendered at Appomattox Courthouse on April 9, 1865, only sixty-eight men were left standing. In three years of hard campaigning, most of the men House fought with were felled, but he survived on morphine.[141] Wartime reliance on emotional palliatives often bled over into the postwar period and fostered addiction.

That is what happened to House. At eight o'clock in the morning on June 17, 1881, House appeared on the steps of the Charity Hospital in New Orleans seeking medical care for his long-standing morphine addiction, having continued to take morphine and opium daily after war's end. The drugs helped drown out the horrible memories of battle and perhaps helped him cope with the economic, social, and political turmoil of Reconstruction. House also needed to take opiates regularly to avoid excruciating withdrawal pains. But after so many years, the toll of addiction began to weigh heavily on him. House's heavy morphine use was financially and physically costly. "He had gradually lost flesh and became weaker until, no longer able to perform his duties, he determined to go to the Charity Hospital," where he told doctors he wanted "to get cured or die." Doctors were dismayed by the veteran's "very weak and emaciated" physical state. His "complexion [was] sully and appearance haggard," his "pupils contracted," and he seemed "nervous" and suffered from "hyperaesthesia," or increased sensitivity to touch, "over [the] entire surface" of his skin, signs that House was perhaps already in withdrawal upon arrival at the hospital. The doctors admired House's determination to quit using morphine, and they wanted to help, so they dosed him with cannabis indica and potassium bromide to dull the terrible chills, diarrhea, vomiting, sleeplessness, and "mental vagaries" of withdrawal. Soon, he broke down and "piteously begged for opium," but the doctors refused to give him any. By mid-July 1881, they deemed the old soldier cured. Doctors were proud of House's apparent redemption, noting that "when questioned upon the subject, he asserts most emphatically that he would rather die than take any more opium."[142]

Opium and Cowardice

House's case illustrates the fraught consequences of opiate use for Civil War soldiers and veterans. Despite its potential benefits, opiates remained fickle, Janus-faced substances that could help and hurt. Although House felt that morphine fortified his mind and transformed him into a model soldier, other soldiers worried that relying on opium to soothe the mind might appear cowardly and even unpatriotic. Benjamin Edward Stiles Jr. of the 16th Georgia Infantry accused another soldier in his regiment of cowardice in June 1862. The man had run from battle, claiming "his powder was wet." Unsatisfied with this excuse, Stiles blamed opium instead, alleging that the cowardly man abused the drug, sapping his will to fight.[143] Even generals were not immune to salacious allegations of opium eating. In June 1864, Union brigadier general Henry Lawrence Eustis was "informed that if he does not resign, charges of neglect of duty and general inefficiency will be preferred against him." "He is said to eat opium," the root of his deficiencies. Under pressure, Eustis acquiesced a few days later.[144] Controversial Union general William Rosecrans also became the target of rumors in 1863. Reeling from the Union's disaster at Chickamauga in 1863, press outlets from *Harper's Weekly* down to lowly soldiers' magazines leveled the scandalous accusation that Rosecrans's apparent lack of aggression on the battlefield was due to opium eating. Even Confederate papers picked up the story, always eager to disparage their enemies. The situation became so uncomfortable for Rosecrans that he was forced to publicly deny the allegation in an 1863 speech in Cincinnati.[145] Rumors of opium eating also haunted disgraced Confederate generals Braxton Bragg and John Bell Hood and even US secretary of state William Seward, although there is little evidence to substantiate these claims.[146]

Rumors of opium eating in Civil War armies served several purposes. Most immediate, allegations of opium abuse provided a convenient explanation for battlefield failures. Discrediting a political opponent with allegations of drunkenness had been a common political strategy before the Civil War, and generals like Rosecrans and Bragg made many enemies.[147] Opportunistic officers hoping to discredit their nemeses found it all too easy to level such scandalous allegations as opium intemperance. These very public accusations also served as implicit warnings to common soldiers that they too must jealously guard their temperance, manhood, and reputation. No soldier wanted to be the next Rosecrans, tainted by charges of opium eating.

It was not merely happenstance that junior officers sometimes warned enlisted men about the risks of opium intoxication. The gathering of young, impressionable soldiers in camps alongside older, uncouth men during the war sparked widespread fears about vice and moral decay in the armies, and many officers took it upon themselves to police their men's behavior.[148] Iowa soldier O. C. Shelton described in November 1864 how his regiment's surgeon gathered the men one night in the dim glow of a campfire. The officer began to read aloud *Confessions of an English Opium-Eater* by Thomas De Quincey. At first glance, this encounter might appear as just another run-of-the-mill camp scene, nothing more than a group of bored men looking to kill time during the monotony of winter camp life. Yet the surgeon's choice of this particular book—one of the most famous morality tales of the nineteenth century—was no mere coincidence. Published to great acclaim in 1821, it traced De Quincey's downward spiral as laudanum addiction ruined his body, mind, and character. Forty years after publication, De Quincey's *Confessions* remained a well-known title. By selecting *Confessions* to read to his men that night, the surgeon sought to impart an important moral lesson: avoid taking opium outside a surgeon's orders, or one risked falling victim to the opium habit like De Quincey or Rosecrans. Shelton might have squirmed as he listened to De Quincey's tale of woe, as the young soldier had already taken opium to ward off diarrhea on several occasions.[149]

Considering the widespread consumption of opiates, it is not surprising that Union army courts-martial frequently turned up evidence of intoxication. Opiates might have been useful remedies for sickness, pain, or stress, but overuse could leave men intoxicated and unable to perform their duties. Although narcotics use was not a crime, opiate intoxication was often cited in charges of conduct prejudicial to good order and military discipline or drunkenness on duty.[150] First Lt. Max Rosenberg of the 54th New York Infantry lost his shoulder straps in December 1864 for "incompetency, habitual drunkenness, neglect of duty, and the constant use of opium."[151] Private Patrick J. Warren of the 7th New York Artillery beat another soldier so badly "as to cover his face with blood" and pleaded guilty to charges of prejudicial conduct. To explain his behavior, Warren said that he was "very sick for three months and using Laudanum, Ether, and Morphine" and guzzled "four or five glasses of beer until I did not know what I was doing." Three months' hard labor and a thirty dollar fine suggested the military did not look kindly on this defense.[152]

Many soldiers tried to absolve themselves by blaming surgeons for prescribing opiates. Sometimes this strategy worked, albeit obliquely. Corporal Patrick Fallon was absent without leave for the Battle of Fredericksburg in December 1862. To explain missing the fight, he claimed to have been given opium pills at an army hospital. Although he was found guilty and sentenced to hard labor for the duration of his enlistment, a sympathetic general remitted the sentence.[153] Private Matthew D. Hankins of the 11th Wisconsin Infantry fell asleep at his post after being prescribed opium by a regimental surgeon. He was convicted, but it was thrown out in February 1865 by a general who determined that "the accused was improperly placed on guard duty, and while under the influence of opiates, administered by the proper medical officer" and thus "could not be held accountable."[154] However, the "surgeons made me do it" defense was inconsistent because sometimes it failed to satisfactorily explain intoxicated soldiers' behavior, as sergeant Augustus Hayden of the 11th US Artillery learned the hard way after falling asleep on duty in June 1862. In his defense, Hayden argued that opium, taken in "the presence" of a surgeon, had made him drowsy. The surgeon confirmed that he had given Hayden two opium pills, "one to take that night and one in the morning," but refused to concede the notion that opium had made the sergeant sleepy. Consequently, Hayden was convicted and busted down to private. William R. Smith, a Union hospital steward, developed the "constant habit of resorting to powerful narcotics," including opium, after contracting a severe case of diarrhea during the Overland Campaign of 1864. Admittedly, when Smith took opium, he was "considerably affected by them," but when the drugs wore off, his bowels became "languid and debilitated." So, he felt justified in self-medicating with the drugs, even while commanding a fatigue party at a hospital in City Point, Virginia. An army court-martial disagreed, finding Smith guilty of conduct prejudicial and drunkenness on duty, ultimately sentencing him to a dishonorable discharge.[155] Court-martial cases involving opiates stemmed from, and ultimately compounded, the antebellum stigmatization of opium eating by branding users as unmanly, cowardly, and poor soldiers, especially when defendants could not articulate a coherent defense on medical grounds.

Stereotypes about opium eaters often surfaced in trial testimony and evidence, illuminating why the army felt justification for punishing some soldiers who used opiates, despite opiate use not being a crime and often being sanctioned by surgeons. Private Arthur Horner of the 1st Missouri Engineers was by his own admission addicted to opiates, which apparently originated in the Mexican-American War. He deserted in July 1863, blaming the act on the influence of opium. Horner confessed to the court-martial, "I never intended to desert, in spirit, [but] under the influence of opium I do many strange things. I have taken an ounce and a half per week, the effects of which has caused all my misfortunes." He was captured and returned to his unit in April 1864, where guards confined Horner and withheld the opium. Cruel, forced withdrawal "threw me into the most hopeless condition," Horner protested when he was dragged before the court-martial in May 1864. But he found no sympathetic ears, except for his brother, also in the Union army, who asked the court to remand Horner to a mental asylum for the "restor[ation] of his mind" and where the addicted soldier had spent time before the war receiving treatment for the habit. For his part, Horner apologetically told the court martial, "I shall not complain of your sentence—I expect punishment." Perhaps this display of penitence softened the punishment. Horner was ultimately convicted of desertion and sentenced to forfeit pay for the period of his absence ($15.64) and to reimburse the army for the cost of capture and transport ($30) and had his enlistment extended. The army never sent Horner to an asylum, and he mustered out July 1865.[156] Horner clearly recognized, articulated, and seems to have internalized the pernicious stereotypes about opium eaters that provided part of the rationale for policing drug use in the army. By embracing these stereotypes and disciplining opiate-using soldiers like Augustus, Smith, and Horner, the Union army's courts-martial also established a precedent for harsh policing of drug use through military entitlement programs, setting the tone for veterans' experiences in the postbellum decades.

If military discipline relied on and reinforced stereotypes about drug users, court-martial proceedings also risked besmirching the Union's war aims by inviting public scandal. This was especially the case when the defendants were white officers of Black regiments. Captain Barry Lynch of the 86th USCT took six opium pills in six hours on July 4, 1864, in Barrancas, Florida. Extremely intoxicated, he threatened to "beat the shit out of" fellow officers who tried to intervene. When they attempted to corral Lynch into his tent, he screamed, "I am a white man," perhaps to separate himself from the Black soldier he commanded and to protest the perception that opium slavery degraded one's whiteness and manhood. After a "long and wearisome trial" of three days, the captain was found guilty of drunkenness on duty and conduct unbecoming and was dismissed from the army.[157] In October 1864 Gen. Benjamin Butler dismissed a USCT surgeon, Christian Miller, for abandoning the wounded men under his care while he was drunk and high from a cocktail of morphine and whiskey.[158] Soldiers' magazines parroted these cases to a titillated audience of Union troops. These scandals sometimes even circulated in the Confederate newspapers, serving as "evidence" that the white officers who oversaw Black Union soldiers were inferior men serving a morally degraded nation.[159] Confederate nationalism needed this kind of dubious moral currency to survive.

Finally, when the war became too much, some men took opiates to kill themselves. One Union soldier "in an attempt at suicide swallowed two ounces of laudanum," a huge dose, "and smoked one grain of opium" for good measure. Somehow, doctors revived the man.[160] J. C. Taylor, a Virginian in the Confederate Navy, also took an overdose of opium on shore leave in Savannah in March 1861, apparently with intent to die by suicide. His friends attempted to reverse the overdose, but he died the next day. Taylor's motivations are unclear, but perhaps he had seen too much of war.[161] Taylor would have likely understood that opium was an accessible means to end one's life, given that reports of such suicides often appeared in newspapers. Overdose deaths in the army were also part of a broader epidemic among Confederate soldiers and civilians, thousands of whom killed themselves with opium, knives, guns, and nooses during and after the Civil War. The wartime South was a world turned upside down, and many white Southerners simply wanted to escape the region's ruined economy and upended social order. Others were too distraught at the loss of loved ones or the collapse of the Confederacy to continue living.[162]

Addiction on the Rise

Murmurs about the risks attendant to opiate use surfaced among doctors and hospital workers during the Civil War, foreshadowing the crisis to come. In the short term, the risk of poisoning was paramount. The Confederate Army's *Manual of Military Surgery*, which called opium "important to the surgeon as gunpowder to the ordnance," was unambiguous about the value of laudanum but dangerously vague in the dosing guidelines, calling for "doses of from twenty to sixty drops, repeated at intervals of from two to six hours."[163] These guidelines were open to individual surgeons' discretion, which could easily result in an accidental overdose, a possibility that troubled many physicians during the war. In 1862, the year of bloody battles at Shiloh, Antietam, and Fredericksburg, one doctor warned that "opium and alcoholic stimulants" were "employed with much more freedom now than a few years ago," even during the antebellum peak of heroic medicine. "Opium and alcohol, in excessive doses," the doctor warned, would "occasion immediate disorder . . . and may destroy life."[164] Predictably, accidents happened. One Union soldier wounded at Antietam received such a heavy dose of opium that he was "carried to the point of narcotization."[165] Another soldier was advised by his regiment's farrier to take an entire ounce of laudanum at one time for diarrhea. Someone called for a surgeon an hour later. He came running only to find the poor soldier "very drowsy, flush faced, pulse slow, pupils much contracted and hands twitching, with tendency to convulsions," apparent signs of opiate overdose.[166]

The women who worked in military hospitals, who often paid more careful attention to their patients than surgeons, also worried about and objected to heavy-handed prescriptions. Harriet Eaton, a Union hospital worker, was leery about a particularly potent recipe developed by the 16th Michigan Infantry's surgeon, Isaac Wixom, for "congestive fever," or malaria. A batch contained forty grams of calomel, twenty grains of quinine, fifteen grains of ipecac, ten grains of opium, three grains of capsicum, and an ounce of turpentine. Too much of any one of these ingredients could produce violent illness. "I told him that was kill or cure," Eaton wrote in her diary. But Wixom was proud of his recipe, which he named "Wixom's dose," so he ignored Eaton's advice.[167] This encounter illustrates wartime concerns about opiate poisonings and the gendered conflicts that frequently erupted between female hospital workers and male surgeons. The latter tended to view women like Eaton as interlopers bent on challenging male dominance, and they routinely dismissed women's hard-earned medical knowledge and skills.[168]

If accidental poisonings were unsettling, the prospect of soldiers becoming opium eaters was downright horrifying. In March 1863, a doctor warned an esteemed audience at the New York Academy of Medicine that the widespread use of opiates might soon fill the Union army's ranks full of "opium drunkards."[169] The specter of opium eating in the army was especially troubling for Northern temperance advocates, who viewed opium abuse as part of a broader moral crisis afflicting the military. Again and again, temperance activists warned that rough-and-tumble army life triggered an epidemic of vice. They railed about the free-flowing whiskey, drugs, prostitution, pornography, and gambling in army camps and hospitals that sent impressionable young men down the path of sin and immorality. Worse still, hardened soldiers might return home after the war and spread vice like a virus, tearing at the fragile nation's moral fabric during the fraught early days of Reconstruction.[170]

When the guns fell mostly silent in 1865, wartime murmurings about the looming drug crisis burst front and center into the headlines. Demobilizing veterans dispersed around the country, spreading the problem of addiction to all corners of the newly reunited nation. Already primed to spot a moral crisis, vigilant observers reported a sharp increase in addiction among white men. In 1867, Rhode Island's *Providence Journal* reported that "the statements of druggists and physicians in different parts of the country indicate that the practice of opium eating is already wide-spread in this country and steadily growing in extent." Local pharmacists reported a "more or less rapid" increase in "the number of their opium customers." The situation had become so alarming that a group of temperance-minded citizens even talked of creating an "Anti-Opium League" to combat the growing plague.[171] Two years later, Michigan's *Voice of the West* observed that "new forms of intemperance" had spread to the Midwest, and "among them none is more to be dreaded than the opium eating habit."[172] When a former Confederate lieutenant, Francis C. Clewell, died of a suspicious morphine overdose in a St. Louis, Missouri, boardinghouse in 1867, the local paper concluded he must have been in the "habit" of taking the drug. Clewell's fatal morphine overdose heralded an alarming new trend of fatal overdoses among former soldiers. Given "one-hundred thousand victims of the opium habit in the United States," Ohio's *Greenville Democrat* feared that opium poppies might soon displace tobacco as cash crop.[173] Doctors were especially worried. Speaking in 1870 at a meeting of the Vermont Medical Society in Montpelier, Carleton P. Frost—who from 1862 to 1863 was surgeon to the 15th Vermont Infantry before joining a Union army enrollment board in the same capacity until 1865—described the rapid action of hypodermic morphine and warned about the "abuses which result from its use for the gratification of a morbid love for the peculiar intoxicating effects of the drug." After explaining that "surgical cases and chronic conditions of disease" led to many addiction cases, Frost closed with an ominous warning: "Opium debases both the mind and the body. The spirit is constantly crying to be relieved from the dead form it is carrying around; that is dragging it down."[174]

To some observers, the scourge of addiction seemed especially pronounced in parts of the South, where the health of the people and even the landscape had been devastated by years of hard war.[175] In 1878, the *New-York Times* singled out Virginia's Shenandoah Valley as having a "reputation" for opium eating. "It is deplorable to observe how the evil has increased" in the region during Reconstruction. "Staunton," a key economic and transportation hub that was home to the state's Western Lunatic Asylum, "has the name of being the great opium city of this part of the country." The city's druggists, who supplied medicines to much of the region, reportedly sold 100 pounds of opium per week, doled out through prescriptions and over the counter. One pharmacist claimed to have sold 79,593 doses of morphine in the previous year. A few miles northeast of Staunton, in Harrisonburg, an exasperated local druggist claimed, "I don't believe there are twenty people ... who are free from the use of opium." Opium eating was so pronounced in the valley that it seemed contagious, the *Times* warned, drawing implicit comparisons to the cholera, smallpox, and yellow fever outbreaks that also swept the nation in the Civil War's aftermath. "A man sees another using the terrible drug, and before he is aware of it he is eating opium himself." "The evil" of the opium habit "is like an epidemic. It is in the atmosphere."[176]

Although newspaper coverage of the Shenandoah Valley's postwar opiate "epidemic" did not explicitly link opium eating to the Civil War, readers would have recognized that the "atmosphere" of addiction could not be understood apart from the war's devastation. For nearly four years, blue-and-gray-clad soldiers and partisans under generals "Stonewall" Jackson, Nathaniel Banks, David Hunter, John Imboden, Jubal Early, and Philip Sheridan had surged back and forth across the Shenandoah Valley, pillaging and burning "the great granary" of the Confederacy.[177] It is difficult to overstate the human, environmental, and economic damage, which lingered for decades. It took years to replace the barns full of looted grain, fields of crops and houses burned to ashes, and valuable horses and mules driven off during the war. Even more sorely felt were the deaths or maiming of practically an entire generation of white Virginia men. Such hardships provided ample reason for the people of the valley to turn to opiates, thus inextricably linking the addiction epidemic to the region's wartime hardships.

For their part, Virginians living in the Shenandoah Valley were horrified by what they read in the papers. Suddenly it seemed that eyes around the nation were fixed on Staunton and its opium eaters. One small-town Georgia paper even alleged that a Staunton woman was forced to sell two horses to fund her morphine addiction, a shameful state of affairs.[178] Some local residents admitted that addiction was a major problem. Out of Woodstock, sixty miles northeast of Staunton, the *Shenandoah Herald* verified the national media's salacious claims, adding that "the effects of morphine are more serious" than whiskey because "parties addicted to the habit will frequently lie and steal in order to get" the drug. But Woodstock readers could rest assured that "in this place there are but few opium eaters."[179] Many Staunton residents, especially the city's pharmacists, vehemently rejected the "wildest falsehoods about the use of opium in this city." A summit of druggists drafted a statement rejecting allegations from outsiders that they sold too much opium and swore that "there [were] not over fifty persons addicted to the fearful habit of opium eating" in the city. The pharmacists dismissed the presence of these opium eaters by arguing that many of them were dying from cancer. Ten physicians endorsed the statement. Local newspapers sought to deflect. The *Staunton Vindicator* cast aspersions beyond the city's borders, claiming that the opium problem was worse in the surrounding Augusta County, an important local distinction.[180] The rival *Staunton Spectator* admitted that "there are a few" in town "whose great misfortune it is to have been innocently brought under the resistless power of opium." But these concerns were just as bad in Ohio or Michigan, the *Spectator* claimed.[181] For years prior, valley newspapers had loudly denounced opium abuse as a Chinese vice and a "pernicious" sin.[182] Now, they could not bear to do an about-face by admitting the severity of the city's drug crisis. Yet the Staunton newspapers implicitly conceded the seriousness of the valley's opium problem by hawking patent medicines that purported to "cure" opiate addiction and carrying advertisements from local doctors who specialized in treating addiction.[183]

What are we to make of these competing versions of the opiate epidemic in the Shenandoah Valley? On the one hand, if the region actually experienced a more severe addiction outbreak than did the rest of the nation, as the *New-York Times* suggested, one might expect to find widespread evidence of fatal overdoses elsewhere in the historical record. Yet few overdose deaths were recorded in the postwar death registers of Staunton or Augusta County.[184] Given this omission, it is tempting to dismiss claims about "the great opium city" as hyperbole. After all, Gilded Age newspapers often leveled salacious, fictitious claims to sell more copies. Accuracy in reporting was not a paramount concern. Yet historians should not be too quick to dismiss rumors about the opium "evil" in the postwar valley.

Opium slavery was so stigmatized that most addicted people desperately tried to keep their condition quiet, often taking their secret to the grave. Opiates were also consumed in private, so most overdose deaths occurred out of sight, often leaving those who discovered the corpses unable to definitively determine a cause of death. Even when an overdose could be ascertained as a definitive cause of death, family, friends, and local officials were often wary about shaming the dead by publicly attributing their deaths to opium eating. As the *National*

Tribune explained in 1882, "It is too much the habit when persons suddenly fall down dead, to report the heart as the cause." This custom "silences all inquiry and investigation" into the affairs of the dead, so that "many an opium-eater is let off" without a fuss "into the grave that covers at once his folly and his crime."[185] Even doctors sometimes obscured their addicted patients' identities in medical journal articles, recognizing that naming the patient would expose them to stigma.[186] Thus, it is difficult to say for sure whether the postwar Shenandoah Valley suffered a more acute opiate crisis than other regions. But, certainly, the charges leveled by the *New-York Times* touched a nerve among many locals, underscoring how Americans in the valley and around the nation had become hypervigilant about opium eating in the Civil War's wake.

Many observers feared that opiate addiction had become a national crisis, sparing no region, and they were right to be alarmed. Between the Civil War and the twentieth century, the number of Americans who used and became addicted to opiates skyrocketed. Quantifying this trend is difficult, since vital records were not kept in most places.[187] But tariff records concerning imported opium help illuminate the epidemic's growth. According to historian David T. Courtwright, the relatively low volume of antebellum opium imports could support a modest cohort of American opium eaters. Courtwright estimates that the opiate addiction rate stood at no more than 0.72 Americans per thousand in 1842, about 12,000 people. Imports escalated, first gradually then sharply in the 1870s. By 1890, enough opium flowed into US ports to sustain an addiction rate as high as 4.59 per one thousand Americans, more than a sixfold increase. The dramatic increase in opium imports suggests that perhaps as many as 313,000 people or so were addicted to opiates in 1890, including veterans and nonveterans. Courtwright estimates that roughly two-thirds of this population, around 221,000, were medicinal users, and the rest, about 92,000, were opium smokers.[188] The increase in opium imports outpaced the growth of the American population threefold. The United States also imported far more opium per capita than other modernizing countries, like Germany or Italy.[189] Numerous contemporary observers noted with unease how opium imports increased sharply beginning in the 1860s and how this traffic showed little sign of abating given the growth in demand. Newspapers frequently echoed these reports, contributing to the public perception that opium eating was trending sharply upward.[190]

Doctors and other contemporary observers rightfully attributed much of the increase in opium eating to fallout from the Civil War, although the war was certainly not the only cause. "A large number of people must use the drug habitually, in some form, for the gratification of their cravings for a stimulant," one writer reasoned in 1866, describing the surge in opium imports. "The medical business connected with the army is responsible for a portion of this increase since the war began."[191] Two years later, the author Horace Day added that "the events of the last few years have unquestionably added greatly to their [opium eaters'] number." "Maimed and shattered survivors from a hundred battle-fields, diseased and disabled soldiers released from hostile prisons, anguished and hopeless wives and mothers, made so by the slaughter of those who were dearest to them, have found, many of them, temporary relief from their sufferings in opium," he observed.[192] Day's book, *The Opium Habit*, published in 1868, was the first among dozens of similar titles that appeared by 1900. The 1870s and 1880s saw a surge of books about addiction published by American doctors, which illustrated the growing alarm about the addiction crisis in the Civil War's wake. In 1872, a physician and patent medicine dealer blamed "our late intestine war" for the surge in opium addiction. "Anterior to" the Civil War, he explained, "a confirmed Opium-Eater was somewhat of a *rara avis*, but now there are probably a quarter of a million in the country!"[193]

Although thousands of injured and ailing veterans were probably counted among the ranks of postwar opium eaters, most addicted Americans were not former soldiers. Opium eaters came from all walks of life, from "the lady of Fifth Avenue to John Chinaman on Baxter Street."[194] Considering the widespread nature of addiction among Americans in the late nineteenth century, Civil War veterans likely represented only a minority among the broader cohort of opiate-addicted Americans during the Gilded Age. Courtwright argues that white women remained the most likely opium eaters after the Civil War, as in the antebellum era.[195] Some contemporary observers agreed. "Five-sixths of the opium-eaters of the country are women, and this class alone consume[s] 70 percent of all the opium imported into the United States," observed an addiction expert in 1888.[196] This figure was perhaps an exaggeration, according to an 1885 study by the Iowa Board of Health. Surveying the demographics of 235 habituates, the study identified 129 women compared to 89 men.[197] But in any case, there were at least as many women as Civil War veterans counted among the ranks of postwar America's opium eaters.

Like veterans, many, although not all, women traced their addiction to wartime hardships. The hunger, overwork, isolation from kin, and violence experienced by so many Southern women was emotionally and mentally devastating, as historian Diane Miller Sommerville has harrowingly documented. Some women even killed themselves to escape the chaos as the Confederacy collapsed from within.[198] Others took to eating opium and sipping laudanum. S. D. Armstrong, a white South Carolina woman, struggled to endure fraught encounters with Union soldiers during Sherman's 1865 March to the Sea. "I never know what it is to be free from pain," she explained to a friend, and "for the last two weeks I have had no sleep but what was caused by opium, and while awake suffer torture with the pain in my face and jaws, from one temple to the other." Stressed and stricken by debilitating headaches, Armstrong began relying on opium to get by. "I hope you will be able to read this," she added, "but I am so nervous from the opium, I can scarcely hold the pen."[199] Opium became a survival strategy for some Confederate women and a way to dull the sting of defeat. In 1870, Marie DeRosset, a close friend of Confederate first lady Varina Davis, killed herself with a massive laudanum overdose. After fleeing the Confederacy for the safety of London, DeRosset had been unable to piece her life back together.[200]

Gilded Age doctors recognized links between opium eating and women's suffering during and after the Civil War. One woman became addicted to opium after using the drug to self-medicate for "worry and suspense concerning the uncertain fate of her husband, who was in the army," according to her physician. The soldier survived the war, returning home to discover that his wife was addicted. Horrified, the husband ordered her to quit the opium, but she refused. Furious, the man asserted his prerogative over his wife's body by removing all opiates from the house, forcing her into hellish withdrawal.[201] Many families waged these internal battles over gendered authority and addiction in the wake of the Civil War. Although troubling, women's struggles often generated less alarm than those of addicted men, even if women's cases were well publicized in the media and medical press.[202]

Over and over in the postwar era, alarmed observers linked the Civil War to the nation's growing epidemic of opiate addiction, even if veteran opium eaters were a minority among American opiate users. A Worcester, Massachusetts, pharmacist reported in 1872 that the recent "increase [in opium eating] is due, in some degree, to the excitements, suffering and mental disquietude resulting from the late war." A Boston druggist added that "veteran soldiers who contracted the habit in the army hospitals are still addicted to the use of opium."[203] Describing opium and alcohol addiction in 1883, physician T. D. Crothers reiterated that "a large number of persons engaged in the late civil war who suffered hardship and malnutrition, became inebriates years after following the psychical and physical traumatism received at that time."[204]

Although many explicitly linked the Civil War to the late-1860s surge in opium eating, others did not. In a widely read 1867 piece in *Harper's New Monthly Magazine*, Fitz Hugh Ludlow, a then-famous opium eater, reported that "the [opium] habit is gaining fearful ground among our professional men, the operatives in our mills, our weary sewing women, our fagged clerks, our disappointed wives, our former liquor-drunkards, [and] our very day-laborers." He observed, "All our classes are yearly increasing their consumption of the drug."[205] Ludlow made no mention of Civil War veterans in this list. Such omissions have led some historians to suggest that opiate addiction must not have been common among Civil War veterans or more writers would have explicitly connected the war and addiction. But considering that most adult men of his generation had served in the war, Ludlow did not necessarily *need* to spell out the fact that many of the day laborers, "fagged clerks," mill operators, and "professional men" were injured or ill veterans. His readers would have understood the unstated fact that wounded veterans were represented among these other demographics. Similarly, an 1868 article in the temperance magazine *Zion's Herald* noted that alongside the antebellum populations associated with addiction—nervous women, prostitutes, and Chinese immigrant opium smokers—America's opium eaters now included "maimed men." These remarks came only three years after the Civil War, so readers would have recognized these "maimed men" as ailing veterans.[206]

A decade on, the outlook for veterans remained bleak. "The delusive habit of taking it [laudanum] to obtain a fleeting repose of the nervous system has recently grown, as our medical men can testify, to alarming proportions," lamented *Scientific American*.[207] Albert Day, a Boston doctor and temperance activist, agreed, elaborating in 1876 that "during the late civil war, the constant excitement to which the whole country was subjected for four or five years, the recruiting of men for the army and navy, their thrilling deeds upon land and sea, their fatigues and exposure to summer's heat and winter's cold, the breaking up of families, the scattering of households, disruption of business relations, and the numerous other exciting influences that attend the pomp and circumstances of war, developed a propensity and created a demand for stimulants," including opium and whiskey. Foreshadowing the long-term health and social effects of opium eating on veterans, Day warned that "the physical, to say nothing of the moral effects of [addiction] . . . will scarcely be eradicated for generations to come."[208]

There seemed to be so many addicted old soldiers that the very identity of Civil War veterans became fused to the act of opium eating, much like the iconic "empty sleeve" or "bloody shirt." The millions of veterans whose "bodies [were] maimed and mangled in battle, or abused in the hospital or prison," seemed more inclined to rely on opiates than others, even if this notion was merely perception.[209] A Boston druggist observed in 1872 that "returned soldiers are rather prone to the [opium] habit, having contracted it in the army." Indeed, "veteran soldiers, as a class, are addicted" to opiates, noted another pharmacist.[210] A few years later in 1878, the *St. Louis Daily Globe Democrat* profiled one such "champion opium-eater," an "ex-Federal soldier" whose opium use surpassed "even De Quincey." Fifteen years after the Civil War, the formerly distinctive identities of veteran and opium eater had fused on the pages of the *Globe Democrat* and in the public consciousness. Readers might have judged the profile a cliché, as if the former soldier was a stock character whom one would be unsurprised to encounter on a street corner. It may have seemed all too familiar when "champion opium-eater" explained that he had "received a minié rifle-ball in the left leg, just above the ankle" at the Battle of Cumberland Gap in September 1863. Badly wounded, "I was sent to the rear and given in charge, with many others, to a young doctor, who had but one cure for everything." "It was opium," said the old soldier. The surgeon "was not stingy about it, so we got as much as we wanted." Considering that "opium was the only thing that would soothe me in any way, I took all that I could get of it, which leaves me today the confirmed slave to the drug that I am." Although more than a decade had passed, "opium-eating [has] stuck to me."[211] Such stories were so commonly voiced that many readers would not have been shocked by this sequence of events.

Veterans' addiction stories attracted sustained attention from doctors and public health authorities throughout the Gilded Age. The influential Medical Society of the State of Pennsylvania formed a committee in 1868 to investigate the sharp rise in intemperance. If many observers feared that opium eating and whiskey guzzling were on the rise, the Committee on Intemperance as a Disease confirmed these suspicions, concluding that sickness and injury during wartime were major factors driving the increase in substance use nationally.[212] A spate of reports about opiate addiction by state boards of health followed during the 1870s and 1880s. When an 1870 investigation of alcohol use in Massachusetts inadvertently uncovered evidence that "the habit of opium-eating and the use of preparations of opium demands attention," the recently established Massachusetts Board of Health commissioned a study.[213] Published in 1872, a survey of 125 physicians found that 68 percent of respondents believed that opiate addiction had increased since the Civil War's end. The board noted that "the taste for opium eating among soldiers retired from the army is alluded to by a few of our correspondents."[214] The Maryland Board of Health followed suit in 1875. A decade later, the Iowa Board of Health published the findings of its own investigation into opium eating, followed three years later by yet another report from the Massachusetts Board of Health. Concerned individual doctors and "muckraker" journalists also turned their attention to the growing addiction crisis, including Orville Marshall of Michigan in 1877, Charles Earle of Chicago in 1880, and Virgil Eaton in 1888.[215] Collectively, these myriad reports affirmed the widespread perception among doctors and pharmacists that opiate addiction was pervasive among Civil War veterans.

Morphine-injecting amputees and opium-eating diarrheal veterans were such common sights in Gilded Age America that they even became fixtures of period novels. One 1867 hit, *Miss Ravenel's Conversion from Secession to Loyalty* by Union veteran John William De Forest, recounted the story of a fictional Union captain who, after suffering a gruesome gunshot wound, received a furlough to recuperate at home. Leaning on opium, the drug leaves the protagonist numb to pain and fatigue but "heavy and dull with the effects of opium which he had taken to enable him to undergo the day's journey." The soldier's loved ones are alarmed by the transformation. De Forest intended the novel to assuage civilian fears about demobilizing soldiers and the prospects for their successful reentry into civilian life. But in the case of opium intemperance, De Forest might have done more to heighten readers' alarm than alleviate it.[216] Soon veterans' addiction became *the* plot. The first American novel about opiate addiction, Edward Payson Roe's 1881 *Without a Home*, did not sport a middle-class white woman or a Chinese opium smoker as the protagonist. Instead, the author profiled a fictional morphine-addicted Confederate veteran, Martin Joclyn, who becomes hopelessly "enslaved" to morphine taken to alleviate a painful war wound. Roe narrates Joclyn's tragic decline as the addicted older soldier abandons his family, vowing "that he would not return until he had regained his manhood" by quitting the morphine. "Alas!" Roe warned his readers, "that day would never come."[217] De Forest and Roe were Civil War veterans whose experiences at war and their cognizance of opiate use among veterans inspired their novels. Taking his cue from medical societies and boards of health, Roe conducted extensive research before writing *Without a Home* to craft a devastatingly accurate portrait of addiction among veterans. Numerous firsthand addiction narratives supplemented other fictional accounts, including Union veteran and Chicago journalist William Rosser Cobbe's *Doctor Judas*, published in 1895. It recounted the author's personal experiences with the opium habit, for which he blamed doctors, heredity, and hardships endured during the Civil War.[218] The moral of these stories was all too clear: Nearly twenty years after the Civil War's guns fell silent, the problem of addiction among veterans had grown out of hand and demanded the nation's attention.[219]

The Civil War veteran–turned–opium eater remained a recurring character in medical texts, newspapers, and fiction during the 1880s and 1890s, although media portrayals of drug addiction gradually evolved, shifting from veterans to focus on younger users of cocaine and heroin. New stereotypes emerged around the turn of the twentieth century. Campaigners against immigrants and vice developed the "white slave" trope depicting fallen women entrapped within Chinese opium dens. Apologists for Jim Crow obsessed over race-baiting allegations that cocaine-fueled Black men endangered white women.[220] Other writers illuminated the urban underworld of young heroin-injecting male vagabonds who menaced the dark alleyways of the nation's fast-growing metropolises. These stereotypes were largely products of Jim Crow prejudices, American imperialism, and Gilded Age cultural anxieties, and they helped animate the early twentieth-century movement to constrain narcotic use.

Yet by the time that Americans turned their attention to these new "drug fiends," it was universally accepted that the Civil War's medical practices and health conditions had helped spark America's first opiate addiction crisis, even if most users were not actually veterans. Decades of alarmist commentary in medical journals and reports, newspapers, and novels cemented this knowledge into the American public's memory of the Civil War. Even President William H. Taft espoused the notion that the Civil War was a main origin point of drug addiction in American history. A 1909 report on the international opium trade, endorsed by Taft, "pointed out that following the Civil War the abuse of medicinal opium and its chief derivative, morphia, set in and spread thickly, or thinly, but over almost the entire country." There was "abundant evidence that one of the prime causes of the misuse of opium and morphia in the United States was the physical and mental overstrain or breakdown of a large number of our population during or immediately following the Civil War."[221] Addicted Civil War veterans and their struggles loomed large in the popular conception of drug addiction, casting a long shadow that would outlive veterans themselves.

PART II

Experiences

Chapter 4

Opium Slavery

Veterans and the Experience of Addiction

Albert Wymer Henley made an agonizing confession in 1878. "In the army," explained the broken-down veteran of the 36th Mississippi Infantry, "I had to use opiates for a complication of painful diseases." Chronic diarrhea and typhoid fever debilitated Henley for months after Vicksburg, forcing the lieutenant to resign from the Confederate army in November 1863, surely a humiliating experience. He found solace in a bottle of morphine, which alleviated the diarrhea and perhaps his distress at leaving the army so ingloriously. But relief came at a cost. "In short," he explained, morphine "fastened its iron grip on my very vitals, and held me enchained and enslaved for near fifteen years." Henley described these years of morphine addiction as a "cruel bondage" to a "relentless and terrible task-master" because it caused unbearable suffering in myriad forms, physical and social. According to prevailing views of opium slavery, Henley's addiction degraded his manhood and moral character and even debased his identity as a white man. Like habitual drunkenness, to be "enslaved" to opiates entailed a level of dependence that was antithetical to widely held ideals of manhood, character, and whiteness, which demanded independence and mastery over one's body and actions. Overreliance on painkillers also seemed to signal that Henley was too weak, or simply unwilling, to endure pain stoically, as was expected of men in the Civil War era. Years of drug use eventually triggered debilitating side effects, sapping Henley's physical vigor and ability to work. Worse still, on the Civil War–era taxonomy of vices, opiate addiction was classified as a form of intemperance, like drunkenness. To his family and neighbors, addiction thus branded Henley as morally condemnable, and even liable to madness as his condition deteriorated.[1]

In this chapter I investigate the experiences and outcomes of opiate addiction for Civil War veterans like Henley. "Slavery" to opiates dominated addicted veterans' postwar lives, destroying their bodies and health while undermining claims to manhood, good character, and whiteness. The effects of long-term opiate use—which had to be consumed daily, often for decades, for users to prevent the onset of withdrawal symptoms and function on a day-to-day basis—appeared to ruin veterans' bodies, leaving them fatigued, emaciated, impotent, and riddled with ghastly self-inflicted injection scars. Users and witnesses feared that the ever-increasing dosage needed to offset tolerance would lead to accidental fatal overdoses, leaving behind grieving families and deeply troubled bystanders. Long-term opiate use also left many veterans unable to work and dependent on family or friends for subsistence. Many of these risks did not result inherently from the act of taking opium but from other people's perceptions or the context in which the drug was consumed. Most addicted veterans were unable to simply quit taking opiates at will, try as they might. This inability to free oneself from opium slavery, as observers and veterans often described addiction, branded men like Henley as weak, lacking in self-control, and intemperate. Furthermore, because of the racial theories of the day, which linked excessive opiate use with non-white people and even with the feared decline of the white race, addiction complicated and sullied veterans' whiteness. Addiction and its wide-ranging consequences thus spelled catastrophe for veterans' health and identities. Facing such a wide spectrum of suffering, opium slavery ultimately proved to be an intensely traumatic and overwhelmingly burdensome experience in many veterans' postwar lives.

Opium Slavery, Health, and Manhood

Opiate use all too often spiraled out of control until addiction dominated many aspects of Civil War veterans' postwar lives, including reputation, self-image, finances, and relationships with families and communities. Long before it reached the crisis point, however, addiction first presented as a health risk. The most immediate dangers of long-term opiate use—addiction and overdose—stemmed from the habit-forming and poisonous nature of the narcotics, which can damage the body when consumed in high doses for years on end. Addicted veterans ran the risk of developing debilitating, life-threatening physical symptoms from opiate use. At first, the beneficial effects of consuming opiates, such as reducing pain and diarrhea to tolerable levels, outweighed the negatives. But as veterans kept taking the medicines over long durations, swallowing and injecting high doses daily or even multiple times a day, for years on end, addiction often became unhealthy. The cons began to outweigh the pros.

After a while, veterans who used opiates developed physical tolerance to the drugs, a state that, according to contemporary doctors, presented one of the earliest and most acute dangers of opiate addiction. American physicians had long known about the phenomenon of tolerance, but they had never encountered it on such a wide scale as during the Civil War's aftermath. When tolerance built up, one needed to consume ever-higher doses to feel the intended effects, such as analgesia and euphoria. As one doctor explained, "When the increase" in dosage "is made, it is like ascending a ladder and casting away the rounds. . . . The larger the dose consumed, the more the system seems to demand, as the drug multiplies complications." In short order, "a larger dose is taken in a desperate effort to allay disagreeable sensations," including withdrawal pain. One man whose "appetite was acquired from the long-continued prescription of anodynes by his physician, some two years ago, during a painful sickness," explained in 1867 that he "had got past deriving any pleasure from its [morphine's] use; his daily allowance merely serving to keep him out of an intense but vague feeling of wretchedness, which seized upon him when he attempted to go without his doses."[2] Although modern medical research suggests that relapse after a period of abstinence from opiates presents a higher risk of overdose than periods of stable use, nineteenth-century doctors believed that tolerance was inherently dangerous because of the high and often-escalating dosages consumed by some users.[3] "This process is continued until the system can tolerate no more without exciting alarming symptoms of narcotism," or overdose.[4] After this cycle continued, the dosages achieved boggled observers' minds. According to one addicted veteran, "The quantity of opium taken by old practitioners varies greatly. A reasonable quantity, after six or eight years' steady use, would be from twelve to sixteen grains morphia per twenty-four hours." Having developed tolerance himself, the man claimed to consume a hefty dose of twelve grains of morphine—equivalent to about 778 milligrams, a potentially lethal dose for the uninitiated—every morning and evening.[5]

Opium users and observers of the "habit" believed that myriad physical dangers might result as the dosage necessary to maintain addicted people increased over time. Risks included weight loss, fatigue, impotence, fatal overdoses—especially after prolonged periods without exposure to opiates such as withdrawal attempts—and more. These effects of opiate use, in turn, seemed to imperil one's manhood, reputation, self-image, and family life. A physician observed how this chain reaction of addiction brought on a litany of dangers for addicted people in 1889. The opium eater is eventually "completely... dominated by the passion for the narcotic." Life became so hellish that "there are few conditions of misery more poignant." "The morphinist" soon "suffers from insomnia, nightmare, hallucinations, trembling of the hands and tongue, impotence, hypochondriac moroseness, neuralgias, and frequent febrile attacks." The drug left the opium eater "lean and cadaverous, his face is expressionless, his eyes have lost their brilliancy." Addiction eventually overthrew the opium eater's mind, morality, and manhood: "His memory is poor, the power of mental application is absent; he becomes treacherous, suspicious, untruthful, in fact, almost demoralized." A "full injection of morphine for a time relieves him, and brings back a sense of *bien être* and the ability to work, but the relief is of but fleeting duration." When it wore off, "the miserable victim soon again sinks into the abyss of despair."[6] The Iowa Board of Health's 1885 report on the opium habit likewise described the full-blown opium eater as physically and morally ruined. "The face" of the addicted "becomes sallow and soggy, the eyes bleared and expressionless, and the final result is either death or insanity." But by that point, "business is gone, family broken, friends lost, moral sense blunted or destroyed, mind incapable of healthy action, body weakened." At this final stage, opium eaters "will lie and steal—do almost anything to obtain the drugs with which and without which they are truly in a veritable hell . . . gloomy and hopeless, the world and the people in it no longer interest them."[7] Realistically, not all opiate users would have embodied this declension, but most descriptions of addiction framed users' physical, mental, and moral decline as inevitable and condemnable.

Opiate addiction thus had a kind of transitive property. The health effects of addiction seemed not only to destroy the body but also to undermine and erode manhood, morality, and health, intersecting cultural constructions. Americans widely believed that one's body—its shape, cleanliness, countenance, and other features—was linked to morality and intelligence. Threats to one element of this equation thus tended to negatively affect the others as well. In this way, opiate addiction paralleled amputation, the classic Civil War disability because of its visibility, although amputation affected only about 7 percent of veterans.[8] "Empty sleeves" often left veterans unable to work and dependent on wives or the state for physical and financial care, inhibiting one's sense of self. But opium eating could be far more dangerous for veterans than life with a missing arm or even a leg. Amputations damaged the man, but opium slavery seemed to destroy him. Empty-sleeved veterans managed to hold on to a degree of tragic dignity as Gilded Age society slowly adapted to accommodate, and sometimes even celebrate, amputees.[9] Not so for veteran opium eaters. As Roberts Bartholow, former Union surgeon and early apostle of hypodermic medicine, once explained, opium slavery left men not only physically disabled but also totally "indifferent to all the duties and obligations of life, reduced to a state of mental and moral weakness most pitiable to behold."[10]

Veterans drew on the familiar antebellum motif of opium slavery to describe how addiction simultaneously destabilized their health and manhood.[11] Echoing Albert Wymer Henley, Texas veteran Byron McKeen confessed ashamedly that "for twelve long years, I have been a slave to the Opium Habit."[12] Joseph C. Darrow, a veteran of the 4th Michigan Infantry, likewise described himself as "a slave to the Habit of using Morphine, with not a ray of hope of ever being emancipated."[13] In 1878, another veteran described how a wartime encounter with a surgeon who "was not stingy" with opium left "me today the confirmed slave to the drug that I am."[14] For their part, doctors also fell back on the antebellum motif of opium slavery in their clinical studies of addiction, having lacked a distinctly medical vocabulary to describe the horrifying transformations experienced by their veteran patients. According to Roberts Bartholow, morphine users became "slaves to a vice beyond their control" as their conditions deteriorated.[15] A physician at an Indiana mental asylum observed that Union veteran William H. Bradley was "the servant of his appetite for narcotics, and [he] is controlled by the desire to satisfy the appetite."[16] Addicted men were "literally chained to opium," which exerted a "demoniac influence" on addicted veterans by destroying their "ability to maintain mastery" over their bodies and behavior when cravings struck.[17] Indeed, addiction "manacled" the user "'with wristlets of brass, and fetters of iron.'"[18] Opium slavery undermined veterans' masculinity because the label signaled one's physical dependency and the loss of self-control and willpower, among other characteristics. "Everlasting slavery" to opium eventually "humiliates opium eaters by a sense of their own weaknesses," concluded one doctor. According to J. B. Mattison, a prominent expert on opiate addiction, "the subtly ensnaring power of opium" rapidly depleted men's bodies and manhood. "One of the finest specimens of physical manhood we ever saw," Mattison explained, "who survived the horrors of Salisbury prison, when the death-rate averaged 80 percent, fell a victim to morphia after only one month's hypodermic using."[19]

This destruction of manhood when one became "enslaved" to opium was among the most disturbing features of addiction for veterans and doctors alike.[20] Such transformation was especially clear in descriptions of withdrawal, which featured heavily in depictions of male opium eating in the popular and medical press. Many veterans who used opiates feared the prospect of fatally overdosing if they continued taking opiates in high doses, thus many users tried to save themselves by simply quitting the drugs. Most men attempted to do so at first through sheer willpower, trying to evidence manly grit, determination, and volition. But the harsh physical effects of sudden withdrawal—which included goosebumps, anxiety, irritability, chills, pain, insomnia, diarrhea, vomiting, stomach cramps, cravings for opiates, and even death from dehydration—proved unbearable for most men, who very often relapsed. Modern medicine explains this outcome by pointing to the brain. Current understandings of addiction posit that long-term opiate use changes the brain. When these changes occur, the drugs' effects become routinized, leading to a kind of stasis that can be maintained only by consuming doses at regular intervals. Addicted people might no longer experience euphoria or pain relief, similar to when they first took opium or morphine, but they needed to continue taking the medicines to remain functional. When one suddenly stops taking opiates "cold turkey" without first slowly tapering down the dosage, the body responds harshly. Excruciating withdrawal symptoms set in, and the only solution is to reintroduce opiates into the body—or somehow struggle through the long ordeal of detoxification, which can last for days or even weeks.[21]

Because nineteenth-century Americans lacked this modern understanding of addiction and withdrawal, a prevailing explanation posited that any man who could not successfully endure opiate withdrawal without giving in to cravings simply lacked the willpower to quit. Relapses were often interpreted as failures of manhood. Joseph C. Darrow, the Michigan veteran who called himself a "slave" to morphine, recalled in 1869 that "the last year or two I have taken from eight to ten and twelve grains of Morphine per day, enough to destroy life in the same number of persons." Humiliated at his debasement and fearing for his life, Darrow desperately wanted to quit and made several attempts to do so. But each time "I omitted taking Morphine one day, I would become completely prostrated and nerveless."[22] If doctors were horrified at their patients' addictions, then the behavior of men in withdrawal was even more awful to behold because it unraveled the patient's manhood. Physicians at New York's Utica asylum forced a New York veteran to detox in 1875. As withdrawal symptoms set in, he began "crying, moaning, and begging for something to keep him quiet," the doctors noted. "Says he is in pain in every bone and muscle."[23] A doctor observing a Confederate veteran withdraw from morphine in the early 1880s noted that he broke down and "piteously begged for opium" during the ordeal.[24] Such behavior was a far cry from the hospital courage demanded from veterans, in war and in peace. Summarizing such reports in an 1878 essay on "the opium habit," an Indiana doctor concluded that the manhood of those who could not complete withdrawal was forever lost. After all, "nothing is more humiliating to a proud man than the thought that he is a *slave*," and nothing revealed one's slavery to opium like the inability to make it through withdrawal without breaking down and begging for the drug.[25]

Some veterans claimed to have quit the drugs through sheer willpower, but theirs were exceptional—and perhaps dubious—cases. A Connecticut soldier contracted chronic diarrhea during the war and upon returning home "had recourse to laudanum" to bring the eruptions under control. As tolerance mounted, he had to increase the dose to dangerous levels, so he eventually decided to lay off the drug. He entered the care of the physician Albert Day in Boston during the late 1860s. Under Day's orders, "the narcotic was cut off entirely and at once." Terrible withdrawal symptoms ensued: nausea, diarrhea, sweats, body shakes, and pain everywhere. But according to Day, the veteran "held out perseveringly nevertheless," seeing the withdrawal process through to the end. Once he recovered, the man sent Day a letter asking that the doctor pass along some advice "in encouragement of repentant yet wavering sufferers" of the opium habit. "The man who meddles with opium will come to perceive by-and-by he is reposing on something other than a bed of roses," the veteran warned. It would take herculean self-control and willpower to "set him emancipate and free" from opium slavery. Indeed, "only through arduous and painful and indomitable persistence against obstacles well-nigh insurmountable will he with any certainty accomplish his purpose." Only "courage and perseverance... in trials renewed from day to day will effect his disenthrallment at last."[26] Such self-aggrandizing language recalled the hospital courage lionized during the war. But most addicted veterans found it impossible to live up to this standard.

Veterans who were unable to bear withdrawal but who broke down and relapsed were widely condemned for their apparent failure of self-control. It took "great willpower" to quit the "habit," yet most addicted men "cannot make the resolution to stop today, but defers it until tomorrow," according to the *Christian Advocate* in 1880.[27] Relapses were typical, and most men never managed to fully overcome their addictions. As a Boston reporter observed in 1888, "When a person becomes an opium-slave, the habit usually holds through life."[28] Even when addicted veterans managed to go for a few days without consuming opiates, they were likely to relapse. "It is a sad fact that more than half of those addicted to the opium habit relapse" observed an author who had interviewed several users.[29] Men who faltered after abruptly quitting the drugs or relapsed later were usually denigrated. They did "not wish to be cured," according to one observer.[30] "The only lapses" in sobriety, added a second critic, "are those who prefer a dissipated to a sober life."[31]

Such condescension illustrated the widespread belief that the inability to overcome addiction was a matter of personal choice, not the result of unseen physiological forces beyond one's control. Observers who believed that addiction began, at its root, as an individual's choice often referred to the "opium habit" when describing addiction. This label overlapped to a certain extent with other labels, like "opium slavery," and multiple descriptors for addiction often appeared together in the same newspaper column or medical journal article. As the *New-York Times* phrased it in 1885, opium addiction was a "self-imposed slavery."[32] The habit and slavery labels both emphasized the opium eater's supposed unmanliness and immorality. But whereas slavery to opium conveyed a consequence of addiction, references to the opium habit were often intended to describe the origins of addiction and reflected the user's ostensible culpability. One doctor described two male "opium habit" patients in 1878. When the first man tried to quit but relapsed, the physician "attributed his failure to want of resolution." The second patient had "been addicted to the habit for thirty years," but when the doctor "informed him that I could redeem him from his bondage," the patient declined to even attempt a cure. Puzzled by his patients' ostensible choices to keep on taking opium, the doctor reasoned that the men must be culpable in their addiction.[33] The notion that addiction was a choice is also evident in reviews of *Opium Eating*, the addiction narrative published in 1876 by an Andersonville survivor. The book recounted how, after contracting a stomach disease at the Confederate prison, a doctor prescribed opium, planting the germ of opium eating that eventually dominated the veteran's life. Physicians who reviewed the book in medical journals flatly rejected the author's premise that doctors were to blame and instead insisted that only the opium eater's personal choices could cause a man to contract the opium habit. As one reviewer put it, opium eating was simply "an abominably bad habit," a condemnable choice that the addicted veteran "willfully persists in."[34]

A vocal cohort of veterans, their families, and sympathetic doctors rejected the notion that addiction was a "habit" and insisted on describing it as "slavery." They contended that swallowing opium or injecting morphine was something addicted people were bound to do against their will, not an impulse that men could overcome merely by flexing their willpower. Those addicted veterans and sympathetic observers who advocated the "opium slavery" model of addiction did not deny many of the emasculating qualities so often ascribed to addiction. But they strongly rejected the notion that users were culpable for their condition. This debate—Was addiction a "habit," a kind of "slavery," or something in between?—eventually developed into a heated medical rift among doctors and temperance advocates. More broadly, the rift between those who primarily considered addiction a "habit" of choice and those who understood addiction as "slavery" represented a manifestation of a broader cultural crisis in Gilded Age America.

Profound and unsettling changes to men's lives between 1870 and 1900 set the backdrop for these dueling understandings of opiate addiction as "habit" versus "slavery." Before the Civil War, independence, even if sometimes a fiction, stood as a hallmark to which white American men aspired. But after the war, frenzied industrialization upended this antebellum ideal. Postwar American society became more mechanized and urbanized than ever. Cities and factories sprouted up as Americans poured into metropolises such as Chicago and New York City by the millions. Gilded Age men increasingly worked white-collar or factory jobs and lived in cities, which threatened the personal autonomy that yeoman white men had formerly aspired to. Their days now centered around the unyielding demands of the clock or the factory foreman. Every few years, economic "panics" like that of 1873 and 1893 forced many men out of work and into poverty, further challenging the once-sacrosanct idea that white men could ever truly be independent in American society.[35] This postwar social and economic turbulence profoundly disrupted prewar conceptions of manhood that stressed independence. To many Americans, it seemed harder, and maybe even downright impossible, to get ahead in the Gilded Age economy or to retain one's manly independence. One historian has aptly described these developments as "the universal crisis of the individual."[36]

Debates over what to call opium eating—habit or slavery—reflected this broader Gilded Age crisis of the individual. The physicians and other middle-class male observers who insisted that addiction was a habit clung to the notion that individual men still possessed absolute free will. These observers preferred to believe that failures in business or health were an individual's personal fault, not the structural by-product of Gilded Age society and economy.[37] Addicted veterans knew better from personal experience, as did their contemporaries—the grangers, trade unionists, and populists who demanded economic reforms. Addicted men's impulse to describe addiction as "slavery" was, in part, intended to express their sense of having lost a degree of free will, the feeling that one could no more resist opium's commands than the relentless ticking of the clock or the bark of a factory foreman.

Yet the notion that addiction was a choice was deeply rooted in American culture and hard to cast away. That is why so many addicted veterans internalized popular criticisms about opium eaters' apparent lack of willpower. In fact, addicted veterans often came to hate themselves. J. M. Richards, a morphine-addicted former Union surgeon, voiced considerable self-loathing at his failure to break the chains of opium slavery through grit and determination. Writing in 1881, Richards recalled his struggles to quit morphine. He wrote, "Sometimes, (for I made several attempts), I would hold out for four or five days, but at the end of that time the limit of my endurance was reached, and I had to go back into my captivity. I was a confirmed morphine eater—that fact could not be disguised. The only way to avoid insanity, or death from mere intensity of pain, seemed to be to follow the path on which I had entered without ever again attempting to leave it."[38] Richards believed himself too weak-willed to see withdrawal through to the end, so he gave up trying to quit. Dejected and hopeless, Richards's sense of self-worth and estimation of his manhood collapsed.[39] As one doctor derisively concluded, "Nothing is more humiliating to a proud man than the thought that he is a *slave*."[40] A broken-down Union veteran institutionalized at New York's Utica asylum became so despondent over his failure of willpower that he felt he was "such a wicked man that he ought not to be allowed to remain in this asylum but should be removed to prison" instead.[41] Another embarrassed veteran confessed to the Utica doctors that "no one knows how wicked he is" because of his relapses.[42] As a third veteran surmised, "man is completely emasculated" by his failure to endure withdrawal.[43]

A rare late nineteenth-century photograph depicting a Civil War veteran posed as if he is about to receive a hypodermic morphine injection vividly illustrates the notion that users lacked willpower and vigor (fig. 4.1). The anonymous subject, purported to be a former soldier, posed with eyes downcast and body limp. An older bearded doctor firmly gripped the patient's left arm. The camera captures the physician with hypodermic syringe in hand, as if he is about to use the needle to inject morphine into the veteran's left arm a few inches below the elbow. The needle does not connect with the skin, suggesting that the image is a staged version of what most Americans expected to see in morphine users, how they supposedly looked and acted. It is an apt illustration of cultural stereotypes about addicted men. Morphine might ease lingering

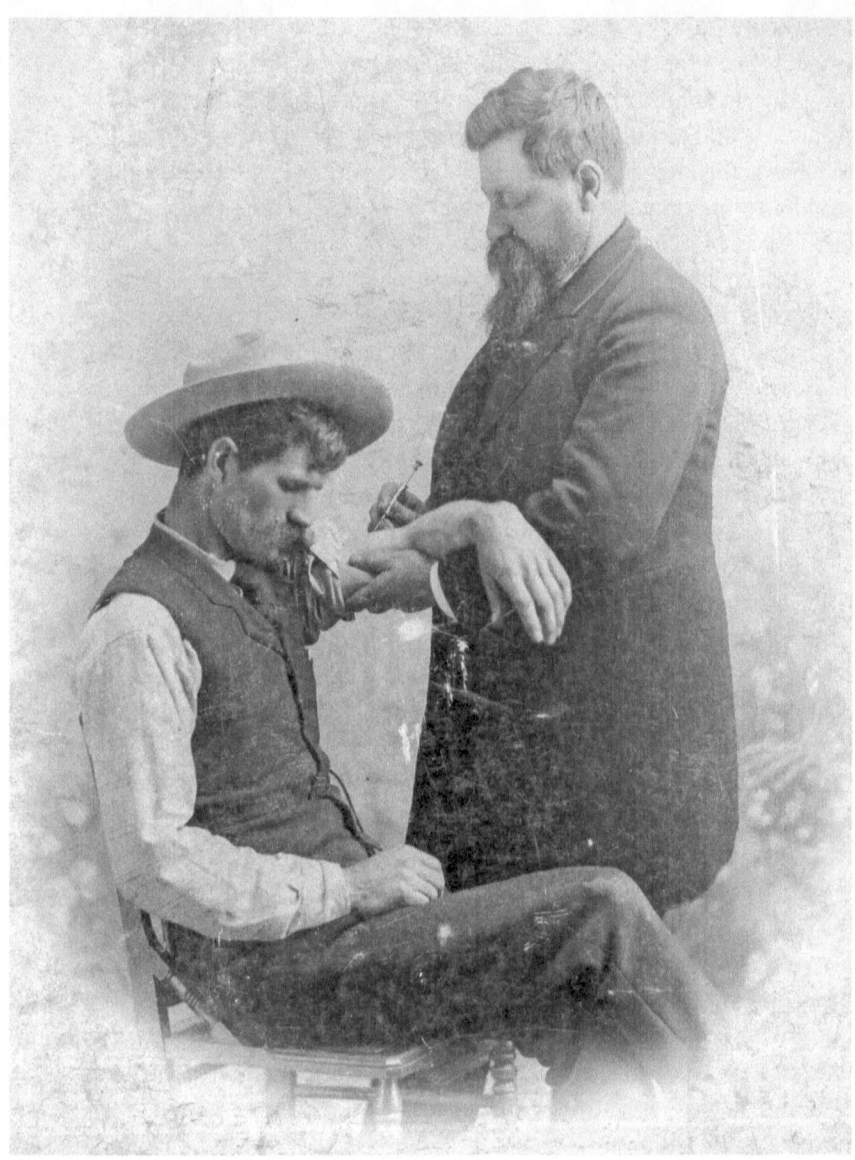

Figure 4.1 Undated cabinet card showing an unnamed Civil War veteran posing as if he is about to receive, or perhaps has just received, an injection of hypodermic morphine from a doctor. The veteran's limp pose embodied how most Americans viewed addicted men—as weak-willed, passive, and unmanly. Courtesy of Stanley B. Burns, M.D., Historic Medical Photography Collection, MS Coll 76, Medical Historical Library, Harvey Cushing/ John Hay Whitney Medical Library, Yale University, New Haven, CT.

pains from the war, but the drug sapped manly vigor and volition in the process. This cabinet card was perhaps intended by the physician to showcase his mastery of the novel technological wonder that was the hypodermic syringe, which increased postwar doctors' capacity to ease pain and suffering far beyond their antebellum forebears; viewers may have taken away this intended message at a glance. Yet if one's gaze lingered, the sorry sight of the passive, downcast, limp veteran, slouching almost lifeless as if under the intoxicating influence of morphine would have struck a nerve too. The subject contrasted sharply, jarringly, with the innumerable, familiar soldier portraits from the war, which pictured stoic men personifying bravery and fortitude as they sat or stood still for the camera's long exposure.

Just as a failure of willpower emasculated opium eaters, so did their apparent inability to endure pain stoically. Men of the Civil War generation were socialized from boyhood to react to pain with stoicism. As boys before the war, they had learned to mercilessly beat each other for sport. The war only confirmed this cult of pain, even if the work of killing and dying took the fun out of it. Many Civil War veterans believed that to shy away from pain was to brand oneself as effeminate.[44] Old soldiers who kept up their wartime "hospital courage" after the war, refusing to complain about pain or take painkillers, were lauded for their manliness. Some wounded veterans even became celebrities for their stoicism, praised by public officials for enduring their "painful wounds" with "uncompromising fortitude" and rewarded with large pensions.[45] By comparison, veterans who admitted they were in pain and openly consumed opiate painkillers revealed an inability or unwillingness to bear pain. They were "weak-nerved people who bear pain badly," according to one observer.[46] Addicted veterans were frequently condemned on these grounds. Despite showing concern for the fate of addicted veterans, Silas Weir Mitchell, the young syringe-wielding Union surgeon at Turner's Lane Hospital in Philadelphia, accused one veteran who had endured multiple amputations of being a "malingerer" because he resorted to morphine to manage his terrible pain.

Mitchell was not alone in condemning addicted veterans for not living up to the expectation that men endure pain stoically. In 1888, President Grover Cleveland impugned the manhood of Clinton Smith, a Union veteran from Indiana, for his inability to endure pain without resorting to opiates. Shot in the arm during the war, Smith became addicted to opiates to cope with the pain. During a bout of severe pain in December 1884, he fatally overdosed in a Union City, Indiana, hotel room. When Congress awarded Eliza Smith, Clinton's wife, a special pension, Cleveland vetoed it on the grounds that the veteran's death was not service related. Explaining his rationale, Cleveland conceded that Smith's wound was "very painful, and that he was in the habit of taking large doses of morphine to alleviate his suffering." But pain was no excuse for resorting to morphine. Many disabled veterans had to live with pain, but most of them did not debase themselves with numbing drugs, as Cleveland believed that Smith had done. Instead of extending sympathy, Cleveland condemned the veteran as an "intemperate" man, "especially when suffering from his wound."[47] Cleveland's negative perception of Smith's manhood and character doubtless influenced his decision to veto the pension. Smith's comrades reacted viscerally to Cleveland's veto message. They accused the president of speaking "disrespectfully of the dead soldier . . . the president not only vetoed the widow's pension, but libeled her husband's memory," according to the Ohio Soldier.[48] Fellow veterans, relatives, friends, and even some doctors often empathized with the plight of veterans who became addicted to opiate painkillers. But allies were few and far between. Theirs was a minority viewpoint, overshadowed by the more frequent condemnation of addicted veterans leveled by Cleveland, Mitchell, and like-minded observers, who clung to prewar cultural expectations that men get by without overreliance on painkilling drugs. Indeed, the denial of pensions for addicted veterans and their widows was typical, a theme explored at length in chapter 6.

Compounding the complexities of withdrawal and pain management, opium slavery also unleashed a host of dramatic physical transformations that simultaneously chipped away at manhood and health. Hypodermic needle puncture marks and abscesses on veterans' arms and legs, for example, served as visual evidence of their total loss of self-control. Physicians stood aghast at the apparent recklessness of veterans who injected themselves over and over, despite the obvious self-harm their injections caused. A. F. Swann injected hypodermic morphine up to twenty times a day for six years. He was "a stout, robust man" when a captain in the 16th Pennsylvania Cavalry but suffered a horrible gunshot wound at Cold Harbor in May 1864. After the war, morphine wrecked Swann's body and manhood. His skin served as undeniable evidence of this horrible transformation. "Both arms are covered with the punctures of the syringe, discolored, and the cellular tissue indurated," Swann's doctor noted with shock.[49] Silas Weir Mitchell, following up on wartime nerve injury patients from Turner's Lane Hospital, wrote to Swann's former surgeon in 1891 inquiring about the captain's postwar health. The surgeon reported that Swann had died in 1878, adding, "I would ask for your private ear that his death was mainly due to bad habits," namely, morphine addiction.[50] The surgeon believed that Swann's recklessness had ruined the captain's manhood and cost his life.

Observers found veterans like Swann to be terrible sights to behold. They embodied carelessness, the antithesis of self-control. From doctors' viewpoints, the ghastly puncture marks that dotted addicted men's thinly stretched skin betrayed their inability, or unwillingness, to abstain from the needle, despite the obvious self-harm that resulted from the injections. When Union sailor

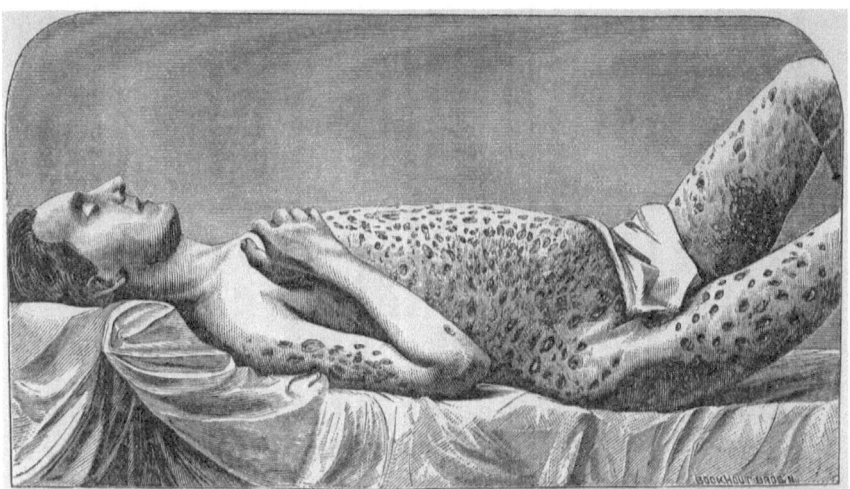

Figure 4.2 "Result of Subcutaneous Injection." Although depicting a nonveteran, the image illustrates the abscesses that often occurred at hypodermic injection sites. To doctors, abscesses signaled the perceived recklessness of men addicted to hypodermic morphine. From H. H. Kane, *Drugs that Enslave: The Opium, Morphine, Chloral and Hashisch Habits* (Philadelphia: Presley Blakiston, 1881), 73.

George W. Gardner appeared before doctors at Indiana's National Military Home in September 1891, needle puncture wounds riddled his skin from head to toe, covering "the whole anterior surface of his body from neck downward and around on his sides as far back as he could reach, his arms down to wrists, and his legs to ankles." (See fig. 4.2.) Like Swann's doctors, Gardner's caretakers were horrified by the sailor's lack of self-control. He simply would not, or could not, stop injecting morphine repeatedly, despite ruining his body and endangering his life. When Gardner fatally overdosed two years later, his doctor subtly condemned the sailor's reckless, self-harming behavior, noting that the Gardner died because he took an "*extra* hypodermic injection of morphia" beyond the bare minimum dose.[51]

Medical reports of abscesses at hypodermic injection sites first appeared in earnest during the Civil War's immediate aftermath. These reports surprised and alarmed American doctors, some of whom had argued that the hypodermic use of morphine was less addictive and dangerous than the oral method.[52] One of the earliest reports appeared in 1870 in the *BMSJ*. It described the terrifying case of an anonymous, veteran-aged man whose hypodermic morphine use had left him "a confirmed slave to the degrading habit of opium-taking, weak in body and mind." His "leg and thigh are so thickly studded with the scars of the innumerable punctures of the syringe that scarcely any healthy appearing integument can be seen." The patient was "enthralled" by still-novel hypodermic

Opium Slavery 119

morphine, "led by it as if he had been an opium-eater, instead of absorbing it through the cellular tissue for all this time."[53] A decade later, the addiction expert H. H. Kane likewise condemned men whose skin bore hypodermic needle puncture wounds like those exhibited by Swann and Gardner. Kane believed these "abscesses" revealed a person's innate recklessness and immorality. Sufferers showed "carelessness in injecting," taking "no care whatever to keep syringe or solution clean"—behavior that underscored their lack of self-control.[54] "Abscess found in the habitues of the syringe," Kane explained, were "due in part to... impure solutions, dirty syringes, and careless injecting."[55] In a culture that widely associated physical uncleanliness with immorality, this rhetoric also branded addicted men as immoral, not just unmanly.

In reality, abscesses were products of unseen microbiological forces, not personal failures. Unbeknownst to addicted veterans or most contemporary doctors, injectable morphine often teemed with microscopic pathogens. Preparing morphine for injection usually involved diluting a tablet of the drug with water. If this water was not first distilled, the solution became contaminated with bacteria. Puncturing the skin with a morphine-laden hypodermic needle thus enabled bacteria to pass the body's external defenses into the tissue and bloodstream. Premixed liquid morphine was available for purchase, but it was no more sanitary. Even these tidy bottles of aqueous morphine solution sometimes sported greenish-brown fungi blooms inside the glass due to contamination during the manufacturing process.[56] Before "germs" became a household word in the early twentieth century, most drug users and doctors had no idea that an injection of morphine could cause bacterial or fungal infections, generating disfiguring pus-filled abscesses. Instead, when judgmental doctors like Kane conjectured that the imprudence, impatience, and innate dirtiness of addicted people caused the abscesses, this victim-blaming rhetoric spawned a moralistic explanation for what historians in hindsight might ascribe to mere microbiological processes. In one sense, these were Civil War scars, just like the amputations that became a symbol of the war's catastrophic human toll and veterans' sacrifices. Yet doctors refused to see it this way, instead choosing to brand men who sported injection scars as unclean, unmanly, and unworthy of sympathy. Ultimately, this nineteenth-century link between needle puncture abscesses and the supposed immorality of drug users helped lay the groundwork for an enduring cultural link between dirtiness and hypodermic drug use.

Abscesses were not the only dramatic, jarring physical symptom of opiate addiction endured by veterans. Severe nausea, indigestion, and constipation were also common, which suppressed appetites and caused severe emaciation. Addicted men suffered from "complete anorexia, wasting, [and] loss of strength," according to a doctor with experience treating opium eaters.[57] A Union veteran of a Maryland cavalry regiment was committed to New York's

Utica asylum in 1877 after long-term opium use. Doctors reported that "for years he has suffered from constipation of the bowels and has been obliged to take strong medicine in order to have a movement."[58] A. F. Swann's "appetite was nearly gone; his bowels were habitually constipated; and the whole man was emaciated" when Silas Weir Mitchell followed up on Swann's case.[59] After years of "using the almost incredible amount of 2 ounces [of morphine] per week," George Gardner, the Union sailor pockmarked with injection abscesses, "declined very much in bodily weight, at one time weighing less than 100 pounds," according to his doctor's notes. "His weight in health was 150 pounds," but morphine had left Gardner's body an emaciated husk.[60] The anonymous Union veteran behind the 1876 narrative *Opium Eating* provided a rare description of this facet of addiction from the sufferer's perspective. Starvation endured at the notoriously unhealthy prison camps at Andersonville and Libby Prison left the veteran with debilitating gastrointestinal issues from the squalid conditions of his captivity, perhaps chronic diarrhea. Returning home, he sought treatment from a "blundering" local doctor, who committed "malpractice" by secretly dosing the veteran with hypodermic morphine injections until he became addicted. The veteran believed the syringe was filled with another drug. The morphine "used to derange my stomach," he claimed, to the point that "the region 'round about' my epigastrium was in a state of communistic insurrection and rebellion. Nothing digested during this time . . . I did not become hungry."[61] Consequently, he withered away. Losing such significant weight posed serious health risks for addicted veterans, igniting a cascade of symptoms associated with malnutrition, from general malaise, fatigue, and irritability to severely weakened immune systems and an elevated risk of death.[62]

Compounding these health risks, emaciation also compromised veterans' physical appearances, an important marker of manhood. Addicted veterans' emaciated frames diverged greatly from the ideal male body of the day, undermining one of the most important facets of manhood. The "perfect man" of the Gilded Age had well-defined, bulging muscles, exuding vigor from neck to calf.[63] An 1888 life insurance manual explained that the perfect man—coincidentally deemed the most insurable man—had a "full" chest, a "well-developed" abdomen, and "limbs plump and tapering." His neck was "short and thick, the shoulders broad, and the head and face inclining to roundness." He ought to have a "florid" complexion, a "countenance pleasing," and, above all, be "physically and mentally active, [and] love fresh air and exercise."[64] (See fig. 4.3.) In contrast, the bodies of addicted veterans like Swann and Gardner were ghastly thin and sickly looking. They lacked the perfect man's sublime physique, and their gaunt faces, bony biceps and thighs, and skeletal rib cages signaled weakness and a lack of vitality (fig. 4.4). As one addicted veteran put it, his body looked "weak and inefficient."[65] Edward Mann, a physician with extensive

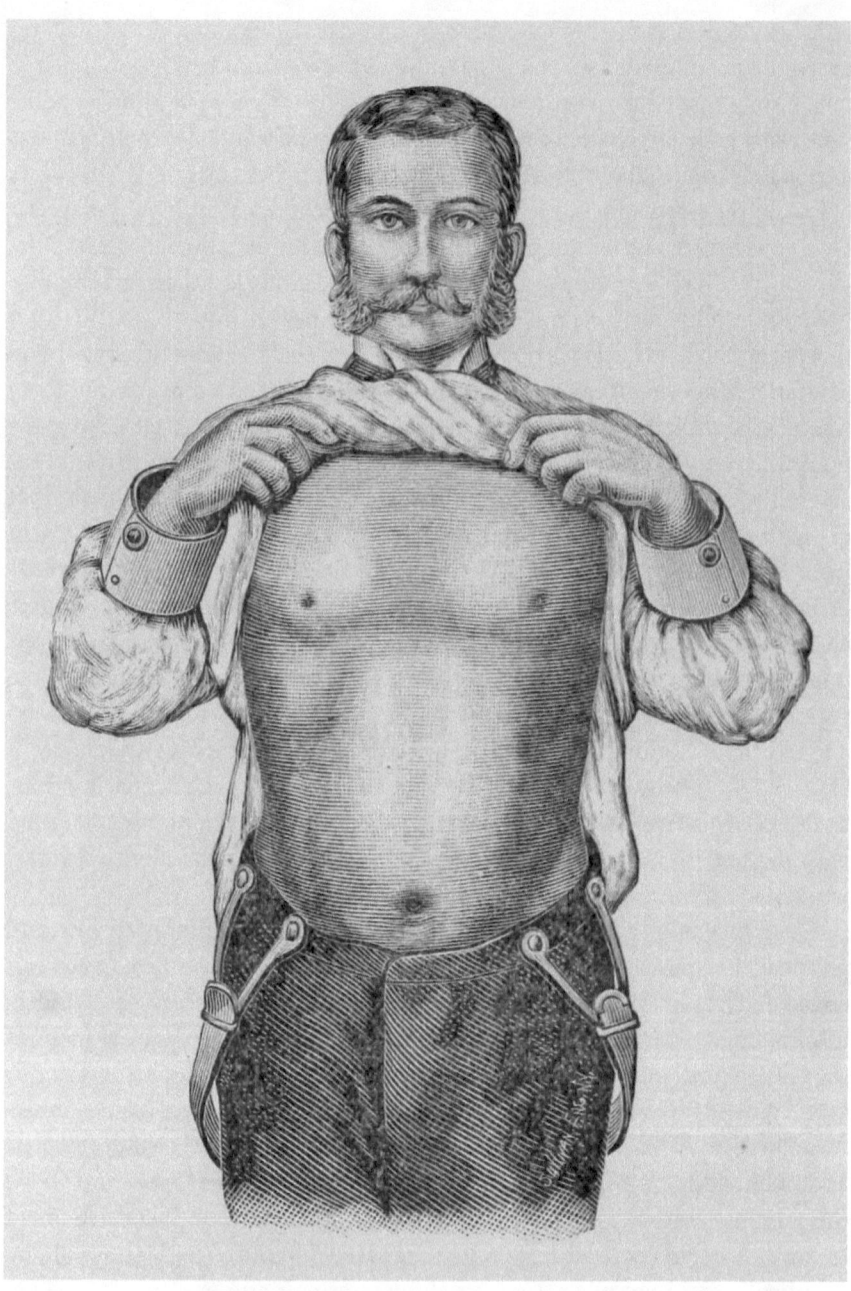

Figure 4.3 Engraving depicting the ideal Gilded Age male physique. The perfect man's stoutness sharply contrasted with the emaciation commonly exhibited by opiate-addicted veterans. Charles F. Stillman, *The Life Insurance Examiner: A Practical Treatise upon Medical Examinations for Life Insurance* (New York: Spectator, 1888), image opposite p. 53.

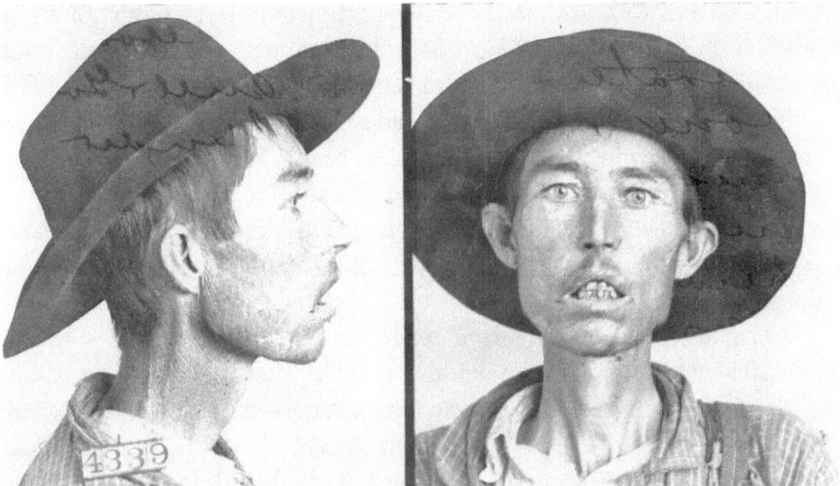

Figure 4.4 Mugshot of Solomon Sivils, an inmate at Leavenworth Federal Penitentiary, ca. 1904. When Sivils was imprisoned at Leavenworth for smuggling liquor into Indian Territory, the prison doctor remarked that the man was "tubercular and extremely emaciated from Morphine addiction. Unfit for manual labor." Although not a Civil War veteran, Sivils's likeness illustrates how emaciated veterans would have appeared to medical observers. Courtesy of National Archives and Records Administration, Washington, DC.

clinical experience treating opium eaters, likewise noted the sapping effects of addiction on his patients' bodies. "The great diagnostic point attending" opiate addiction, Mann explained, "is the strange expression of the physiognomy, the wan complexion, the sunken eyes, the vacant look . . . the eyes lose their brightness; the patient becomes prematurely old. The face sometimes is an expressiveless mask, and the skin takes on an earthy tint. The patient, if not cured, gradually falls into a decline and dies."[66] The bodies of severely addicted men thus deviated markedly from the ideal male body of the day, undermining their manhood.

Emaciated men were desperate to gain weight to offset the deleterious effects of addiction. Advertisements for patent medicine remedies for opiate addiction reveal the great lengths veterans took to gain weight. Samuel B. Collins, an Indiana veteran who became a patent medicine magnate, capitalized on this desperation to gain weight to drive up sales of his Painless Opium Antidote. Collins hawked the product in classified advertisements in veterans' periodicals and through pamphlets brimming with testimonials by supposedly satisfied customers, many of them former soldiers. George Kirk, an Indiana veteran who was physically debilitated by opium addiction, claimed in an 1871 testimonial that after taking Collins's antidote, "I rapidly gained strength—so rapidly that my friends all noticed, and remarked the change." J. C. Ketchum, a Michigan veteran, also took Collins's cure, happily reporting that "I weigh thirty pounds more than I did a year ago. My wife thinks I had better consult you about substitute for ham and eggs; she says I keep her very busy cooking. . . . I feel so different and so much more like my old self; and, above all, feel myself no longer a slave," having been "restored to life, health, and manhood again" by Collins's antidote.[67] Such testimonials indicate a desire among addicted men to mitigate, and even reverse, the risks that opiate addiction posed for health and manhood, as well as an awareness on Collins's part that a large market for his product existed among veterans.

Physical debility stemming from opiate addiction often became so severe that it prevented veterans from working and left them dependent on family and friends for support. Union veteran John J. Patterson, a former Union army surgeon who was dismayed by his inability to quit morphine through sheer willpower, described how opiate addiction left him bedridden and under the constant care of his wife. "I could not sleep until an injection was administered," Patterson wrote. "My wife would get up at all hours of the night and use the syringe on me. My health was so poor that I was confined to my room, and at last to my bed. I could not eat until I used the morphine"—nor could he practice medicine or financially support his family.[68] A veteran of the storied 69th New York Infantry suffered a similar fate. The man, who was ultimately committed to a mental asylum in Utica, New York, in 1882, "suffered from chronic diarrhea" as a soldier during the Civil War. "For its relief [he] used hypodermic injections of morphia and in this way formed the habit," according to his asylum medical records. "After the war he practiced dentistry in Burlington, Iowa, and also in Rock Island," his physician noted, "till seven years ago when he lost his practice mostly through his morphia habit," which had ostensibly left him unable to focus and prone to erratic behavior.[69] Addiction, by this accounting, ruined the veteran's business and made him a burden on family and friends. Countless veterans suffered the same fate, left physically unable to work after years of opiate use.

Ironically, abstaining from opiates also left some men unable to work. The anonymous Union veteran author of *Opium Eating* lamented his inability to perform clerical work without hypodermic morphine injections at regular intervals throughout the day. "I found that the taking of my medicine had settled down into something like regularity," he wrote. Morphine injections set the rhythm of the day and enabled him to focus for a few hours. But when "the time came around" to take another shot, "I was restless, lacking spirit, and unable to do anything to any purpose till I had an injection."[70] Gilded Age addiction doctors frequently reported similar anecdotes, remarking with dismay that their male patients were damned if they continued in the opium habit but were left unable to work if they abstained from their usual dose. According to

Edward Mann, "It is an invariable rule that work is impossible except when the patient is under the influence." But the "steady increase of poison injected, means, of course, a progressive cachexia, both moral and physical."[71] Addicted men thus found themselves in a difficult bind: they could not keep up their work without opiates, but prolonged drug use also rendered them unable to work, with severe repercussions for their masculine identity.

To many contemporary observers, chronic opiate use also seemed to undermine intellect, ambition, focus, and mental acuity, preventing addicted veterans from performing the white-collar work that was increasingly associated with bourgeois masculinity in the late nineteenth century. Such work demanded mental prowess and an aptitude for numbers that severely addicted veterans could no longer muster.[72] Indeed, disabled veterans were often steered toward white-collar clerical positions as an alternative to private charity or government welfare. Yet opiates left veterans unable to function in the fields or behind a desk. The New York veteran whose morphine addiction cost him a successful dental practice was "incoherent in speech" and "forgetful" to the point that he could not even "recognize his own mother," let alone keep accurate records, according to the Utica asylum doctors.[73] Another Union veteran recalled in 1870 his experience with opium. He had been discharged late in the war after becoming too severely wounded to be useful to the army any longer. "I was returning to it [home] and to them [family] a mere wreck," the veteran lamented, "an arm left upon the well-fought field of Shiloh; a bullet near my spine, the parting compliment of the day at Stone River; constitution broken, ambition gone, wasted to a shadow, and only sustained by the wonderful power of Opium."[74] His war wounds robbed the veteran of his ability to do manual labor, but opium stole away the man's potential to succeed at white-collar work. Another veteran, a forty-three-year-old banker in New York, also reported being unable to concentrate on his work because of drug and alcohol addiction.[75] As addiction progressed, the "business ability is gradually weakened," one writer claimed, "and a morbid indifference assumes the place of former ambition until the despondent brain too frequently tries and hopes to find relief in an 'overdose.'" The habitué's "mind cannot be fixed upon anything whatever in a business way; reading, writing or study."[76] Describing William H. Bradley, a morphine-addicted Union veteran, a physician dryly noted that "his business matters are unattended to."[77] These descriptions carried a double meaning. Taken at face value, such remarks conveyed how opiate addiction disabled veterans and left them unable to perform business activity. In this way, the health consequences of opiate addiction led to ripple effects like decreased incomes and the loss of professional identity, important markers of manhood.[78]

Commentary about addicted veterans' lack of business ability also conveyed a deeper, even more unsettling meaning. To the ears of Gilded Age observers, accusations of opium eaters' lack of business capacity doubled as a condemnation of addicted men's manhood on the grounds that they had ceded total control over their person and affairs to others. "Minding one's business"—or, maintaining control over one's own body, dependents, and financial affairs—was a crucial component of manhood in the late nineteenth century. Habitual intoxication opened one's affairs up to the control of others, exchanging manly independence for unmanly dependence.[79] Moreover, against the backdrop of the Industrial Revolution, so much of a man's worth to society seemed rooted in his productive capacity, a by-product of the Gilded Age's increasingly capitalistic economy. Consequently, when dependency to morphine left men idle and unable to work, the drug seemed to ruin his productive capacity and ability to contribute to society, let alone support himself and his family. Thus opium's effect on productivity not only damaged addicted men's claims to manhood but also directly challenged the capitalist ethos of the postwar United States.[80]

Opium Slavery, Family Life, and Community Relations

The complications and consequences of opiate addiction often pushed veterans' relationships with families and communities to the brink. Ruined marriages and opium slavery seemed to go hand in hand. "The great majority of opium-takers," veteran and nonveteran alike, "are or have been married," the *Christian Advocate* reported in 1880. But "many of both sexes who have occupied this relation are now separated, the unreliability and loss of respect, and untruthfulness, which the habit usually produces, being the cause."[81] For their part, veterans worried that opium eating was an unavoidable marriage killer. William Rosser Cobbe, a noted Chicago journalist and former Union sailor, hated what his "long night of opium slavery" did to his marriage. Throughout years of addiction, Cobbe put his "innocent" wife through hell. Despite the many hardships Cobbe endured himself, she still "suffered the *most* for my transgressions."[82]

The inability of addicted veterans to work was a major point of contention in their families, who endured poverty and the inability to live up to bourgeois cultural norms. Addiction prevented veterans from fulfilling the masculine familial role of breadwinner, a central expectation for Victorian men that many disabled veterans were unable to meet.[83] In some cases, opiate addiction even brought about the total inversion of gender norms by forcing wives to become caretakers and wage earners. Robert B. Warburton, formerly of the 25th New York Cavalry, was "very intemperate and addicted to the excessive use of opium and morphine," which made him unreliable and "disposed to roam about the country." Warburton abandoned Mary, his wife, who was forced to take up "sewing at a disreputable boarding house"—a thinly veiled euphemism for prostitution—according to her unsuccessful application for a widow's pension.[84]

Opiate addiction thus profoundly disrupted gender relations within veterans' households. Considered in this light, addiction can be understood as another dimension of the Civil War's broader "crisis in gender" identified by historian LeeAnn Whites.[85]

The 1896 separation of Frances B. Goolrick, a Virginia high-society woman and great-great-granddaughter of George Mason, from her husband, Confederate veteran John Tackett Goolrick, provides a rare window into the disruption that addiction caused for veterans' families (fig. 4.5). John had been a teenaged soldier in the Fredericksburg Artillery. He was shot through the left thigh at Petersburg in October 1864 and spent time recovering at Chimborazo, where he was likely treated with opiates. He developed a long-standing but secret addiction to morphine at some point in the ensuing decades, perhaps to cope with the lingering pain from his war wound.[86] He later became a lawyer, local judge, and a notable Lost Cause author and was even invited to meet President Warren G. Harding during a 1921 Marine Corps reenactment of the Battle of the Wilderness (fig. 4.6). Meanwhile, John's secret, known only to his wife, exacted a terrible toll. His law practice, the family's finances, and the Goolricks' marital happiness deteriorated, and Frances blamed the morphine. John promised her over and over that he would quit, but his perpetual failure to break off the morphine "habit" nearly imploded their marriage.

One afternoon in the winter of 1896, the Goolricks' tense situation exploded in drama. Upon returning home to the couple's Washington, DC, townhouse from an outing on February 5, 1896, Frances discovered her husband slumped over in a morphine daze. With John yet again under the drug's influence, breaking his vows to quit, Frances snapped. She scrawled a frank, emotional letter to her brother in Fredericksburg voicing her disgust at John's latest relapse. She was at her wit's end over his "weakness and folly." Soon, Frances wrote, John "will have gotten over the effects of whatever it is that he took and will then beg and implore me not to do this. but I *must*, I *must*, I can bear neither for myself or the children, this life any longer." "I am in constant terror of I don't know what happening," she added, alluding to the risk of fatal overdose or the public disclosure of his morphine use. But "what can I do? He can do anything if only he could break off this horrible habit. But it seem[s] he can't and it's his mind and brain clouded by drink, or whatever it is he takes, there is no dependence to be put in him."[87] Frances was far from alone in her mixed exasperation at John's relapse, her desperation to get away from him, and her concern about his fate. Women in the orbit of opium eaters often vacillated between sympathy, rage, and the desire to simply wash their hands of addicted husbands, sons, and friends. Leaving a temperance meeting one night in 1881, a young woman accosted a male friend she encountered on the street while he was high. He told her he was seeking to "kill his blues" by habitually using

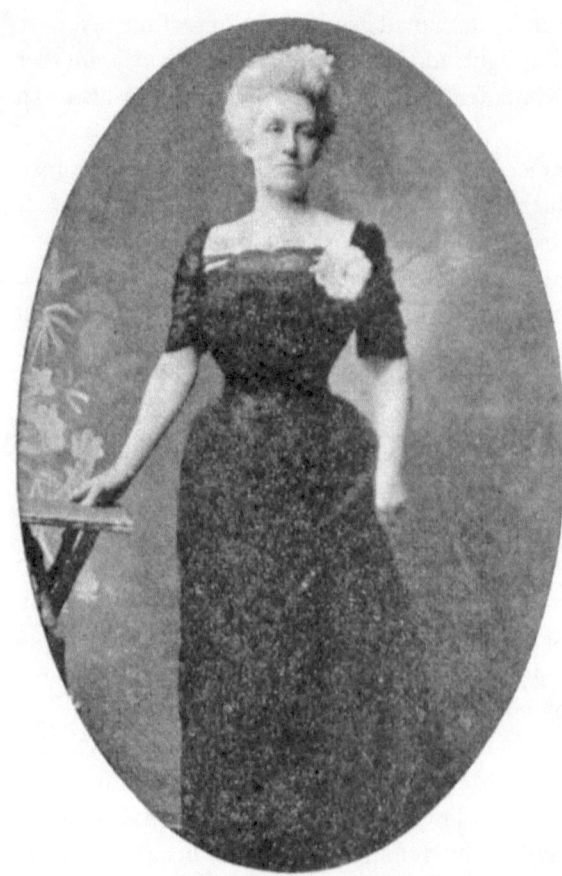

Figure 4.5 (top) Portrait of Frances B. Goolrick. Undated photograph in *Confederate Veteran*, December 1917, 573.

Figure 4.6 (bottom) Photograph depicting an elderly John Tackett Goolrick (*right*) meeting President Warren G. Harding in 1921 on the Wilderness battlefield. From John T. Goolrick, *Historic Fredericksburg: The Story of an Old Town* (Richmond: Whittet & Shepperson, 1922).

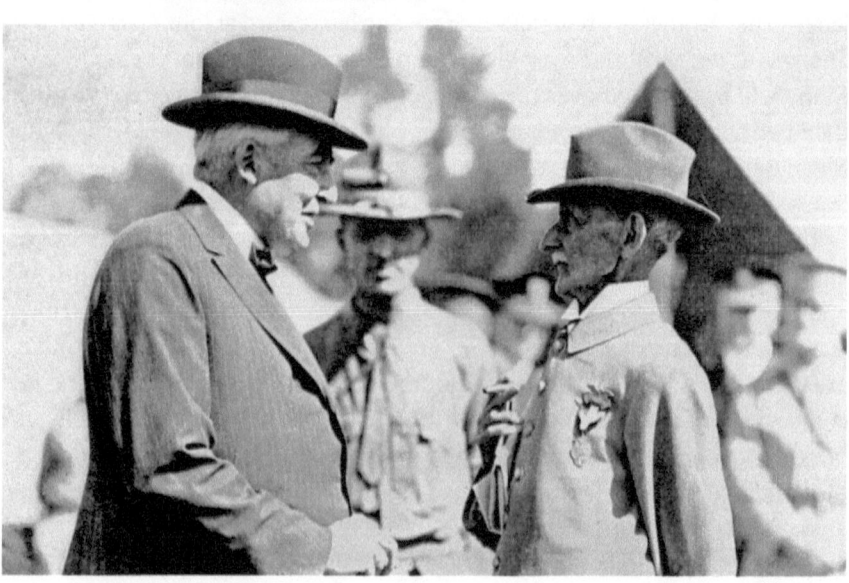

morphine. When she confronted him about the drug use, he lied and deflected, but the woman would not relent. She called him a "coward" with a "selfish" and "wicked" addiction that "disgraced" his family and bereaved his friends.[88] Frances and many other wives, mothers, daughters, and sisters of addicted Civil War veterans shared this sentiment.

Enraged and distraught by John's unreliability and failure to uphold his obligations, Frances seized control over the Goolrick family's affairs and announced her intent to divorce John. This scenario would not be totally unprecedented. A decade and a half earlier, a Missouri court had granted James Dawson of St. Louis the right to divorce his wife, Eva, because of her "habitual drunkenness produced by opiates" and her concealment of the "habit" from him.[89] Frances may or may not have been aware of this case, but certainly she shared James Dawson's impulse. Yet such a scandalous divorce would invite public scrutiny. Although contemptuous toward John, relatives soon talked Frances down and proposed a solution.[90] To give her space, the family quietly shuttled the ailing veteran off to Fredericksburg, Virginia, to stay with his brother William, a physician, and sister-in-law Nora. They would ultimately care for John for several months in 1896. During this convalescence, William and Nora locked John in the house under around-the-clock guard and denied him any morphine, which he attempted to steal to ease the terrible withdrawal symptoms that soon began. His screams echoed throughout the house, haunting his relatives.[91] Costs soon added up, and with John, a lawyer by trade, incapacitated and unable to generate income, the family's financial resources dwindled. Realizing Frances was unable to pay her expenses, John and Frances's firstborn son, Charles O'Conor Goolrick, a cadet at the Virginia Military Institute, offered to quit school, return home, and look for work to support his mother, an embarrassing prospect for all involved. He dropped out shortly thereafter.[92] The effects of addiction often cascaded down from veterans to their children and extended families.

Frances and John eventually reunited, but his addiction never ceased taking a toll on her. In January 1915, Frances was forced to resign the presidency of the local United Daughters of the Confederacy chapter after receiving a letter from the chapter's vice president that implied that John had relapsed yet again. The group's members believed his addiction reflected badly upon the "dignity" of Frances's office.[93] When John died in September 1925, an obituary claimed his "path was not strewn with roses," obliquely hinting at his struggles with morphine and its disastrous effects on the Goolrick family.[94] Even John's death certificate hints at the lingering effects of addiction, indicating his death resulted from myocarditis, a rare consequence of a heart infection caused by mycobacterium. Twenty-first-century researchers have linked such infections to chronic morphine use, which suppresses the immune system, giving opportunistic bacteria a beachhead in the body's internal organs.[95] As the

Goolricks' experience suggests, when opiates disabled veterans by "clouding" their minds—as Frances remarked of John—this state prevented men from minding their business, degraded one's manhood, and caused major financial disruptions, emotional turmoil, and embarrassment for families.

If the Goolricks' saga illuminates the ordinarily private complexities of addicted veterans' family lives, then John's fate also speaks to broader questions about how to interpret Civil War veterans' postwar lives. John's story does not fit neatly into prevailing scholarly understandings of veteranhood. By outward appearances, he was everything that Confederate veterans aspired to be: John was praised for his successful career, and his Lost Cause writing and stumping elevated him from just another teenaged Confederate into a regional celebrity during the Gilded Age.[96] Frances appeared the genteel wife, and their boys had promising futures. Crucially, John did not appear to bear any unpleasant physical scars or disabling wounds from his army days, given that his addiction to morphine was a closely guarded family secret—at least until the couple could no longer maintain the facade of health and normalcy. For decades, few casual observers could have spotted that skeleton lurking in John's closet.

However, to the historian, John's collapse in 1896 and the drama that ensued shatters the image of his "successful" return to civilian life after leaving the army. Thus, the Goolricks' case reveals an important, but often overlooked, perspective on the ultimate fates of Civil War veterans and how historians have understood these men's postwar lives. To understand the war's long-term impact on veterans, scholars have often relied on useful dichotomies. Veterans who survived the slaughter and made it home were either traumatized or not traumatized. They were successful later in life despite the war, or they were unsuccessful because of it. They struggled to pull their postwar lives together, or they moved on from the war and became well-adjusted veterans, proud of their military service and physical sacrifices. John existed somewhere in between these neat categories. Morphine addiction left him unable to fully leave the Civil War in the past, even if he wanted to, but the family's discretion also meant that most of John's peers did not identify him as a broken-down old soldier stuck in the past. Most Civil War veterans were in-between men, like John.

The Goolricks' tragedy also illuminates how opiate addiction, like other war-related disabilities, crossed class lines but hurt the poor more than the wealthy. Rich and poor veterans both suffered from addiction's physical and social agonies, yet the Goolricks could afford to pay for John's long-term convalescence at his brother's farmhouse. They kept all knowledge of John's addiction in the family for as long as possible, even marking letters "strictly private," to avoid any harsh judgments of their communities.[97] After a few weeks, they began making quiet inquiries to doctors, asking about the possibility of commitment. But the Goolricks feared that "if sent to Williamsburg," the location of Virginia's Eastern Lunatic Asylum, "from here (a small town) such would be commented upon and asked about."[98] Instead, they opted to keep John discreetly locked up at his brother's home. The addictions of wealthy veterans often went unnoticed until a crisis point, like John and Frances's near-divorce in 1896.

Sometimes the crisis came only after death. Albert Ferry, a former Confederate captain on the staff of P. G. T. Beauregard, also became addicted to morphine after falling ill during the war. Ferry was a Creole princeling born into a wealthy family of Louisiana sugar planters, far above the upper-middle-class social station of the Virginia Goolricks. Still, all the money in the South could not save Ferry from an overdose death. Despite his standing at the pinnacle of Southern society, in 1883 Ferry died unglamorously from a morphine overdose in a room at the Germania Boarding House in Houston, alone and far from his sugar kingdom. No one seems to have known about his "habit of taking morphine" until it was discovered by a coroner's inquest.[99] Certainly, addiction was often hard on wealthy men like Goolrick and Ferry, but poverty meant that addiction meted out unique forms of humiliation. The wealthy could afford to purchase opiates with discretion and keep their addictions private, but poorer men had to humble themselves before friends and neighbors to get opiates.

Addiction often left poor veterans at the mercy of their neighbors, straining relationships with their communities. Impoverished, addicted men often had to beg for charity or prostrate themselves to obtain public welfare, a fraught proposition considering the stigma of addiction. Alpheus M. Chappell, the former Confederate captain shot through the knee while leading his men across the killing fields at Pickett's Charge and who subsequently became addicted to morphine, lived in poverty after the war.[100] Decades after Gettysburg, his debilitating wound left him in chronic pain and unable to work. Chappell, a modestly wealthy man before the Civil War, had become desperately poor. His station was so badly reduced that he could not even afford to buy morphine, a basic need for the addicted veteran, as necessary as food, water, and shelter. That is why Chappell told a would-be benefactor in a May 1886 letter, "I can't stop" taking morphine, but "can't get it often except people give it to me." He hoped the recipient of the letter, former Confederate general William R. Terry, could help him obtain a pension from the commonwealth of Virginia. Disclosing his condition was surely a humiliating experience for Chappell.[101]

Some addicted veterans were even forced to seek public welfare, straining the goodwill and resources of their local communities. Union veteran Joseph D. Depoy was a carpenter in Delaware County, Indiana, before the war, worth a mere $135 in 1860 in personal property and real estate. Thirty-six years old with a wife and five hungry children to feed, Depoy lived on the edge of poverty, an accident or injury away from ruin. Older than most early-war volunteers, perhaps money was a motivating factor for Depoy when he enlisted as a private in the 12th Indiana Infantry for a one-year enlistment term in May 1861. At some point, Depoy must have been severely injured, perhaps in the army or after the war, but the details are unclear. In any case, he became addicted to laudanum. By the 1880s, the out-of-work carpenter could no longer support himself or his family. He was unable to afford $1.50 to buy shoes for his daughter, let alone pay for the seventeen ounces of laudanum he needed per month, which cost twelve and a half cents an ounce.[102]

With nowhere else to turn, Depoy fell back on county poor relief. From at least September 1878 through November 1886, Delaware County officials paid Depoy's wife five dollars a month to "board" him. They also paid a local merchant, Joseph LeFavour, as well as the firm Lockhart & Stright, who supplied the Depoy children's shoes and Joseph's morphine. The Delaware County Board of Commissioners, who administered the county's poor relief, showed a remarkable amount of goodwill toward the addicted veteran and his family. But charity came with strings attached. Depoy was forced to confess his shameful, intimate secrets, down to the last drop of laudanum, to the county auditor. Every item the family needed—from the three yards of muslin they used to make winter clothes in September 1879 to sixty-six ounces of laudanum Joseph Depoy swallowed to self-medicate between January and May 1881—was scrutinized by the family's social betters. Even when these necessities were approved by the county, the bureaucratic intrusion into their lives must have been humiliating. Moreover, it is hard to imagine that the local merchants would have continued to furnish drugs and supplies to the veteran or tolerate his family without a guarantee of recompense from the county poor relief officials.[103]

Yet all things considered, the Depoys were lucky. Poor, addicted veterans often experienced homelessness, sometimes ending up in almshouses, a fate few Americans would envy. George M. Barber, a veteran of the 3rd New York Infantry, was shot at Dennis Bluffs in May 1864 and "lay in the rain and was wet for four days after before wound was dressed by a surgeon." He also suffered from gonorrhea, typhoid, and pneumonia during the war, conditions that were often treated by opiates. Consequently, by his own admission, Barber was "addicted to the use of opium from 1864 to 1882." After mustering out, he could find no place to lay his head except a poorhouse near Chicago, where he lived in 1869–75 and again in 1890–93 before being hospitalized for locomotor ataxia in 1893.[104] Such a fate must have been humiliating for the veteran, even as it ostensibly validated classist Gilded Age theories that charity only encouraged dependence.

Opium slavery thus compounded the economic inequalities of the Gilded Age and reflected the intense class biases of Victorian society. Addiction made the poor even poorer. Communities also scrutinized the addiction of the poor more closely than they did the wealthy. Since reports of opium slavery surfaced during the antebellum decades, Americans had considered middle-class opium eaters as more worthy of sympathy and medical aid, whereas lower-class users were dismissed as the "wrong" sort of people, unworthy of aid or sympathy and subjected to additional scrutiny beyond that experienced by middle or upper-class people.[105] The cultural milieu of the Gilded Age magnified this long-standing classist perspective on addiction. Addicted veterans received far less public scrutiny if they could keep their conditions secret and continue to approximate bourgeois ideals of behavior and appearance, yet this was possible only when one had money. Thus, the John T. Goolricks of the world could be politely ignored by their communities, their wealth becoming a shield. The Joseph D. Depoys were not so fortunate. Still, the Goolricks' story also reveals a paradox. Bourgeois veterans had further to fall in terms of social and economic standing than did men already living in poverty, so opiate addiction uniquely threatened the social identity of upper- and middle-class veterans. Gilded Age observers often attributed such men's fall from wealth and social prominence to opiate addiction. "A large number of those who have formerly occupied high social positions and enjoyed wealth, but have become reduced in circumstances and position, are taking the drug," according to an explanation given in an 1880 newspaper article.[106]

The notion that the condition involved trickery and deception made it even more difficult for addicted veterans to live up to the bourgeois norms of Victorian society. F. Baldwin Morris, once a surgeon in the 78th Pennsylvania Infantry, took great pains to keep his postwar morphine use secret from his beloved wife. He feared she would reject him if she discovered his "evil habit," which he believed would make him "repulsive to his own flesh and blood." But secrecy meant emotional isolation, such that Morris's attempts to quit the drug were all the more difficult and contributed to his self-loathing. The "torment that was secretly endured by me," Morris later confessed, "is beyond description."[107] According to Edward Mann, a Gilded Age doctor who specialized in treating addiction, most men took great pains to conceal their conditions, fearing that the stigma of addiction would lead to harsh repercussions. "We have treated many cases in eminent men," Mann reported in 1887, who have, "except to a professional eye, nothing betrayed the hidden vice to which they were addicted."[108] Some opium eaters were sniffed out by sharp-eyed physicians. "Unless the habit [sic] have been of long continuance," explained one doctor in 1868, "and the moral sense so seriously enfeebled that all feeling of shame is lost, the patient will often persist in denying the fact, although the indications of it are unmistakable" to the well-trained physician.[109] Like doctors, life insurance companies grappled with the problem of deception. Opium addiction was so unhealthy and stigmatized that early life insurance firms barred their agents from selling policies to addicted men. "The habitual opium-eater, should, as a rule, be rejected," because "opium-eating lessens the expectation of life." Yet the prevailing belief that opium eaters were liars and frauds convinced life insurance companies that they would try to hoodwink the company by hiding their addictions, or claiming they used only "occasional doses of opium," when applying for policies. So as not to be fooled, agents should inquire into the habits of the applicant and closely inspect his "contracted pupils, quick, rapid movements," and "general dullness, lassitude, sleepiness . . . and husky voice."[110] Applications required would-be policyholders to disclose any opiate abuse, and life insurance companies sometimes refused payouts or sued for damages when they suspected a dead policyholder had covered up addiction.[111]

Efforts to conceal addiction often proved successful, however. Not all addicted veterans became emaciated or had injection scars on their arms and legs, and many people were able to keep their opiate use private. As one doctor remarked in 1872, some men's addiction was "so unobtrusive as often to pass unnoticed by the casual observer, the professional eye alone detecting the secret."[112] The strategy of concealing opiate use to avoid detection underscores how much the negative social repercussions of opium slavery were tied not to the act of taking opium but to observers' perceptions of drug users. Moreover, so many individuals successfully concealed addiction that it is difficult to ascertain the scale of opiate addiction in the nineteenth century. Because most opium eaters tried to go unnoticed, they were often reticent to speak openly about addiction in the letters and diaries that historians have traditionally relied on to investigate the Civil War era. Additionally, when addicted veterans successfully avoided public scrutiny, it meant that they did not come into contact with state bureaucratic apparatuses that generated the paperwork that makes up much of the medical-historical record of the era. Many addicted men did come into contact with the state, thus generating historical records—public health reports, commitment records, coroners' inquests—that reveal much about the experience and outcomes of opiate addiction for veterans. But these cases likely represented the tip of the iceberg and were merely a fraction of the total number of addicted Americans in the postbellum decades.

While maintaining a veil of secrecy around one's addiction had pragmatic benefits, it could have profoundly negative repercussions for veterans' interpersonal relationships and standing in their communities. Most nineteenth-century Americans believed that deception, even under the guise of individual privacy, was immoral. The active measures of deception needed to keep addiction secret thus detracted from one's moral standing. "Opium-using is a secret vice," explained the Committee on Intemperance as a Disease, the body convened in 1868 by the Medical Society of the State of Pennsylvania to investigate the alarming increase in opium eating and drunkenness in the Civil War's wake. According to Edward Mann, the widely published Gilded

Age addiction expert, addicted men sought to "defy detection" by attempting to appear normal at a glance. Only when confronted by a knowledgeable physician did most opium eaters "reluctantly acknowledge their hidden vice."[113] With opium slavery increasingly a topic of national conversation, a growing number of Americans came around to the view that opiate-dependent people were inherently deceitful. As one doctor quipped in 1888, "'All men are liars,' said the writer of ancient days, and the revised version of modern times is, 'All men—who take opium—are liars.'"[114]

Observers frequently remarked about an apparent link between theft and opiate addiction, as well, fulfilling the antebellum notion that addicted men were "ready to sell wife and children . . . for the continuance of his wretched and transient delight."[115] One writer noted in 1872 that "it is a well known fact that persons addicted to this habit are as careful in endeavoring to conceal the fact from their friends and the world, as a criminal is desirous of covering up all traces of his rascality."[116] Bourgeois observers believed that addicted men stole because drug use rendered them morally inferior or perhaps revealed an inherent immorality. According to a correspondent of the Massachusetts Board of Health, whose 1872 report concluded that opiate addiction was alarmingly on the rise, "enfeeblement of the mental powers, as well as of the moral sense, follows" opium eating, and "among the more common evidences of moral deterioration, are kleptomania . . . and a marked propensity to untruthfulness."[117] But without question, some men were forced to steal out of necessity, being otherwise unable to maintain their addictions and stave off withdrawal. A thirty-one-year-old veteran from Buffalo, formerly a captain in the 10th New York Infantry, became so enthralled to opium that he ultimately had to steal to pay for the drug. According to the man's doctors, while on "campaign in Virginia" during the Civil War, "he contracted a severe neuralgia for which he was directed to take opium in small quantities. As pain was severe he enlarged the dose until he had a strong taste for it." After leaving the army, the captain returned to Buffalo, where he found work as a clerk, all the while addicted to opium. But his wages were not enough to pay for the "2 to 3 drachms of crude opium a day together with large quantities of liquor & tobacco" he consumed as tolerance mounted. Despite his "good reputation," background as an officer, and "collegiate" education, the captain, who "handl[ed] large sums of money" at work, began "pilfering" from his employer to pay for his opium habit.[118]

The cultural association of addiction with thievery and criminality meant that addicted Civil War veterans often landed in jails, despite the absence of laws against opiate possession or use. Newspapers routinely reported that people accused of crimes like theft had been motivated in part by a need to fund the opium habit or procure drugs.[119] Brutal police and prison wardens had little sympathy, abusing prisoners by forcing them to withdraw cold turkey.

Wirt Morris, formerly a lieutenant in the 14th West Virginia Infantry, spent an awful night in a Boston jail after he was "found in a violent condition in a cheap lodging house" in December 1897. Believing that Morris was suffering from delirium tremens, police locked him in a padded cell, where he "died a violent death." He had only just arrived in Boston a few days before after a stay in a Maine soldiers' home.[120] Another Union veteran, Cyrus Harmon of Akron, Ohio, suffered a similar fate. He "had been a user of morphine ever since the war," becoming addicted to the drug after a physician prescribed it to deaden the pain of a half-healed Civil War gunshot injury. At age seventy, Harmon still carried the bullet in his body and "could not live" without the fifteen dollars of morphine he took each month—not a crime but certainly a "habit" that many of his neighbors looked down on. After being convicted of receiving stolen goods alongside his son in 1901, Harmon was sentenced to a year in an Ohio state penitentiary. The warden promptly forced Harmon into sudden withdrawal, an agonizing and life-threatening process. Yet the warden denied medical assistance, leaving the elderly veteran writhing in agony on the floor of his cell until he fatally seized a few hours later. An autopsy revealed that "the excessive use of morphine had utterly shattered many of his vitals," ostensibly exonerating the warden. But Harmon's old army comrades and many community members were livid. Evidencing the undercurrent of sympathy sometimes extended to opium eaters like Harmon because of their veteran status, local newspapers fired off a volley of articles denouncing the cruelty of the warden and reminding readers of veterans' wartime sacrifices. Harmon had been a member of the local Grand Army of the Republic post, and its membership appointed a committee to visit the governor and protest the veteran's "inhuman" death.[121]

Characterizations of opiate addiction as deceptive and criminal in nature underscore the ways in which opium eating violated bourgeois ideals of good moral character, which demanded honesty and forthrightness about one's actions and identity. According to the nineteenth-century constellation of beliefs that historian Karen Halttunen has called the "cult of sincerity," deception about one's inner character and actions constituted a "social offense that threatened to dissolve the ties of mutual confidence that bind men together."[122] By this rule, hiding injection scars beneath long sleeves, swallowing laudanum only when alone in the shadows, or stealing money to pay for drugs—actions merely intended to protect addicted men from public scrutiny—were thought to be acts of outright deception and hypocrisy. Many observers of the opium habit saw this violation of the cult of sincerity as unavoidable, yet unforgivable. One doctor observed in 1877 how "opiamania and morphiamania sets aside the character of the individual," who "eschew[s] no means, no trick, to deceive the physician, and secure this drug."[123] Such deception profoundly altered doctors' and communities' perception of addicted veterans, taxing relationships to the breaking point.

Compounding the strain of addiction on veterans' marriages, prolonged use often caused impotence, a hidden complication of addiction that men could easily keep secret from the public, if not their wives. Years of morphine use left Royal F. West, a New York veteran, with "no venereal desire or power."[124] Another New Yorker, George M. Barber, suffered the total "loss of sexual appetite," having "no erections for a year or more."[125] Their fates were typical. A physician with extensive clinical experience treating opiate-addicted men claimed in 1881, "The ability to desire or accomplish the sexual act has been completely destroyed in 98 percent of all cases observed by us."[126] Impotence triggered harsh social and emotional consequences. Some impotent men were subjected to the embarrassment of having their genitals scrutinized and sexual performance criticized by doctors.[127] Impotence also undermined addicted veterans' marriages and intimate relationships because the inability to have an erection limited couples' range of sexual expression and fulfillment. Furthermore, because sexual ability was a key criterion for measuring one's manliness, impotent veterans could not live up to idealized expectations of sexual performance. Opiate addiction thus literally and figuratively emasculated veterans. The inability to have sex also meant that addicted men could not father children, a consequence of addiction that was particularly jarring given the racial context of the Gilded Age, in which many observers linked impotence to the supposed decline of the white race in the United States.[128]

Family members were often privy to secret opiate addictions, even when veterans managed to stave off public scrutiny. In the often-cramped quarters of nineteenth-century houses, wives, children, parents, and siblings witnessed addicted veterans swallow opium or inject morphine multiple times daily, sometimes for years on end. This physical and emotional proximity to opiates and opiate addiction left these relatives at heightened risk of becoming addicted themselves, not unlike the spread of a contagious virus within households. A writer in *Century Illustrated Monthly Magazine* observed this phenomenon, describing how a husband's opiate addiction might spread to his wife: "All the husband's ills and annoyances reappear in the wife in an exaggerated form. She is more sleepless than he is; more addicted to blue pills and morphia."[129] Addicted veterans usually stored their drugs within the home, perhaps tucked away in medicine cupboards or dresser drawers. The presence of opiates in the home heightened the potential that veterans' family members might one day begin injecting or swallowing opium too when they inevitably faced pain or sickness.[130]

Diversion might explain how Amanda E. Jones, the wife of Confederate veteran Andrew J. Jones, became addicted to morphine, although this conclusion is only one possible scenario, considering that opiates were largely unregulated. After the war, the Joneses settled on a farm in Halifax County, North Carolina. At some point, the pair became addicted to morphine. On September 21, 1898, after displaying wildly erratic behavior, they were committed to the state lunatic asylum in Raleigh. The couple had threatened suicide and violence against others, including their children. Andrew, who injected some fifteen grains of morphine a day, also bore the deep scars on his skin from hypodermic needle injections, and Amanda had developed a "disposition to wander from home." The asylum doctors attributed these troubling behaviors to "toxic insanity" brought on by the couple's morphine habits.[131]

If opium eating broke apart such families as the Goolricks and the Joneses, it also strained veterans' relations with their social networks and communities. Addiction sometimes forced veterans to ask other people for favors, including Thomas B. Chaplin, a Confederate veteran and formerly wealthy sea island planter of St. Helena, South Carolina. Addicted to opium, with no money to his name and a plantation ruined by the war, Chaplin needed help procuring opium from his druggist, G. W. Aimar of Charleston. Every month or two, Chaplin ordered a few dollars of opium. On February 3, 1877, he begged the druggist to "send the article," two dollars' worth of opium, "as soon as possible on night of this" letter.[132] The time-sensitive nature of the plea illustrates how many poor veterans were unable to afford to keep stockpiles of opium on hand, despite the drug being relatively cheap, and hints at Chaplin's desperation to avoid falling into painful withdrawal by running out of opium. Thankfully for Chaplin, who could not pay even such a small amount of cash up front, Aimar generously extended credit. Perhaps the druggist sensed a long-term customer in the making if Chaplin's financial fortunes ever improved. Addiction could be good for druggists' businesses. But before long, Chaplin proved unable to pay any of his bill. Aimar grew frustrated and began stamping the veteran's letters as "arrant."[133]

Aimar must have threatened to cut Chaplin off, because in the summer of 1877 his orders for opium became more delicate in tone. On June 16, Chaplin wrote to Aimar to "request the favor of a supply of the drug[,] say the same quantity sent me last." Chaplin was careful to phrase his request politely, yet firmly, telling Aimar "if doing so inconveniences you—tell me so in your reply and I will hurry up the money, but please not to disappoint me in the article for you *know* I *must* have it." The veteran added, "I consider my [illegible] actions with you as an old acquaintance and friend to be strictly private and confidential."[134] Such a request was fraught, because if a frustrated Aimar let slip the news that the insolvent Chaplin, formerly a slaveholding planter, was now himself enslaved to opium, the scandal might have ruined what little remained of the veteran's reputation. Aimar eventually supplied the opium to Chaplin, who racked up a hefty twenty-two-dollar debt by August 1878. At that point, Chaplin sensed that he might have pushed Aimar's graces too far, and he apologized for "disappointing" his "friend" by not settling the account promptly. "Please do not be uneasy, I will soon do something" to make payment, Chaplin promised.[135] A few weeks later, he wrote again to thank Aimar for his "kind patience," which was clearly wearing very thin.[136] The emotionally laden letters between the addicted old soldier and the fed-up druggist illustrate the strain that opium eating put on veterans' relationships with their communities. Aimar had the power to destroy Chaplin's standing by exposing him as an opium eater and a deadbeat. At any moment, Aimar could also cut off Chaplin's credit, forcing the veteran into painful, dangerous withdrawal. Chaplin eventually got a job as the local census taker for the 1880 federal census in hopes of paying his balance.[137] It is unclear whether the two men ever fell out hard or if Aimar disclosed Chaplin's secret, but the temptation to reveal the indebted veteran's opium eating must have been powerful.

Opium Slavery and Racial Decline

Besides the personal toll of opiate addiction for many veterans, more broadly considered, the phenomenon also threatened white Americans' place within the tumultuous racial order of Reconstruction and the Gilded Age. A particularly distressing facet of the addiction crisis was that white men comprised a growing number of American opium eaters. And addiction did not stop with the opium eater himself but seemed to run in the family, afflicting veterans' children. In the context of Gilded Age scientific theories about heredity and race science, the familial transmission of opiate addiction was deeply troubling because it threatened to erode the whiteness of the fragile United States during a time of racial upheaval marked by powerful movements for Black equality and heavy immigration from China.

Several influential Gilded Age intellectuals loudly voiced concerns about the cumulative effects of opiate addiction on the future of the white race. George Miller Beard, the medical and racial theorist who coined the Gilded Age disease known as "neurasthenia," argued that white racial superiority had left the bodies of overly "civilized" white Americans, especially white-collar "brain-workers," more susceptible to the ill effects of opium than were Chinese opium users, whom Beard deemed racially inferior. Beard predicted a looming crisis in 1871, warning that white Americans' sensitivity to intoxicating, addictive opiates, the primary drugs used to treat nervousness and neurasthenia, would spark a national racial crisis. Addiction and neurasthenia went hand in hand, and with cases on the rise, Beard feared for the nation's future.[138] His colleague Albert Day agreed, expanding on Beard's theory. Day alleged in 1876 that "we need not look further for the cause which is degenerating the race.... Why all of this neuralgia? Why all the sleeplessness and nervousness which physicians now meet with?" The answer to these questions, Day argued, was "the use of narcotic drugs" like opium. Doctors and patients alike acted as if "the only relief" for nervousness "to be found is in a little more opium; a little more chloral." Other doctors chimed in with purported evidence to support the notion that opiates acted more powerfully on overcivilized white bodies. As a Richmond clinician observed in 1883, "I have noticed that thin, dark-complexioned persons of either Southern or Semitic races usually require more morphia to affect them hypodermically than the fresh, rosy, light-complexioned individuals who are more common among our Anglo-Saxon race."[139] Considering the unique health risks that opium posed to overcivilized white bodies, race scientists warned that the widespread use of opiates would only hasten white racial decline by facilitating addiction. As Day explained, opium slavery was a chief "foe of our race."[140]

With the addiction epidemic spiraling out of control, Beard's and Day's warnings about opium slavery and the decline of white America became alarmingly salient. Opium abuse, long associated with the racial other, now seemed to muddle users' whiteness and even threaten to snuff out the potential of future generations of white Americans, who Beard and Day hoped would continue to dominate American society. Their warnings also reverberated with emerging medical and scientific ideas about the hereditary transmission of disease. Opium eating thus became a form of what Teddy Roosevelt would later describe as "race suicide," a manifestation of overcivilization that might erode white dominance by thinning white Americans' numbers.[141] Familial transmission of nervousness or, alternatively, impotence that prevented white births would bring about this much-feared racial collapse. Doctors widely voiced the belief that addiction left white men impotent and unable to father children or propagate the race. Moreover, doctors warned that even if a white male opium eater could still father children, they would be debilitated in body and mind—infirmities that seemed to cascade down by heredity to one's offspring. Addicted white fathers meant fewer and less capable white children. As one observer noted in 1879, "Should children be born to the opium eater, their vitality is less than ordinary, and should they survive to maturity, they are, as women, barren, and, as men, sterile." Within a generation, the families of white opium eaters faced "complete extinction," as did the race by extension if the addiction epidemic continued to spread unchecked.[142] One physician explained that a "family where for three generations whisky and morphin [sic] were both used, the third generation is almost extinct, without offspring; the one representative has never used either drug, but suffers for the sins of his ancestors."[143] Ultimately, with the revelation that opiate addiction might bring on the demise of the white race, the outcomes of addiction seemed to some observers even more important than the fates of individual veterans and their families. Opium slavery now threatened the future of the American republic.[144] As *Scientific American* warned, such "degeneracy . . . cannot go on indefinitely. . . . The excessively feeble and nervous [white] stocks must perish."[145]

Considering these alarming and widely believed theories about the role of opiate addiction in hastening white racial decline—even if such theories were racist and dubious—it is unsurprising that opium became a target of white supremacist lawmakers. Yet iatrogenic opiate addiction among whites, a far more pressing problem by the numbers, attracted much less scrutiny from opportunistic race-baiting politicians than did opium smoking among Chinese immigrants. Heavily influenced by accounts of antebellum missionaries in China, Americans had long associated this form of consumption with the allegedly inferior Chinese. In the postwar decades, as an unprecedented influx of Chinese men and women migrated to the United States to find work in cities, on railroads, and in goldfields, anti-immigration voices began loudly blaming Chinese for spreading opium abuse, which followed from racist rhetoric first developed in 1850s and 1860s. The operators of Chinatown opium dens allegedly ushered in white customers off the street. After sampling a free puff of opium, white men soon became "opium slaves" for the benefit of Chinese purses, and white women transformed into "white slaves" for sexual pleasure.[146]

These scandalous allegations profoundly shaped public perceptions of the opium "problem" in the Gilded Age. As the *New-York Times* observed, "Statements of the vicious influence of the Chinese . . . have had the effect of revising newspaper discussions of the opium habit."[147] The *Brooklyn Daily Eagle* warned that opiate use among whites was so widespread that New England was "becoming almost Asiatic."[148] *Frank Leslie's* published an opulent full-page woodcut of a Chinese opium den with an ominous warning. Lest the euphoric opium smokers and curling wisps of smoke strike readers as romantic, the paper noted that "a stranger might seriously ask himself whether the mania for the drug be not as strong in this civilized country as in China." Indeed, "while alcoholic intoxication is decreasing throughout the United States, opium drunkenness is increasing" in the Civil War's wake. Legislation banning over-the-counter purchases, mail orders, and unlimited refills were urgently needed to "check the vice."[149] Further still, xenophobes warned that to check the spread of addiction among whites, reverse racial decline, and save the republic, something had to be done about Chinese immigration.

In reality, the "problem" of opium smoking was badly overblown. The number of opium smokers was relatively small. In the 1890s, they comprised no more than about 92,000 users out of a total opiate-addicted population of up to about 313,000. The number of whites who learned to use the drug in Chinese opium dens was infinitesimal compared with the hundreds of thousands of whites who learned to swallow or inject medicinal opiates from their doctors. Rather, the anti-opium smoking hysteria was a truer reflection of Jim Crow racism and xenophobia than the demographics of the addiction crisis. Heated media coverage about opium smoking was often intended as ammunition to justify anti-Chinese immigration measures. This strategy was effective, helping inspire passage of the Chinese Exclusion Act of 1882, which effectively banned an entire race of immigrants for the first time in US history.[150]

The 1870s and 1880s also ushered in a wave of Jim Crow laws and ordinances aimed at restricting opium smoking and interracial gatherings in opium dens. Dozens of measures were passed in states and cities around the country, starting with San Francisco in 1875 and moving eastward. In 1887, the Texas legislature sought to ban opium smoking by defining opium dens as "disorderly houses."[151] By 1915, a year after the passage of the first federal law restricting the flow of medicinal opiates, twenty-seven states and numerous cities had passed anti-opium smoking measures. Enforcement was spotty, however. Intermittent public panics about interracial fraternization between whites and Chinese immigrants in opium dens prompted police raids and mass arrests.[152] When the scare receded, smoking resumed, underscoring the true purpose of anti-opium smoking laws. Considered in the context of Jim Crow efforts to enforce racial segregation between white, Black, and Chinese Americans, Gilded Age measures against opium seem to have been aimed more at preventing interracial gatherings than stamping out opiate use. Texas labeled opium dens "disorderly houses" for this reason: it was not drug use but the mingling of races that these laws were intended to prevent. The same Jim Crow logic undergirded contemporaneous efforts to regulate or ban cocaine. According to white supremacists like Senator Ben Tillman of South Carolina, cocaine fueled the rape and murder of vulnerable white women by black men.[153] During the late nineteenth century, American missionaries, imperialists, and temperance activists also emerged as loud critics of the British-dominated international opium trade, lobbying for such prohibitionist laws as the 1909 Smoking Opium Exclusion Act. Its passage signaled a federal effort to ban opium smoking in the new American empire in the Pacific. The measure fostered the veneer of American moral superiority over the British, who for decades had sanctioned the opium trade and used its profits to underwrite their sprawling empire.[154] Yet the very existence of domestic white American "opium slaves" blurred racial lines and undercut Jim Crow anti-opium posturing. Each time an addicted white Civil War veteran's story appeared in the newspaper, his existence defied, and threatened to upend, the prevailing racial order of the day. Race scientists, doctors, and politicians struggled to reckon with this reality.

Even still, the Civil War veteran opium eater's experience diverged markedly from that of Chinese opium smokers, powerfully illuminating the hypocrisies that underwrote Gilded Age drug policies. Opium smoking among Chinese immigrants was criminalized and used as fodder for xenophobic exclusion campaigns and racial segregation, whereas the public outcry about opium eating among white Americans paled by comparison. Medicinal opiate addiction among whites generated much hand-wringing, as we have seen. But addicted Civil War veterans did not become the target of systematic racial persecution, unlike Chinese immigrant opium smokers who were subjected to harsh punitive measures like mass arrests and immigration bans. Instead, the emerging American carceral state was content to police addicted veterans indirectly, not through laws but with pension programs, soldiers' homes, and mental asylums, each explored in subsequent chapters. Juxtaposing the harsh treatment of Chinese opium smokers against that of white Civil War veteran opium eaters underscores the twisted racial dynamics of the postwar decades, when threats to white dominance, even imagined ones, warranted overwhelming state responses to maintain white supremacy, while actual public health crises garnered relatively little public resources.

Opiate Addiction and the Long Health Crisis of the Civil War

If racist Gilded Age fears about the hereditary transmission of opiate addiction reflected contemporary scientific "truths," modern understandings of opiate addiction dispel these ideas. Addiction was not actually transmissible by heredity, yet the multigenerational impact of addiction on the post–Civil War generation should not be overlooked or dismissed. Even when the children of veterans did not develop opiate addictions themselves, they suffered because of their fathers' conditions. The postwar opiate addiction epidemic really did represent an intergenerational health crisis, even if that crisis manifested in veterans' families differently from how race scientists expected. In fact, opium eating was merely one example of the broad, intergenerational health disaster triggered by the Civil War. Seeking to quantify the health and socioeconomic outcomes of the Civil War for veterans and their families, modern economists compared nearly 40,000 Union army draftees' 1864–65 military medical examinations with the corresponding medical examinations conducted at the behest of Pension Bureau during the Gilded Age.[155] Linking this health data to Gilded Age census records reveals how veterans' sicknesses and injuries negatively affected the health of their children for decades. Researchers identified a correlation between veterans' war-related disabilities and the diminished health and socioeconomic status of their adult children in the nineteenth and early twentieth centuries. In an era in which the US economy was still primarily based on manual labor, war wounds left many men unable to work at full capacity, often permanently reducing their socioeconomic status. Pensions helped, but not enough. Unshakable, grinding poverty left many disabled veterans unable to feed, clothe, and care for their children, who often grew up malnourished and exposed to environmental risks. Consequently, in adulthood, the children of disabled veterans faced an elevated risk of early death.[156]

It stands to reason that the same intergenerational health pattern held true among the families of opiate-addicted Civil War veterans. One New York veteran self-medicated with morphine, opium, and paregoric for chronic diarrhea. In 1880, he was committed to the state asylum at Utica, where physicians remarked that self-medication had left him "incapacitated to care for himself in any way" and a burden to his family. "I think," the doctor added, "all this has been caused by the inordinate use of opiates and stimulants."[157] Coupled with war wounds and sickness, addiction also left John J. Patterson, John Tackett Goolrick, and many other users too disabled to work at full capacity, diminishing their socioeconomic status. In some extreme cases, such as that of Robert B. Warburton, addiction led veterans to abandon their families. Poverty ensued, and the long-term health of veterans' children surely suffered.

While some veterans managed to survive addiction for decades, countless lives were cut short by fatal overdoses, accidental and intentional. Observers struggled to understand opaque overdose deaths, and in hindsight, it is difficult to say with certainty why some individuals died from overdoses. Not all deaths were related to addiction. Millions of Americans used opium, morphine, and laudanum for all sorts of maladies, and sometimes people accidentally took too much. Some addicted men appear to have overdosed after periods of abstinence, and the loss of tolerance provides a plausible explanation for such deaths.[158] Other individuals may have fatally miscalculated a dose of morphine, a potent drug. Such errors, even by long-term experienced users, could easily cause an overdose. In any case, sudden overdose deaths proved jarring for families, friends, and onlookers, contributing to the stigma surrounding opiate use and the tragedy that characterized the addiction epidemic. William Ogle Key, formerly a Confederate quartermaster, died of a morphine overdose a decade after leaving the army. He had traveled to Baltimore on business in November 1874, where his corpse was discovered one morning in a posh hotel room. According to the city's *Press and Messenger*, "he died from taking morphine to excess, whether for the purpose of suicide or from accident, unknown." Either way, Key died alone in a strange bed, thousands of miles away from his grieving family in Mobile, Alabama.[159] Coroners' reports from Gilded Age cities are rife with similar cases of men who fatally overdosed under mysterious circumstances.[160] Some veterans who died from opiate overdoses had been using them since the Civil War for sickness and injuries contracted in the line of duty, whereas other victims were one-time users looking to treat run-of-the mill maladies contracted long after leaving the army. It was often impossible to distinguish between the two. Either way, the opaqueness of unexpected overdose deaths horrified observers, contributing to the stigma surrounding drug use.

Against long odds, many veterans managed to survive with opiate addictions for decades. They quietly endured opium slavery's harsh physical, emotional, and social consequences for years, only to have their addictions revealed when, in old age, they could no longer care for themselves. One Confederate veteran was shot in the head during the Civil War, prescribed morphine for the pain, and became addicted. He apparently worked out an arrangement with a family doctor, who supplied the veteran with regular morphine for decades. More than fifty years after the Civil War—sometime between 1919 and 1923—the veteran showed up at Shreveport, Louisiana's short-lived Progressive Era morphine maintenance clinic, seeking morphine to avoid going into withdrawal.[161] Another old former Confederate, William Blankenbaker, was committed to the Western State Lunatic Asylum in Staunton, Virginia, at age seventy-eight in March 1906, more than forty years after leaving the Confederate army. According to asylum doctors, Blankenbaker suffered from "senile dementia" caused by "old age and opium habit" of "six months or more" in duration. He "uses tobacco & opium to a great extent," the doctors noted, usually "a piece the size of a grain of corn is his dose." Blankenbaker seemed to know where he was but not "when he is." He seemed "quite cheerful and very fond of talking about the War Between the States." Blankenbaker died at the asylum in February 1907.[162] A morphine-addicted Union veteran, Perry Bowser, likewise used the drug for fifty years, the majority of his life. As he recalled, "I first used morphine at the Marine hospital in Vicksburg and coming home in Nov. 1865. It is impossible to do without it and remain sane." In December 1865, Bowser's family doctor "found him suffering from chronic diarrhea accompanied with chills." "He was very weak [and] scarcely able to sit up" and "had been in the habit of checking" the chronic diarrhea "by the use of morphine," to which Bowser was "obliged" to use "constantly . . . until he formed the habit." At the height of his addiction, Bowser took 60 grains of morphine a day, once attesting that he could "not live without its use unless with the most terrible suffering." Yet using morphine often left Bowser in bad straits. Doctors attributed "all of his physical disability," including intermittent insanity, "irregular bowels," and emaciation, to "the excessive use of that drug (opium)." Bowser continued taking morphine until 1915, when he died of "chronic morphinism" and complications from a fractured right hip after an accidental fall at the Marion, Indiana, branch of the National Home for Disabled Volunteer Soldiers.[163]

The cases of elderly opiate users such as Blankenbaker and Bowser offer a glimpse into the surprisingly long-term health consequences of the Civil War for many veterans. Members of the Civil War generation often considered the war to have been the most important formative event in their lives.[164] This also held true for health. Having become addicted to opium and morphine as young men, they grew old with their "habits." To addicted veterans, the urge to swallow an opium pill, gulp down a swig of laudanum, or inject a syringe of morphine was a constant, unwanted reminder of Civil War service. In this sense, addicted veterans had much in common with elderly veteran amputees, whose "empty sleeves" served as individual and community reminders of wartime sacrifices. For many veterans, opium did not release its bondage until death, often decades after the Civil War ended. The epidemic thus calls attention to the very long term health fallout of the Civil War, which lasted well into the twentieth century. Scholarship on the war's health legacy in postwar America has more often focused on the shorter term, like the smallpox outbreaks that swept through communities of refugees and freedpeople, or the cholera and yellow fever epidemics that erupted across the nation in the late 1860s.[165] Yet veterans like Blankenbaker and Bowser serve as reminders that the Civil War's health crisis did not quickly fade within a few years of the guns falling silent.

Elderly veteran opiate users often spent their final years in conflict with Gilded Age bureaucracies, which were staffed by men who objected mightily to drug use. Some addicted veterans ran afoul of the law, winding up confined in almshouses and jails. Other men were deemed insane and sent to mental asylums. Many veterans who managed to avoid these fates attempted, often unsuccessfully, to secure pensions or lodging and medical care at soldiers' homes to support them in old age. The next chapters follow these threads, focusing on the contentious interactions between addicted veterans and the bureaucrats who made their lives intensely difficult. These especially well-documented cases underscore the myriad negative outcomes of opium slavery for veterans and, crucially, reveal how the Gilded Age state sought to police addiction in the era before the criminalization of narcotics.

Chapter 5

Opium Mania

Addiction as Mental Illness

William Blankenbaker drew his last shallow painful breath in a mental asylum, forty-two years after the Civil War. The bitter end came precisely at 2:15 in the morning on February 17, 1907, in Ward 11 of Staunton, Virginia's Western State Hospital. Blankenbaker, unlike some opiate-addicted Civil War veterans, did not die from an overdose in his youth. He had lived on "a little opium; a piece the size of a grain of corn," taken daily for as long as he could remember. Perhaps it began at Chimborazo Hospital, where he was treated for the gruesome leg fracture that led to his medical discharge from the 13th Virginia Cavalry in January 1865. Decades later, the painful wound still gave Blankenbaker such "a great deal of trouble" that "he walks with difficulty on that account." The ailing, silver-haired old soldier survived his addiction for decades. But Blankenbaker's family and physicians believed the morphine had driven him insane, warranting institutionalization in March 1906.

At the Staunton asylum, psychiatrists described Blankenbaker as "depressed," "senile," "filthy in habits," "disposed to wander," and unable to recognize the loved ones who traveled to visit him. According to the asylum doctors, Blankenbaker's insanity stemmed directly from his advanced age and "opium habit." The veteran's opium-wrought delusions, psychiatrists observed, centered on his Civil War experiences. Indeed, he did not "know when he is" but was "very fond of talking about the War Between the States" while limping through the asylum wards. Blankenbaker was, according to the medical logic of the day, a psychiatric casualty of the Civil War by way of opiate addiction.[1]

Opium slavery represented an intersecting physical, social, and cultural crisis for Civil War veterans. Making matters worse, as Blankenbaker's case illustrates, the negative outcomes of addiction did not stop at poor health, ruined manhood, muddled whiteness, or isolation from family and community. Medicine also framed addiction as a kind of insanity. This chapter explores the nineteenth-century notion that opium "slavery" could cause a mental health crisis—how contemporary psychiatrists understood the phenomenon. Psychiatrists believed that many addicted people like Blankenbaker were driven "insane" by opium. In their fits of melancholy and mania, disorderly opium eaters often threatened violence against themselves and others, straining relationships to the brink, leaving their families and communities in search of solutions. Consequently, hundreds of veteran opium eaters, and perhaps more, were institutionalized in American mental asylums during the late nineteenth and early twentieth centuries. These veterans usually arrived at asylums at the behest of families or neighbors who, often after years of caring for their loved ones, ultimately pursued institutionalization to ease the burdens of managing addicted men at home. Psychiatrists treated opium eaters at the asylums because of addiction's classification as a form of insanity, one of the many complex modes of understanding drug dependence in this era. Although families ordinarily initiated the commitment process, the state also had a vested interest in controlling opium eaters' aberrant behavior to uphold public safety and order.

Public mental asylums, important components in states' carceral apparatuses, served this purpose well. Veterans caught up in these facilities suffered tremendously during their ordeals. Held in asylums against their will for years, even decades, addicted veterans endured physical violence, unsanitary and unhealthy living conditions, prolonged separation from loved ones, and forced, uncompensated labor under the guise of medical therapy. The treatment that "inmates" received at these asylums compounded their suffering. In America's Gilded Age asylums, opium "slavery" was transformed into a more literal form of unfreedom, costing veterans not only their bodies, reputations, and self-esteem but their personal liberty as well.

Uncovering the harrowing stories of the opiate-addicted veterans who were confined within the bars and walls of these asylums makes clear the personal costs of addiction for veterans and their families, underscoring themes sketched out in previous chapters. Investigating the fate of institutionalized veterans also reveals new insight into how the Civil War generation thought about mental illness and trauma, as well as the war's role in causing it. Historians recognize that insanity and trauma are not transhistorical entities. Historical context, not just biology, informs how Americans have defined mental illness, what experiences they have found to be traumatic, and how they have responded psychologically, emotionally, and culturally. Nineteenth-century Americans inhabited a different cultural and medical world than ours. Considering the historicity of trauma, it is difficult for modern historians to get inside the heads of the Civil War generation. Thus, contemporary asylum doctors' insights become especially valuable for scholars. Nineteenth-century psychiatrists had their thumbs on the pulse of Civil War–era understandings of mental illness and trauma, and they articulated addicted veterans' stories within this framework.[2]

Considering opiate addiction by its nineteenth-century medical classification, as a variety of insanity, enhances historians' understanding of the Civil War's mental health fallout in postbellum America. When veterans like Blankenbaker were institutionalized, they encountered asylum doctors with unparalleled expertise in insanity. Psychiatrists assessed patients' mental state and crafted a restorative or custodial medical plan, a process that often generated remarkably detailed case histories replete with articulate medical explanations.³ These rare, hard-to-access, and, until recently, largely untapped historical records give unparalleled insight into how contemporary observers understood the Civil War's mental health crisis, especially their conviction that the war drove many survivors insane. As scholars have lately sought to more fully account for the terrible human suffering unleashed by the Civil War, historians have increasingly recognized that mental illness experienced by veterans represented, at least in part, an extension of the war's carnage into the postwar era. Innovative recent studies on veterans' wartime and postwar lives have revealed the widespread prevalence of mental illness. Contemporary observers attributed many, although certainly not all, cases of insanity to physical, psychological, and emotional distress experienced during the war.⁴ Collectively, the recent wave of war trauma studies has significantly enhanced historians' understanding of the suffering engendered by America's bloodiest war. Twenty-first-century historians are much closer to understanding the Civil War's health, social, and cultural consequences than ever.

Yet some historians are reticent to embrace the findings of trauma studies, criticizing this scholarly turn on several grounds. Critics allege that studies of mental illness in the Civil War era employ "retrospective diagnosis," anachronistically projecting present-day diagnoses like post-traumatic stress disorder (PTSD) into the past, when these labels and their undergirding psychological concepts were unfamiliar. This critique implies that modern medical insights should be off-limits to historians seeking to gauge the mental health aftershocks of the Civil War. Other scholars contend that the Civil War generation held premodern views about death and suffering and consequently lacked the cultural sensibilities to articulate or even experience psychological distress in a manner approximating what is today understood as traumatic. According to this line of reasoning, because death was so routine and culturally prominent in the nineteenth century, the Civil War generation would have been immunized from emotional or psychological trauma stemming from the war's maelstrom, even if they did have a label for this kind of mental illness. Thus, the argument that the Civil War directly or indirectly caused trauma-induced mental illness is both anachronistic and lacks sufficient historical evidence.⁵

Such critiques miss the mark when it comes to opiate addiction. Almost all nineteenth-century American medical and lay observers believed that chronic opiate use could, and often did, cause insanity, although not among all users.⁶ Civil War–era psychiatrists repeatedly voiced this conviction in asylum records and medical journals. The voices of asylum doctors—who in their day were the primary government and medical authorities tasked with diagnosing mental illness—have much to offer historians interested in Civil War veterans and mental illness.[7] Asylum admissions logs, case files, annual reports, lunacy inquests, and medical journal articles convey in unparalleled detail psychiatrists' unique eyewitness perspectives on the mental health consequences of the Civil War. These sources frequently described psychological and emotional trauma stemming from wartime military service and health conditions, including, but not limited to, opiate addiction. Thus, reframing opium slavery as a mental health crisis, the way nineteenth-century psychiatrists understood it, not only provides a unique angle from which to witness the effects of addiction on veterans and their families but also yields fresh evidence of the war's often catastrophic effects for many veterans' mental health and well-being.

Opium Mania and Commitment Patterns

American physicians remained puzzled by many of opium's mysteries after the Civil War, as antebellum doctors had been. Widespread addiction among white men had raised vexing questions about the racial future of the nation, and doctors still could not agree on why so many men relapsed after being ostensibly "cured" of their addictions. By the 1870s, many doctors would question the classification of addiction as a form of intemperance, instead theorizing that the locus of addiction was simply diseased brain cells. This theory—called "inebriety" and explored in chapter 8—challenged decades of moral-medical dogma. Yet if much remained unknown and in flux about the nature of opiate addiction against the backdrop of the Civil War era's broader mental health crisis, one characteristic of opium eating remained clear beyond the shadow of any doubt: practically all doctors accepted the notion that abusing opiates could drive a person insane. Some clinicians described this condition as "opium mania," although it went by various labels during the Gilded Age.[8] Other physicians concocted more scientific-sounding names, keeping up with the "scientific medicine" of the day, also partially a product of the Civil War. Antebellum labels like "opium eater" and the "opium habit" remained common but were now joined in the medical lexicon by newly developed diagnoses such as "opiomania," "opiophagism," "opium inebriety," "opium psycho-neurosis," "papaverism," and "morphinism."[9] One popular medical textbook explained in 1899 that "morphine is next to alcohol the poison most frequently regarded as a cause of insanity.... It gives rise to insane habit (morphinomania), loss of moral sense, of truth, honesty, and all altruistic feelings. It gives rise to sensory illusions and hallucinations, which may originate various forms of delusional insanity, resembling those produced by alcohol." Users were thus liable to "mania or active melancholia of a very violent or suicidal type," especially when deprived of their accustomed dose.[10] While such scientific-sounding labels for opiate addiction emerged late in the century, the textbook's matter-of-fact summation of drugs' destabilizing effects on the mind reflected a century of American medical consensus. The Civil War did not fully destabilize the antebellum idea that opium eating caused insanity but provided even more evidence to support the thought.

It followed that opiate addiction often resulted in veterans and other opiate users being institutionalized on the grounds of insanity. Considering how hard it was to get a bed in overcrowded Gilded Age asylums, it stands to reason that only the most severe and unmanageable cases of addiction culminated in institutionalization. Opium and morphine "maniacs" likely represented only a fraction of the broader population of addicted Americans, which means asylum records are not necessarily an accurate gauge of addiction patterns in the nation at large. Yet the records made it clear that these facilities became de facto treatment centers for addiction in the nineteenth century. This phenomenon emerged long before the Civil War, but commitments for opium mania increased sharply as the addiction rate spiked in the war's wake. During the Gilded Age, asylums around the nation were littered with individuals who psychiatrists believed were driven mad by opium and morphine. Opium mania and morphinomania became so widespread that some asylums even adapted their admissions processes and criteria to accommodate the surge. Asylum doctors began screening would-be patients for addiction before agreeing to admission. The premise was that identifying patients' opium and morphine "habits" early on would enable asylum doctors to treat their insanity more effectively. Alternately, it might help weed out the incorrigibly addicted. W. J. Conklin, superintendent of Ohio's newly established Longview Asylum, first became concerned about prescription opiate addiction during the Civil War, when he observed that "a drawback to its [opium's] use is the liability to the formation of the opium-habit."[11] Consequently, he rewrote Longview's admission questionnaires, to be completed before potential patients could be admitted. Were the insane "addicted to the use of opium, tobacco, or spiritous liquors? Are they used moderately or intemperately?"[12]

This screening practice soon spread to other asylums. New York's State Lunatic Asylum at Utica—among the most prominent asylums in the nation because of its famous superintendent, John P. Gray, who in 1881–82 served as a witness in the insanity trial of the presidential assassin Charles Guiteau—also adopted the practice. Gray wanted to ascertain if his new patients were "addicted to the use of liquors, opium or tobacco." In one February 1887 Utica questionnaire, a respondent admitted that the veteran in question "was addicted to the youse [sic] of Opium." The asylum doctors diagnosed the older soldier, a physician himself, with dementia caused by the "constant use of opium." For years he had taken "enormous doses of morphine and cocaine." The spiral of addiction cost the veteran his medical practice, however. Despondent and with "no friends" to help, the man tried to end his suffering by cutting his femoral artery. When the attempt failed, he was committed to Utica. Gray and his fellow doctors described the addicted veteran as "very feeble minded and childish," "indolent," and "very fond of taking Dover's powder." Indeed, "almost daily" he asked "for some drug or other." Doctors eventually took him off the opiates, and in March 1888 he was released.[13] Such pointed queries and detailed responses did not appear in the commitment forms or medical casebooks of antebellum asylums. The sudden appearance of questions about opiate use in asylum paperwork during the Civil War underscores how the addiction epidemic refracted through postwar medicine.

Asylum doctors observed a shocking increase in opiate addiction cases during the immediate aftermath of the Civil War, although not all were linked to the conflict. Thomas Greene, superintendent of Georgia's state asylum at Milledgeville, reported to the state legislature in 1868 that "there is a terrible evil abroad in our land, and prevailing to an extent, that few persons have any conception of: It is the habitual and excessive use of . . . opium or its salts." Greene posited opiate use was a frequent cause of insanity.[14] Physicians from Minnesota to Massachusetts made similar reports in the *American Journal of Insanity*. As the official periodical of the Association of Medical Superintendents of American Institutions for the Insane, the journal served as an essential means of communication between asylum doctors and represented a major forum for American psychiatry.[15] In 1869, Peter Bryce, superintendent of Alabama's Insane Hospital at Tuscaloosa, reported an increase in opium eating in his state. The *Journal of Insanity*'s editor, John P. Gray of New York's Utica asylum, echoed his colleague's alarm, adding that "the habit of opium eating . . . is so much more common in this country than would generally be supposed," spawning ever more psychiatric admissions for opium mania.[16]

Gray believed that the Civil War was behind some, although not all, of the increase in opium mania, and he angrily chastised colleagues who refused to see this connection. In 1867, Gray even called out the esteemed Pennsylvania asylum superintendent Thomas Kirkbride, whose Kirkbride Plan provided the architectural and therapeutic model for most mid-nineteenth-century American asylums. Kirkbride was a towering figure in psychiatry, but Gray believed the Pennsylvanian was not doing enough to combat substance use stemming from the war. "But has not Dr. Kirkbride failed to notice the most important cause of the late increase of drunkenness, at least among men? According to our observation," Gray explained, "this is to be found in the idleness and abandon of camp life, alternating with the exposure and other hardships, to which so large a proportion of our young men were subjected during the late war. Tobacco and opium are also used to a greater extent than formerly, and this fact is probably to be accounted for in the same way."[17] The

Civil War, Gray concluded, had caused an outbreak of opiate addiction and insanity. This unusually frank attack on Kirkbride underscores the urgency of the situation after the war, illustrating how out of hand the epidemic felt to some observers. Elite nineteenth-century American psychiatrists like Gray and Kirkbride were reticent to criticize their colleagues so openly, even in professional journals, which could be reprinted in lay periodicals and used to attack physicians' reputations.[18] That Gray so publicly rebuked Kirkbride illustrates how thoroughly convinced many asylum doctors had become that the war was behind the recent alarming increase in opiate addiction.[19] Gray's fears soon found eager ears, Kirkbride notwithstanding. Beginning in the late 1860s, state medical societies, boards of health, legislatures, newspapers, medical journals, and opium import duties presented compelling evidence that an epidemic of opiate addiction was afoot. Predictably, as more Americans than ever before went mad from opium, asylums saw an influx of commitments for opiate addiction–related insanity.

In antebellum America, a trickle of opium eaters found themselves committed to America's asylums every year. But in the postbellum decades, demand for addiction care increased exponentially, so that a deluge of morphinomaniacs flooded into asylums. Thousands of Americans, veterans and civilians alike, found themselves trapped behind padlocked doors and barred windows for little else than the persistent medical belief that addiction should be treated within asylums. With this postwar influx of opium eaters, new demographic patterns of institutionalization emerged. Most opium eaters treated in antebellum asylums had been white women, with only a handful of addicted men committed to prewar asylum wards. Many women opium eaters continued to face institutionalization after the Civil War. Sarah J. Alexander was committed to the Western Lunatic Asylum in Staunton, Virginia, in October 1869. She had been taking opiates since 1849, when it was originally prescribed for childbirth. She had taken her "usual dose" of an ounce of laudanum "freely ever since (except when deprived by her husband) without the power of self control." "During the war when she could not procure" opium because of Confederate medical supply shortages, she "used tinc. of ginger and such things." Despite, or perhaps because of, her husband's efforts to keep her from using laudanum, Alexander became despondent and suicidal. Frustrated, her husband took her to the asylum, where doctors intervened by tapering down her dose slowly over the course of two years and substituting chloral, quinine, and strychnine for opiates. Alexander vacillated between shame and agony, once telling her doctors that she "felt as if she could break her neck to get opium" and on another day admitting to "disgrace[ing] her husband and family." In agony, she even attempted to escape the asylum, although doctors discovered the plot and had her locked in a room.[20]

Women like Sarah Alexander could be found in asylums well into the twentieth century, but they were no longer a majority among institutionalized drug users. In the later 1860s, male opium eaters flooded into asylums, and by the 1880s, many facilities reached parity between white male and female opiate addiction patients. Rarely were Black Americans committed to asylums that housed white patients, with such notable exceptions as St. Elizabeths in Washington, DC, and Virginia's Eastern Lunatic Asylum.[21] Asylum doctors reported few cases of addiction among Black "inmates," considering the racial disparities of the addiction epidemic and the prevailing racist theories that Black people were immune from addiction for several reasons. At New York's Utica asylum, between the Civil War and 1888, at least seventy-five men and women whom the asylum doctors recorded as suffering from opium and morphine habits were admitted. Forty of these patients were men and thirty-five were women. Of the male patients, at least sixteen were Union veterans, or 40 percent.[22] Between 1868 and 1889, Virginia's Western Lunatic Asylum admitted at least nineteen patients whom doctors reported as having previously abused opiates, including eight women and eleven men. All but three of the men were Civil War veterans.[23]

Identifying Civil War veterans among the broader population of asylum patients is a difficult task for historians, given that most asylums' admissions registers and medical casebooks do not identify patients as veterans. Among other minutiae, nineteenth-century asylum doctors typically recorded their patients' names, sex, age, and classification of insanity, usually in the pre-Freudian categories of mania, melancholia, and dementia, which came in acute or chronic varieties. Although asylum records varied widely in detail, scope, and preservation, admissions logs and patient clinical records often provided additional factors that ostensibly contributed to insanity, including "habits," such as alcohol or opiate use. Sometimes this information was neatly laid out on preprinted forms, and in other facilities doctors kept long, detailed—or, at times, frustratingly short—chronological notes. Yet for all these assorted demographic and medical details, useful as they are to historians, asylum doctors often failed to identify former soldiers as such.[24] Perhaps some practitioners considered this backstory unnecessary because veterans were ubiquitous in postwar asylums, especially in places like Virginia, where about 90 percent of adult white males had fought in the war.[25] Thus William Blankenbaker was not identified as a Confederate veteran in his admission records of the Western State Hospital, despite doctors' clinical casebook notes describing the old soldier's penchant for rambling about his Civil War days. Some asylums, like the New York State Asylum at Utica, inquired in commitment paperwork: "if a man, state if he was in the army, to what regiment he belonged, etc."[26] This request frequently went unanswered, however, because patients were often unable or unwilling to describe their histories to prying doctors. Thus, one patient admitted to the Utica asylum in 1886 was not identified as a Union veteran in his medical chart, even though the man's doctors described his affinity for proudly wearing a Grand Army of the Republic membership badge. Patients' possessions were usually confiscated at admission, but when doctors confiscated this badge, the man protested bitterly. Only when his wife wrote the superintendent to plead her husband's case, however, did the asylum doctors finally relent and return the badge to the proud veteran.[27] In this instance, discerning that the patient was a Union army veteran was straightforward upon reading the casebooks. Yet the piecemeal nature of nineteenth-century asylum records complicates historians' ability to source large samples of institutionalized veterans. In recent years, however, the mass digitization of Civil War military service records has made it more feasible to discern Civil War veterans from nonveteran asylum patients, despite the absence of military service markers in asylum records.

Utilizing the records of nine mental asylums in New York, Virginia, Indiana, North Carolina, South Carolina, Georgia, and Washington, DC, I investigated the cases of sixty-nine Civil War veterans who were committed to these institutions.[28] The subset of asylum cases included twenty-six Union veterans committed to St. Elizabeths Asylum in Washington, DC; five Union veterans committed to the Indiana Hospital for the Insane; three Union veterans committed to New York's Willard Asylum for the Chronic Insane in Ovid; fifteen Union veterans committed to New York's State Lunatic Asylum in Utica; eight Confederate veterans committed to Virginia's Western Lunatic Asylum in Staunton; one Confederate veteran committed to Virginia's Eastern Lunatic Asylum in Williamsburg; ten Confederate veterans committed to the North Carolina Hospital for the Insane in Raleigh, often referred to as the Dorothea Dix Hospital; and one Confederate veteran committed to the South Carolina Lunatic Asylum at Columbia. These asylums offer a broad geographic perspective, encompassing North and South. They also generated some of the most complete, extant Civil War–era asylum records available to historians. In some cases, opiate addiction was the stated reason for veterans' insanity, whereas in others, asylum doctors identified opiate addiction as one of several factors that negatively affected veterans' mental health and precipitated commitment.

The Decision to Institutionalize

Once a Civil War veteran exhibited signs of opium mania, his family faced the terrible choice between institutionalization or home care. Most families preferred the latter option—committing a loved one to an asylum was a measure of last resort, an emotionally and socially taxing ordeal that families usually chose only after exhausting all other options. Countless opiate-addicted veterans thus avoided institutionalization. Some families could not bear the prospect of separation from their addicted fathers, husbands, brothers, and sons. Others felt searing guilt at the thought of subjecting loved ones to the horrific conditions in Gilded Age asylums, which were overcrowded, unhealthy, violent, and often medically ineffective by nineteenth-century standards. Many families also tried to ignore their loved ones' addictions, unable to come to grips with the notion that their cherished son or husband might be an opium maniac.[29] The stigma of the asylum and the unwanted gossip invited by commitment processing also thwarted some families. Most public commitments required a court order and the involvement of local authorities to execute the order. Every step in this process necessitated that families expose their most intimate and shameful secrets to judges, sheriffs, juries, and other community members. Yet the alternative, home care, could also bring about the same result and was often cost prohibitive.

The specifics of the commitment process varied by state, yet the medical, legal, and social processes of institutionalization shared commonalities no matter the jurisdiction.[30] Some well-to-do families pursued private-pay commitments, writing directly to asylum superintendents, often after consulting a local physician. If the institution had open beds, the superintendent might welcome private patients, but public asylums were frequently too crowded to spare a private-pay bed. Most commitments were thus court ordered, taxpayer-funded affairs. Families or community caregivers initiated public commitments by obtaining a physician's assessment of the addicted man. If the case was too severe to manage at home or it was thought that institutionalization might benefit the addicted individual, the doctor would recommend commitment. The family or physician might then send an application for commitment to the asylum, usually in questionnaire form or via letter. Alternately, one could go to a local or county judge for a lunacy inquest. Sometimes juries were assembled to weigh in. Once the court issued a commitment order or a superintendent accepted a private patient's case, the hard work of transporting the patient to the asylum began. Violent, unwilling patients had to be captured or corralled by families or sheriffs before being spirited away to asylums, often hundreds of miles away. This traumatic event might involve fighting, yelling, and tears. It was often a terribly public spectacle. Patient confidentiality was not paramount in the late nineteenth century, and the families of addicted veterans often dreaded the public scrutiny that would occur when neighbors or the local newspaper learned about their plight through the court proceedings or transportation ordeal.

The experience of the Goolricks of Virginia illustrates why families were reluctant to institutionalize their addicted loved ones and reveals the calculus that families worked through when considering doing so. After John Tackett

Goolrick's 1896 separation from Frances Goolrick, his beleaguered wife, the Confederate veteran spent months confined in his brother's farmhouse outside Fredericksburg, Virginia. There, John's family forced him into sudden withdrawal from morphine, a traumatic and dangerous experience for all parties involved. While he withdrew from opiates, John had to be monitored around the clock, at grave risk to his health and great financial and emotional expense to his family. A constant stream of watchmen and nurses was hired to keep John from dying, running away, or sneaking morphine when no one was looking. Such a breach of protocol would force his frustrated caretakers to restart the harrowing withdrawal regimen anew. The family needed to trust the staff to keep a secret and paid well for their tight-lipped vigilance. Moreover, if John failed to improve quickly, his fed-up wife might finally divorce him. Throughout the ordeal, Frances fielded numerous letters from her brother urging an end to the marriage. "I am but sorry and disheartened about Goolrick," although "I am not at all surprised," he wrote. "Were I in your place," he added, "I should sensibly put [John] out of my life as it is now a matter of self-preservation with you and your children."[31]

Meanwhile, John's brother and sister-in-law, William and Nora Goolrick, quickly grew tired of hearing the pitiful man's moans and screams. "He is not like himself," Nora reported to Frances.[32] John "cries a good deal and is very dependent," the antithesis of the manly stoicism and independence to be expected of someone in John's station.[33] "My heart aches to look at him," a horrified Nora added.[34] An asylum offered a tempting but fraught solution. In letters to Frances during March 1896, William and Nora repeatedly voiced their desire to ease the emotional and financial burdens of home care by having John committed to an asylum. But the Goolricks' calculus had to weigh the potential shame of institutionalization against the potential benefits for John's health. A prominent family of socialites and public figures, the Goolricks feared the social repercussions of having John committed in Northern Virginia, not far from where the family lived. The nearest option was Virginia's Eastern Lunatic Asylum in Williamsburg, about a hundred miles southeast of Fredericksburg, but the family's reputation would be ruined if word about John's addiction got out during the commitment process or after he arrived at the asylum. The family had already taken great pains to keep John's condition under wraps, literally marking their correspondence as "strictly private."[35] To further avoid unwanted gossip, William, Nora, and Frances even considered spiriting the ailing veteran off to an out-of-state urban asylum, where he might remain anonymous. As William warned Frances, "I believe it would be best that he should be sent to St. Elizabeths . . . as this would be very little noticed in a city whereas if sent to Williamsburg [Virginia's Eastern Lunatic Asylum] from here (a small town) such would be commented upon and asked about."

If William worried about the Goolrick name, Nora was more concerned about depositing John in an overcrowded, loud, unhealthy, and violent asylum. Such a fate would be a worse "horror" than withdrawal.[36]

Moreover, the numerous physicians consulted by the family gave mixed recommendations about how to help John. According to one doctor, if John were "put in an asylum it would more than likely *produce* insanity," instead of a cure.[37] With few good options, Nora added, "We must continue to pray." The family ultimately elected to keep John locked up in his brother's farmhouse until he either improved or died, whichever came first. With his health rapidly deteriorating, doctors were finally called in to supervise John's withdrawal, adding to the expenses of home care and widening the circle of people with intimate knowledge about the Goolricks' private affairs. "Stimulants and opiates have been withheld and nervines and sedatives substituted," reported one doctor, "but still his [John's] mental aberrations continue and his extreme weakness is out of proportion to the amount of food he consumes." John remained bedridden for months with little prospect of short-term recovery. "From his present appearance," the physician informed Frances, "it will take at least six months for him to be able to do anything."[38] Yet despite the mounting emotional and financial expenses, the Goolricks still felt that home care outweighed institutionalization, which could fatally ruin the family's social clout. Finally, with the spring thaw in April 1896, John began showing signs of improvement. He felt well enough, and brave enough, to muster a letter to Frances, hoping to reassure her with the news that "the doctor says that the treatment here is having a splendid effect on me." John added, "I feel like a different man," summoning as much of his former dignity and manliness as he could now muster.[39]

The Goolricks' tortured calculus was shared by countless other families and communities, although few caregivers could muster the upper-class John Goolrick's considerable financial resources. Eventually, the ability and resolve of families to care for addicted loved ones broke down, and they turned to asylums for relief from the overwhelming emotional, physical, and financial burdens involved in home care. Yet once the decision to institutionalize was reached, it did not necessarily provide speedy relief. The commitment proceedings for Robert B. Andrews aptly illustrate the lengthy, arduous nature of the process, as well as the desperate circumstances that drove families and communities down this path. Formerly a private in the 18th North Carolina Infantry, Andrews was wounded during the Civil War and spent time in a Union prison camp. At some point in the ensuing decades, Andrews developed an opiate addiction, which eventually grew out of hand, driving him mad, according to his neighbors. Andrews neglected his affairs and left his Wake County, North Carolina, farm untended. Sympathetic friends stepped in, attempting to run his farm and care for the "demented" veteran, as they described him. But they soon reached their wit's end. Andrews's behavior was simply too erratic, his demeanor too volatile, to bear. He even threatened to murder his caregivers, who lacked the resources and energy needed to simultaneously keep watch over Andrews, run his farm, and protect themselves from his sporadic threats of violence, all while tending to their own affairs and families.

With all other options exhausted, the neighbors were forced to initiate commitment proceedings against Andrews in January 1888, remarking in their petition to the Superior Court of Wake County that the veteran had become too burdensome and was "entirely incapable of understanding or attending to his business" or "the minor affairs of life." Petitions for commitment required sustained community action to settle and could be time consuming, given the need to convey petitions and court orders to their destinations. Rural court sessions occurred only periodically. Assembling a large jury was also a complicated process, involving negotiating farmers' schedules, travel time, and the weather, among other variables. In January 1888, as per a court order, the Wake County sheriff called a twelve-man jury to conduct a lunacy inquest and establish Andrews's "mental capacity." A month later, on February 14, 1888, Valentine's Day, the jury finally assembled, found Andrews insane, and had him committed at age fifty to the Dorothea Dix Hospital in Raleigh. Yet for reasons not disclosed in the extant court record, the Wake County sheriff did not actually deliver Andrews to the asylum until December 1889—nearly two years after his neighbors petitioned for commitment. Perhaps the asylum had no room for Andrews or the paperwork had been filled out improperly. Andrews's community was thus forced to provide the veteran with food and shelter, clean his body, and occupy his attention in the long interim, all the while enduring the veteran's threats of violence and erratic behavior. Ultimately, commitment did not prove a quick, easy solution for Andrews's neighbors, nor for most people in their situation.[40]

The many deficiencies of home care for addicted veterans' inability to attend to "the minor affairs of life" were not the only reasons why families resorted to initiating commitment proceedings. Compulsive lying and deceitfulness, actions and character traits long associated with opium eating, exacerbated tensions between addicted veterans and their loved ones. Sometimes emotions became so raw that families opted for commitment as recourse and even as punishment. One young veteran from Greene, New York, apparently lied about his age to enlist underage in the First New York Veteran Cavalry in 1863. Fifteen years later and racked with painful neuralgia in his legs, the young man had become addicted to hypodermic morphine, which he regularly injected into the right leg to obtain "freedom from pain and mental quiet." Doctors believed that the veteran's usual dose of morphine, ten grains daily, was so powerful that it transformed a once-studious person into a restless, irritable, hallucinating insomniac. This veteran had once resolved to quit. But knowing the severe withdrawal symptoms would overcome his willpower, the young man locked himself in his parents' house and insisted that they refrain from giving him morphine, no matter how much he begged and pleaded. This ad hoc detox plan might have worked, had the veteran not stashed morphine bottles around the house. In secret, he continued taking morphine to spare himself from the excruciating withdrawal pains. By the time the parents stumbled on their son's hidden morphine reserves, they had reached their wit's end. This level of deception undermined bourgeois codes of morality and thwarted treatment efforts, to say nothing of destroying trust between family members. The man's family simply could not tolerate the situation any longer. Exasperated at their son's deception and unable to cope with his hallucinations and erratic behavior, the family broke down and sent the young veteran to the Utica asylum in October 1878.[41]

Domestic violence was one of the most common triggers for institutionalization. Most opiate-addicted veterans who ended up in asylums exhibited extreme, terrifying, and violent behaviors, making these men particularly difficult to manage at home. Realistically, violent behaviors probably did not stem exclusively from opiate use, and often veterans exhibited comorbidities that affected their mental health. Still, when violence became overwhelming, families and communities had little choice but to seek institutionalization. A morphine-addicted New York veteran was committed to the state asylum at Utica in March 1886, driven "insane from the use of whiskey and morphia" according to a physician's commitment certificate. Doctors believed that drug abuse transformed the veteran, who became not only burdensome to care for at home but also downright "dangerous to himself and family," especially his wife, whom the man "has beaten several times." Seeking protection from domestic violence, his wife involved the local authorities, who acted together to have the veteran committed. In this case, family and local authorities linked his opiate addiction not just with his insanity and inability to care for himself but also to wife beating and the unraveling of domesticity.[42]

Another young New York veteran was "attacked" by mania in June 1867, just a day after his wedding. When it became apparent his condition would not improve, he was committed to New York's Willard Asylum for the Chronic Insane, where he remained until at least 1890. The doctors at Willard attributed the veterans' mania to opiate abuse. He guzzled "spirits and paregoric by the bottle. Morphine. It is possible, opium in other forms," according to his medical record. Opiate abuse, the doctors believed, brought on a slew of deeply troubling symptoms of insanity that must have terrified the man's wife and made it impossible for her to manage her husband at home for long. He was "excitable and violent on some occasions . . . showed a disposition to injure himself . . .

has threatened to shoot imaginary persons who, as he supposes, abuse him." Some of his delusions reflected his time in the army. He even "says this asylum is West Point and that he is commander in chief of the army" and "imagines his head is cut off some nights."[43] Samuel Martin, formerly a musician in the 18th Indiana Infantry, was committed to the Indiana Hospital for the Insane in Indianapolis in 1895. According to asylum doctors, Martin was "distructive, suicidal, homicidal," and "sleepless and violent at times." He had also "attempted to kill his daughter with a hatchet."[44] D. Z. Swisher, a morphine-addicted veteran of the 3rd Battery Virginia Artillery, could no longer be contained by his elderly wife, thus she had him committed to Virginia's Western State Lunatic Asylum on December 21, 1906, decades after he served in the 3rd Battery Virginia Artillery. Despite his advanced age, within the ten days prior to arriving at the asylum, Swisher had "threaten[ed] violence," been "excited, homicidal and suicidal," even "attempt[ing] to castrate himself" by cutting off his left testicle with a pair of scissors then refusing medical care for his injury.[45]

Addiction, Suicide, and Asylums

Opium mania drove some veterans to the point of suicide, prompting their commitment. Considering the powerful stigmas surrounding addiction, men often internalized the notion that slavery to opium degraded their moral character and manhood, leaving them hopeless about the future. Most veterans' attempts to quit the powerful narcotics failed, and relapses left men feeling embarrassed, emasculated, and confused. The dreadful prospect of never emancipating themselves from morphine led some men to consider killing themselves. One veteran explained that "I would give the world to be able to discontinue it [opium]. Many a time I have had a pistol to my mouth to blow my brains out, and I have my forebodings that . . . my career" as an opium eater "will end in suicide."[46] Perhaps his suicidal anxiety was performative. Yet some men certainly felt this impulse in their bones, enough to act on it. Milton M. Wishard, a veteran of the 53rd Indiana Infantry, worked as a hospital steward during the war before becoming the superintendent of the Indiana Soldiers' Home in Indianapolis. On Valentine's Day, 1877, he died by cutting his throat in a water closet at the St. James Hotel in New Orleans. Wishard was despondent because his friends and colleagues had noticed personality changes, which they attributed to his long-term opium addiction. Even Wishard thought he had become "half crazed" from withdrawal attempts and relapses. In his pocket, Wishard left $1,728 for his family and a note explaining his motivations. "Opium is the cause of it all," he wrote. "God only knows how I have fought this terrible habit, but whenever it gets hold of the system it is too late. . . . God pity the opium eater." The shocking opium-fueled suicide was picked up by newspapers all over the country.[47] Such cases appear to have been common, although it is impossible to know how many veteran opium eaters committed suicide.[48]

Yet if some veterans believed that suicide offered a tempting, even rational escape from the bondage of opium slavery, psychiatrists and families disagreed, insisting that suicidal behavior was an irrational manifestation of opium mania. Suicidal veterans and the doctors who tried to prevent them from the act disagreed about its meaning, although all parties agreed that opium played a part. Psychiatrists believed the drug drove veterans mad, making them so dependent and despondent that they could not resist the drug-fueled impulse to harm themselves. Men who wanted to kill themselves because they could not quit taking opium were diagnosed as melancholic, whereas those who attempted suicide during withdrawal were labeled manic. One New York veteran was admitted to the Utica asylum on May 20, 1882, after attempting to kill himself several times. The asylum doctors believed that morphine, originally prescribed by a family doctor, had driven the veteran mad. Psychiatrists described how morphine had left the man "fully consumed with the idea that his life was not worth living" and paranoid that "something was going to happen" to him. The doctors were also shocked to witness the physical effects of long-term morphine use, which had left the man emaciated and constipated. Once, "while in a very despondent state [he] took an ounce of tr. of opium but measures were taken to prevent fatal results." When the laudanum failed to end his life, he "took 25 cts worth of morphia and at another time took 25 cts worth of opium." The asylum doctors sought to treat the suicidal urges and underlying mania by slowly withdrawing the veteran from morphine. Soon, he "gained much in flesh and strength" and became "more cheerful and hopeful," having "realize[d] that he had been not right in his mind." Finally, in September 1887, after five years in the asylum, the veteran was finally discharged as "recovered" and sent back to family in Owego, New York.[49] His remarkable recovery served as convincing proof to the asylum doctors that morphine addiction could drive one mad to the point of having suicidal impulses and that, under the right care, such men might become sane again.

The pattern of suicides that emerged among opiate-addicted Civil War veterans was not unprecedented. Swallowing a fatal dose of opium, morphine, or laudanum had long been a quick, cheap, and relatively painless way for individuals to leave their world and its many hardships behind. Yet intentional overdose deaths appear to have become even more common in the war's wake, when suicide rates among Southern whites skyrocketed as they struggled to come to grips with the collapse of the antebellum racial order, the loss of a generation of military-aged men, and the obliteration of personal wealth through years of war and emancipation.[50] Reeling from the myriad traumas of war, countless Civil War veterans died by intentionally swallowing fatal doses of opium, morphine, and laudanum.

Facing a growing postwar outbreak of opium mania and suicides, the asylum offered a solution. The medical belief that suicides were an expression of insanity made the asylum a natural venue for mitigating the opium mania crisis. When veterans expressed the desire to kill themselves and the willingness to act on it, families often felt they had little recourse but to have their loved ones committed. Practically speaking, families hoped that institutionalization would not only cure veterans' addictions but also prevent them from dying by suicide. It was much more difficult to kill oneself in an asylum, where patients were prohibited from possessing knives, guns, ropes, and poisons. James R. Boyd, a sixty-year-old farmer from Louisa County, Virginia, and a former Confederate artillerist, was committed to Virginia's Western Lunatic Asylum in May 1883 for melancholia. He exhibited bizarre behavior before his commitment, using opium and attempting suicide repeatedly. The doctors attributed Boyd's insanity to heredity and "use of opium," and they dosed him with bromide and chloral hydrate shortly after admission, likely to mitigate opiate withdrawal symptoms. Under close medical supervision, Boyd became "much improved both mentally and physically," and he was released from the asylum in August 1883. But upon returning home, he relapsed into opium addiction and resumed his attempts at suicide, precipitating a second commitment in June 1884. In Boyd's case, his history of opium use coupled with his suicide attempts made him unmanageable at home, resulting in institutionalization.[51]

Many Union and Confederate veterans ultimately came to feel that their lives were unbearable in the Civil War's aftermath. The Civil War frequently set the backdrop for veterans' suicides, having contributed to their distress and resulting desire to die. The hardships and stresses of military medical practice wore down Frank B. Williams, surgeon to the 4th New York Artillery, to a deep depression. As an army surgeon, Williams had, without doubt, performed countless bloody surgeries. He had witnessed far too many men scream and writhe in agony in military hospitals, only to succumb to post-operation infections, despite Williams's best efforts to save their lives. The weight of these experiences apparently became too much for the doctor to manage. So, in October 1865, just a few months after leaving the service, Williams visited a dear friend, Napoleon Dalton, in New York City. Upon entering the parlor of Dalton's home, the surgeon shook his friend's hand and declared that "it was the last time he should thus greet him as he had taken about 50 grains of morphine, which he thought would kill him in a half an hour." Horrified, Dalton rushed Williams to the New-York Hospital, but to no avail. The former Union army surgeon died there of a morphine overdose, at just thirty-eight years old.[52] "Colonel J. G. P.," a Union officer formerly of the 139th Pennsylvania Infantry, suffered a gunshot wound in the right wrist in July 1864. The hand was so badly mangled that it had to be amputated. In the process of the gunshot wound or the surgery, several of the colonel's nerves were severely damaged, leaving him in excruciating pain. No treatment seemed to help, including a follow-up surgery to remove nerves from the stump. The veteran's muscles "incessantly . . . quiver[ed] in a singular manner, night and day, whether asleep or awake," and eventually he went insane. The man's doctors did not attribute his insanity to the wound or the war but rather to postwar business troubles. But the veteran himself located his trouble in the unceasing pain emanating from his wartime injury. Eventually, in 1880, he was committed to an asylum after threatening suicide and violence against his family. The asylum doctors reported that he "groans most of the time. Wants opium to kill himself." In both cases, the Civil War set in motion the series of events that drove Williams and "Colonel J. G. P." to the point of suicide.[53]

Tragically, some addicted veterans apparently committed suicide to avoid commitment to asylums. Potentially spending the rest of one's life in an asylum was a horrible prospect for veterans who did not consider themselves insane, and men sometimes took extreme measures to avoid such a fate. Edward Sylvester Matthews (fig. 5.1), a US Navy surgeon during the Civil War, apparently killed himself to avoid being committed. Matthews had contracted yellow fever and malaria during the war, and after returning home to Providence, Rhode Island, in 1865, he continued suffering from lingering effects of the diseases. He had his wife, Mary, dose him with morphine, and he soon became addicted. Horrified, Mary "read up a book upon the opium habit, [and] commenced to try to cure him myself," she recalled, by substituting chloroform for morphine. But her efforts failed, and in 1881, Mary and her father tried to commit Matthews. Terrified, Matthews refused to cooperate. On the way to the asylum, while being escorted by his father-in-law, the sailor snuck away and swallowed a fatal overdose of morphine on the night of August 15, 1881. A police officer tried to revive him, but it was too late. Matthews died a few hours later.[54]

When addicted veterans like Matthews overdosed to death, the circumstances that led up to their deaths were often murky. Matthews had taken too much morphine—that much was clear to his loved ones and the police. But his intention was opaque. Considering his impending institutionalization, it appears that Matthews died by suicide. But veterans like Matthews who fatally overdosed often died alone. They rarely explained their intentions to friends or left suicide notes, the cases Milton M. Wishard or Frank B. Williams notwithstanding. Intent being elusive, loved ones and coroners struggled to ascertain whether the deceased had intended to die or if they had simply taken too much opium by accident.[55] This inability to cut through the fogginess of overdose deaths compounded the misery of loved ones, many of whom were

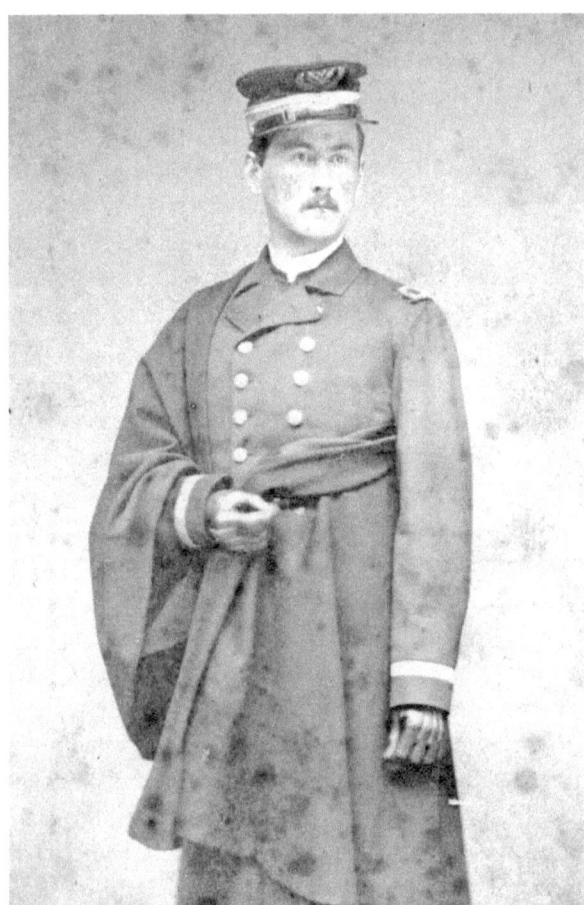

Figure 5.1 Edward Sylvester Matthews's carte de visite, ca. 1864. Matthews died from a morphine overdose while traveling with family to a mental asylum in 1881. Courtesy of Ron Field Collection.

left grieving and without financial support after the husbands, fathers, and sons died.

This was especially true when the dead had been addicted to opiates. Observers struggled to ascertain if the dead had intended to kill themselves or, having developed tolerance to opiates' effects, had accidentally taken too high of a dose. Seeking to explain such deaths, to make the unthinkable act thinkable, families, friends, and newspapers scrutinized veterans' deaths from every possible angle, from the medical history of the deceased to their emotional state, manner of death, and even the moment when the corpse was discovered. Francis C. Clewell—a down-on-his-luck former Confederate captain turned fugitive hiding out from the law after killing a freedman in Mississippi—died of a morphine overdose in St. Louis in April 1867. The coroner ruled the act a suicide. But Clewell's friends and family vehemently contested this verdict, insisting that the veteran, who was addicted to morphine, had overdosed accidentally.

The ensuing debate received national attention, being covered by no fewer than seven newspapers as far afield as Memphis, Atlanta, and Chicago.[56]

Some papers reported Clewell's death as merely the latest example of the rash of suicides among Confederate soldiers and veterans during the 1860s and accepted the conclusions of the St. Louis coroner, as the *Chicago Tribune* reported of Clewell's death: "He had been in the Confederate army; came to St. Louis; loafed round the Southern hotel till he became penniless.... In vain he tried for work, and a settled fit of despondency finally took possession of him, and one day he announced to one of his fellow boarders his wish to die. ... Upon his room-mate coming home that night, he found Clewell stretched on the bed—his eyes rolled far up—his limbs stiffened and cold."[57] Other accounts took issue with the St. Louis coroner's verdict, siding with Clewell's loved ones, who insisted that the fatal overdose was simply an accident. "The suicide was an inference [by the coroner], and nothing in the way of proof was adduced, save that the young gentleman at one time remarked to a companion that he was disheartened and tired of life, and was tempted to put an end to it," according to an editorialist writing in the *St. Louis Daily Dispatch*. The paper even expressed sympathy for Clewell, who "died like a brave fellow, whatever troubles of mind he may have been harassed with."[58] A friend from the St. Louis boardinghouse where Clewell had been staying also contested the coroner's ruling, insisting in a letter to Clewell's mother that her son had been ill and, in a feverish delirium, accidentally swallowed too much morphine to quell his chills.[59] Clewell's untimely death by morphine illustrates how the Civil War left many veterans in desperate emotional and mental straits, sometimes culminating in suicide. The frenzied public debate over Clewell's death—Was it suicide or accidental overdose?—illustrates the difficulties that observers faced when trying to ascertain the meaning behind veterans' overdose deaths. The dueling accounts of Clewell's suicide also indicate that observers sometimes felt great sympathy for the victims of overdoses, despite little charity being extended to opium eaters in life.

Experiencing the Asylum

Despite the perceived necessity of institutionalizing unmanageable veterans, the physical and emotional distance resulting from commitment proved traumatic for many families. Most families lived far from asylums, so visits had to be few and far between. Distance sometimes proved unbearable. Shortly after arriving at the Utica asylum in 1874, an addicted thirty-three-year-old Union veteran found himself missing his wife. "I have now been here 24 hours. I need not say that it has been a long time for me and I don't doubt also for you," he wrote in a love letter that was ultimately intercepted by asylum workers. Even this short separation proved emotionally taxing.[60] The sadness of separation often cut both ways. Another New York veteran, a devoted forty-eight-year-old father and husband, was committed by his wife and brother to the Utica asylum on November 13, 1877. A decade before, "opium was prescribed by a physician for a severe diarrhea which he had at that time," the asylum doctors noted. Like many former soldiers, "after the diarrhea was controlled, he continued taking opium, gradually increasing the amount until he was taking one drachm of morphine a week." Such a dangerously high dose, coupled with on-again off-again attempts to quit the morphine, left the man with a bad case of melancholia—so bad, in fact, that his family believed the asylum was his best bet at recovery, despite the family separation that institutionalization would entail. Yet after navigating the complex and lengthy commitment process, they immediately regretted their decision. The veteran's children and wife missed him so dearly that they begged the asylum superintendent for his release, despite the long-standing history of depression and addiction. A heartfelt letter addressed to the asylum superintendent by the man's brother also pleaded for the veteran's release "on account of his wife and family [for] had I have known the great sorrow it was to bring to his family I would never have placed him there." Indeed, "his wife will certainly die if he is not brought home . . . believe me we are in great earnest about this." The letter must have tugged at the heartstrings of the ordinarily stern superintendent, who recognized the severe emotional and financial burdens endured by the families of committed veterans. On December 1, 1877, just two weeks after arriving at Utica, the superintendent released the veteran, despite his addiction being "unimproved."[61] While this soldier managed to leave the asylum quickly, most men were not so lucky.

Addicted veterans often spent years and even decades in asylums. Once they set foot on asylum grounds, many addicted veterans never left. Robert B. Andrews, the fifty-year-old North Carolina veteran whose neighbors had attempted to care for him, entered Raleigh's Dorothea Dix Hospital late in 1889. Institutionalization spelled the end of his personal freedom, for Andrews would never leave the institution. He died there in 1919, having lived thirty years in the asylum, nearly half his life.[62] Charles Y. Sturgeon, a veteran of the 140th Illinois Infantry, was admitted in May 1895 to St. Elizabeths in Washington, DC, for "acute mania," which the doctors chalked up to "morphinism." Doctors held him there for nearly seventeen years until he died on February 14, 1912.[63] The New York veteran whose paregoric use ostensibly left him delusional and admitted to the Willard Asylum not long after his wedding spent at least twenty-three years in the asylum beginning in 1867.[64]

Such lengthy stays were typical not only for addicted Civil War veterans but increasingly also for most patients. Changing conditions within American asylums resulted in an increased number of long-term commitments during the

Gilded Age, as asylums transformed from curative institutions into custodial facilities. During the antebellum years, most American asylum doctors held a positive outlook on their patients' prospects, and psychiatrists believed they could be restored to sanity under the proper circumstances. After the Civil War, the outlook for insanity became increasingly gloomy. Rather than attempting to cure and release patients, pessimistic asylum doctors believed that most individuals were incurable. Some states, such as New York, created long-term asylums for the "chronic insane," like that at Willard. Psychiatrists witnessed an apparent increase in insanity the last thirty years of the nineteenth century, stemming not only from the Civil War but also from the rise of neurasthenia and nervousness foretold by George Beard. The census of 1880 confirmed what Beard had warned about. Some 91,997 Americans suffered from insanity out of a population of 50 million. The rate of addiction had more than doubled since 1850, when a mere 15,610 out of 21 million Americans were insane in 1850. Admissions to asylums skyrocketed, and the prospects for restorative treatments seemed even more unlikely.[65] By 1900, most asylums transformed into custodial centers, where "inmates" were held for long stretches of time, often for life. Thus, veterans who were committed nearer to the turn of the twentieth century risked longer-term asylum stays than had those who were admitted closer to the Civil War. Additionally, those men who were committed during the 1880s, 1890s, and beyond were often elderly. They tended to exhibit, according to asylum doctors' contemporary reports, signs of senile dementia and other infirmities of old age, diminishing prospects for recovery. Finally, for reasons that asylum doctors found to be murky, some veterans simply never got better. Try as they might to cure morphine mania with sedatives, diet, bucolic settings, work, or confinement, some doctors simply could not assuage the delusions, violent outbursts, and hallucinations so often attendant to opiate addiction or comorbid mental illnesses.

Lengthy confinements in asylums were all too common, but not a given. Some veterans appeared to improve quickly and were discharged after relatively short stints in the institutions. Veterans fortunate enough to be released from asylums quickly were usually those men who did not act violently toward others or themselves. In most cases, patients who were not physically aggressive or suicidal, and who did not evidence other signs of mental illness had good prospects for release. But they had to be cured of the opium habit first. To that end, asylum doctors experimented on their patients throughout the late nineteenth century, seeking to identify the best clinical method for curing opiate addiction.

In many cases, doctors gradually reduced patients' opium or morphine dose over the course of several days or weeks while administering chloral hydrate and sometimes low-dose opiates to mitigate withdrawal symptoms. Once patients recovered their wits enough to convince asylum doctors that they had sworn off the drugs, they were often released to their families' care. However, these men relapsed frequently. Unknown to nineteenth-century medicine, opiates' effects on the brain can cause cravings that can reoccur for years after withdrawal ends. Although they did not understand precisely why cravings occurred, doctors and veterans recognized the psychological toll. Cravings for opium and morphine—which were powerful, even irresistible—often landed supposedly "improved" veterans right back in the asylum from where they came. Michael Hoare, a veteran of the 3rd and 5th Michigan Cavalry, was admitted to St. Elizabeths on April 19, 1895, for "acute melancholia" of six months' duration brought on by "morphinism." He did well in the asylum, and soon doctors felt confident enough about his behavior and prognosis to let him go. Hoare was discharged on February 10, 1896, and his case was marked as "recovered" in the asylum record. But Hoare soon relapsed, and on September 15, 1896, seven months after first leaving the asylum, he was readmitted to St. Elizabeths from a local soldiers' home. The asylum doctors noted that he was, yet again, suffering from "acute melancholia" caused by "morphinism." The cycle repeated once more, and Hoare was discharged on May 22, 1897. His subsequent fate is unknown.[66]

Asylums and the Carceral State

The institutionalization of opiate-addicted veterans and other Americans was a solution that served multiple purposes at several levels of society. Many families, doctors, and even some addicted veterans genuinely believed that asylums could help opium eaters recover. Institutionalization also served the pragmatic financial, emotional, and physical needs of the families and communities who initiated most commitments in the nineteenth century.[67] They sought to "transfer" the "burden of dependence" of caring for severely addicted loved ones to asylums, as one historian explains.[68] In the case of Robert B. Andrews, the North Carolina veteran committed by his neighbors, the weight of caring for the aging, infirm, and demented veteran eventually proved unbearable. The same pattern is evident in the case of John Tackett Goolrick, whose family strongly considered commitment to ease the great financial and emotional expense involved in caring for him.

On the other hand, when institutionalization is considered within the context of the growing nineteenth-century carceral state, the increasingly commonplace commitment of opiate-addicted people in the postwar decades suggests a secondary function for asylums. These facilities formed an integral part of many states' carceral apparatuses in the nineteenth century. Institutionalization allowed the state, by way of courts and asylums, to police ideas and behaviors that were widely seen as morally or culturally deviant without passing laws expressly criminalizing these acts and characteristics.[69] This was particularly true after the Civil War, when opium eating among white men appeared to be a more dangerous social threat than ever, hastening the much-feared decline of the white race. It was not a coincidence that commitments for white male opium eaters skyrocketed against the backdrop of "race suicide," neurasthenia, and Chinese immigration. Locking up addicted veterans and other male opium users within asylum walls helped cover up the growing epidemic and assuage cultural and medical fears stemming from mass addiction. It was this facet of institutionalization that former US surgeon general William A. Hammond was referring to in 1891 when he remarked that "the victim" of alcohol or narcotics "may be subjected to actual imprisonment, either in an inebriate asylum, a hospital, or a jail," despite the absence of criminal laws against drug use or possession outside the context of interracial opium dens.[70]

Consequently, in the aftermath of the Civil War, states began pouring resources into asylums, which were now tasked with policing opiate addiction. Legislatures chartered new kinds of asylums to house opium eaters and people addicted to other substances like alcohol while also passing laws expressly calling for their institutionalization. In March 1865, New York State enacted a law for the institutionalization of "inebriates," namely, heavy users of alcohol or opiates who had become "lost to self-control, unable ... to attend to business, or thereby dangerous to remain at large," to the New York State Inebriate Asylum at Binghamton. Chartered in 1859, it was one of the nation's first medical facilities dedicated to the treatment of addiction.[71] According to the asylum's charter, the institution served dual purposes. It was to provide "medical treatment" to help inebriates recover. Equally important was the task of maintaining social order. The asylum also existed for the "control of the inebriate," whose deviant behaviors violated bourgeois social mores and even threatened public safety.[72] In the Civil War's wake, several states enacted similar measures to use public mental asylums to police opiate addiction, which many Americans believed to be a rapidly proliferating problem that presented a clear public danger. In 1872, the Kentucky legislature passed a bill "to check the practice of opium eating ... which is greatly on the increase." The new law allowed for the involuntary commitment of "any person who, through the excessive use of opium" or other drugs, "has become incompetent to manage himself or his estate."[73]

Virginia followed suit in March 1876, when the legislature passed a bill incorporating an asylum for "the reclamation and care of inebriates and opium eaters." The Pinel Hospital, located in Richmond's western outskirts, was to serve as the state's main facility for treating opium eaters.[74] Former Confederate soldier James Dunlap Moncure served as superintendent until 1884, when he assumed the same post at Virginia's Eastern State Lunatic Asylum, also home to many veterans deemed insane.[75] Once opium eaters became "lost to self-control, and unfit to attend to any business," a local justice of the peace or two relatives or friends could pursue commitment. After a brief investigation involving a physician's testimony, opiate-addicted Virginians could be sent to Pinel, even against their will, until the hospital's doctors deemed it "safe to allow [them] to go at large" or until a year passed, whichever came sooner. After commitment, counties that sent patients were entitled "to take charge of" the committed person's personal property and real estate. The legislature believed these measures would protect Virginia's communities from dangerous, deviant opium eaters, while also freeing up beds in the state's public asylums for forms of insanity thought to be incurable, such as senile dementia. Through Pinel Hospital, the commonwealth and its growing carceral apparatus ultimately found a means of policing opiate addiction, despite the absence of laws criminalizing narcotic possession or use. Such a facility was long overdue, according to Virginia's physicians. The *Virginia Medical Monthly* applauded the creation of Pinel Hospital because "for many years Virginia has felt the need of an establishment wherein the unfortunate victims of alcohol and opium could be reclaimed." Men like John Tackett Goolrick or the opium eaters of the Shenandoah Valley were a plague, draining their families' financial and emotional resources and that of the commonwealth's overtaxed asylums. After receiving treatment at Pinel, opium eaters might even one day "resume their places as useful members of society."[76] As this optimistic language suggests, Pinel Hospital simultaneously illustrated the state's desire to control and reform addicted people, as well as an emerging belief in some corners of society that opium eaters deserved medical assistance. Pinel Hospital remained a small-scale affair until it shuttered in the late 1880s or early 1890s, treating only a few dozen patients at a time.[77] Yet the facility heralded a growing national trend.

New Hampshire, Massachusetts, and Ohio also passed or considered similar measures in the 1880s and 1890s. In 1885, the Massachusetts legislature provided for the commitment of inebriates to the state's mental asylums. But when a flood of drunkards and opium eaters overwhelmed them, the legislature established a separate hospital at Foxborough for inebriates in 1889, followed by the opening of a larger state inebriate asylum at Norfolk in 1914. Both hospitals operated until 1920.[78] The Massachusetts plan soon attracted nationwide attention. Calling for a similar publicly funded inebriate home in 1887, the frustrated superintendent of New Hampshire's public mental asylum remarked that opium and alcohol inebriates were taking up far too many beds in his institution, which detracted from the asylum's ability to admit more severe cases of insanity. Still, he conceded, "it is none the less a fact that these unfortunate persons must at times be detained somewhere," lest the state lose its ability to police dangerous, deviant behaviors. "Unfortunately," the superintendent noted, "the asylum is the only suitable place." He wished New Hampshire would pass legislation along the lines of a Massachusetts law that allowed for the commitment of drunkards to asylums. The only major difference that needed correction in New Hampshire's law was that the Massachusetts statute "does not allow, as it should, mild compulsory labor for this class of persons."[79]

New York did not pass laws expressly for the purpose of institutionalizing opium eaters, but the state's ad hoc mental health practices served that purpose. As New York's public asylum system expanded beginning in the late 1860s from one facility at Utica to a hulking five-institution system by 1870—not including the nation's first inebriate asylum in Binghamton, which began admitting patients in 1864—the state's asylums increasingly ensnared opiate users, many of whom were committed after spending time in local jails. This pattern only fueled the perception that opium eating was linked to criminality. One New York veteran committed to the Utica asylum in 1875 had, according to his jailers, grown irrational and deceptive because of extended opiate use. Working as a clerk, the man had been forging checks and using the money to buy morphine. When he was discovered, the man was arrested, and he spent time in jail before being transferred to the asylum.[80] Some observers lauded asylums as the only effective check on the alarming spread of opiate addiction in the postwar decades. As a doctor explained in 1881, "The victims of opium eating, though in the same category as the dipsomaniac, can be more easily committed to an asylum, because there is no other legal method of restraint, the opium habit not having yet been made a crime."[81] Although opiates, and opiate addiction by extension, were not formally criminalized until the Progressive Era, the targeting of opium eaters by state criminal and asylum apparatuses suggests that addiction fell far outside behavioral norms and had to be policed by the state so as to safeguard public safety, according to some Americans. Asylums thus served the needs of the state alongside those of addicted veterans' families.

Regardless of the motive behind commitment, addicted veterans suffered a profound loss of personal liberty in asylums, and they were often exposed to dangerous, violent, and unhealthy living conditions in the overcrowded facilities. During the late nineteenth century, American asylums effectively transformed into custodial institutions. They were no longer tasked primarily with treating mental illness in the expectation of recovery and release, as had been the central mission of antebellum asylums, but were charged with confining the dangerously mad, both for the individual's personal protection and that of communities. American psychiatrists became increasingly pessimistic about the prognosis of the insane as the nineteenth century progressed. This intellectual evolution in turn animated the evolving medical and social functions of asylums, negatively affecting opiate-addicted Civil War veterans' experiences within asylums.[82]

As the purpose of asylums evolved in the Gilded Age, living conditions and standards of medical care within the institutions deteriorated. Custodial care meant that the number of insane patients confined within public asylums grew precipitously across the country, far outpacing the number of beds available in mental institutions. Thomas Kirkbride, in his influential mid-nineteenth-century plan for asylums, put the ideal number of patients in state mental institutions at 250. In most asylums, this target was quickly surpassed; in 1850, the average American asylum held 333 patients. Although crowded asylums were not ideal, in the decade before the Civil War, asylum populations were relatively stable. In 1860, the average patient population stood at 369, a marginal increase spread over the span of a decade. But by 1870, after the Civil War had helped trigger a crisis of insanity that translated to increased demand for psychiatric care, the average patient population of American mental asylums grew dramatically to 473 patients, nearly double Kirkbride's ideal.[83] Many asylums experienced even more precipitous growth as admissions surged during and immediately after the war. St. Elizabeths asylum in Washington, DC, founded in 1855, admitted 95 patients in 1860 and had a total patient population of 262. The asylum, sometimes referred to as the Government Hospital for the Insane, was the federal government's repository for insane soldiers and veterans. After four long years of alternating war excitement and heartbreak, institutionalizations in the nation's capital skyrocketed. In 1865 alone, St. Elizabeths admitted 512 patients. By 1875, the total patient population had surged to 912. Simultaneously, the institution's "cure" rate plummeted, signaling a shift to custodial care. In 1860, St. Elizabeths' doctors had discharged 48 out of 262 individuals as "recovered." In 1875 the number of "recovered" patients discharged stood at 78 out of a population of 912. In other words, the cure rate at St. Elizabeths declined from 18.3 percent before the Civil War to a mere 8.6 percent a decade after the war's end.[84]

Demand for asylum beds was even higher in some parts of the war-torn South, despite the general lack of funds to support expanding their capacity. Demand for mental health care in Georgia became so overwhelming that, in 1869, the state asylum in Milledgeville totally halted admissions, being "crowded to its utmost capacity." Even still, the superintendent reported, Georgians kept appearing at the facility with loved ones in tow, stating "that they had no means whatsoever of taking them back, and could not possibly do so, or [that] the patient was a very violent[,] dangerous [one] who if returned must necessarily be confined, perhaps ironed, in the county jail greatly to the affliction of their friends and injury to the patient." "Additional means of accommodation must be established," the superintendent told the governor with a sense of urgency.[85] In 1869 and 1870, doctors at Staunton, Virginia's Western Lunatic Asylum admitted merely a quarter of applications, rejecting 149 requests for admission while approving just 59. That year, the superintendent reported that recovery was "favorable" for a mere 13 patients under his care, while "doubtful" or "decidedly unfavorable" for

322 patients.[86] Meanwhile, despite skyrocketing patient populations, shrinking state budgets meant that fewer funds were available to support asylums. Most institutions lacked the money to expand or keep pace with the influx of admissions, so spending on traditional medical therapies for insanity—such as good housing and food, bucolic landscaping, and entertainment to occupy and recover the mind—began to fall by the wayside as the number of admissions increased and discharges decreased.[87] Postwar asylums thus faced severe overcrowding, underfunding, and sharply diminished therapeutic success.

Terrible living conditions resulted from these problems. Overcrowding made for loud, smelly, sickly, and violent living quarters. The cloying odor of feces emanated from patients' quarters, where they often slept multiple bodies to a room. Some individuals could not bathe or use sanitary facilities, so bunkmates were exposed to filth, stink, and contagious diseases. The shrieks of people confined in painful "Utica cribs," a controversial boxlike restraint designed to make patients compliant by preventing them from sitting up, threatened to wake one up at all hours of the night. The smells, sights, and sounds of the asylum surely worsened veterans' emotional and mental state. The conditions were so bad at John P. Gray's Utica asylum that the legislature of New York launched an investigation that lasted from 1879 to 1882. Patients, staff, and doctors sat for interviews, providing a shocking account of the dangerous, unsanitary living situations at Utica, as well as the daily, sustained use of violence by asylum staff to control patients.[88]

Violence plagued asylums, in part because underfunding translated to understaffing. Patients usually interacted only with each other or attendants on a day-to-day basis. Psychiatrists, who commanded much higher salaries, were few and far between. Patients often suffered extreme violence at the hands of attendants, who meted out beatings for even minor disciplinary infractions. The threat of violence came from other patients as well. In most facilities, patients were supposed to be separated by perceived degrees of mental illness, but in practice, opiate-addicted patients were forced to mingle with violent and delusional patients.[89] At New York's Willard Asylum for the Chronic Insane, one aggressive patient grabbed a hapless resident and forcefully pulled the man's leg perpendicular to his body, extending the limb to such an extreme angle that it literally split open, requiring stitches to repair the "badly torn" flesh. The next year, in April 1877, an "inoffensive" patient "happened to pass by" and accidentally touch a violent patient, who lunged and pinned the passerby to the floor with a chokehold that nearly killed him and left severe bruises on the face and neck. There were no attendants nearby to prevent the attack, which ended only after a third patient retrieved a staff member from another building.[90] Omnipresent violence, whether at the hands of attendants or patients, was part of daily life in many asylums.

Therapy for addiction also entailed a kind of violence. To make up for budget shortfalls and as a therapeutic exercise, doctors often forced inmates to work without pay or with subpar wages, meaning that opiate addiction could effectively result in forced labor.[91] One addicted veteran committed to the Willard asylum was forced to work off and on throughout the 1870s and 1880s, without wages and with little hope of ever being released.[92] Mary Walsh was enraged to learn that her veteran husband Redmond—who was institutionalized at St. Elizabeths in Washington, DC, for causes unknown from 1867 until he died in 1908—was being forced to work at his prewar trade, boiler making, without pay in 1873. She wrote to the superintendent demanding the end of Redmond's forced labor. "He is surely entitled to compensation," she argued. If the offense continued, Mary threatened to have her congressman "exert himself" on her behalf.[93]

Critics of asylums were deeply troubled by such stories. One American neurologist lamented in 1880 that "to be pronounced insane by physicians, by a judge, or by a jury, means imprisonment months, years, or for life." For addicted Civil War veterans and other patients, asylums resulted in "the loss of liberty, property, and unhappiness."[94] They had little recourse to extricate themselves from these harrowing conditions, as "inmates" were legally confined in asylums until doctors ordered their release. Escape offered little hope because authorities often captured and returned fugitives to the asylum. Occasional furloughs for patients on the mend offered minimal respite. Conditions at Virginia's Western Lunatic Asylum were so bad that one patient, nearing the end of a monthlong furlough in 1875, apparently killed himself rather than return to the asylum, which had recently taken to confining suicidal patients in "cribs, neatly made of stained pine" and wire.[95] Conditions at St. Elizabeths were also grim enough that some men tried to escape. George W. Long was admitted to St. Elizabeths on August 29, 1891, for "general paralysis" of six months' duration that doctors attributed to "morphia and alcohol." Long could not bear life in the asylum, so he somehow managed to escape on March 30, 1892. Tragically, he did not find peace outside the asylum either, dying in a New York City hospital nine days later.[96]

Asylums represented a powerful mechanism for policing addiction in the Gilded Age carceral state, long before addiction was formally criminalized in the Progressive Era. Yet the growth of the welfare state in the post–Civil War decades also provided authorities with new avenues to police addiction among veterans. Historians recognize federal and state pensions for Civil War veterans, along with veterans' homes, as important expressions of state development in the Gilded Age. Yet the Americans who ran these programs, from the lowly Pension Bureau special investigators who hunted for fraud to presidents like Grover Cleveland who dictated national policy, stamped their personal judgments on each and every pension claim or admission application they processed. Military entitlement programs thus buttressed state efforts to check the growth of opium eating. Chapter 6 analyzes the protracted battles between veterans and the government over entitlements. Government officials and veterans differed sharply on whether drug users deserved pensions and access to soldiers' homes, leading to harsh consequences for addicted men, despite their fierce self-advocacy.

Chapter 6

Vicious Habits

Addiction and Military Entitlements

Civil War veteran Perry Bowser spent much of his adult life trying to claim military entitlements, without much to show for his efforts in the end. In 1864 as he lay injured in a Vicksburg military hospital, Union surgeons gave the young soldier morphine, which he continued to take to stave off debilitating chronic diarrhea after the war. Returning home to Indiana, Bowser became addicted, and he ended up living the rest of his life dependent on the drug. During five long decades of addiction, Bowser's largely unsuccessful attempts to claim entitlements for his Civil War military service caused nearly as much heartache as the morphine itself. First, when doctors discovered Bowser's "vicious habit" of morphine abuse, Pension Bureau agents declared that the disabled old soldier was unworthy of a livable pension. Stubborn and undeterred, Bowser tried again and again to obtain a decent pension. In fact, he plied the Pension Bureau with so many appeals for pension increases over a forty-year period that his astonishingly thick pension file spans nearly 350 pages.

Little came of these attempts, to Bowser's dismay. He grew despondent, even attempting suicide three times. Eventually, Bowser's wife got a divorce and headed for California, leaving him penniless, unable to work, and too poor to afford his daily morphine, much less food or rent. As a last resort, unhoused, impoverished, and addicted, Bowser turned to the National Home for Disabled Volunteer Soldiers (NHDVS), hoping to find a hot meal and a warm bed. But, like the Pension Bureau, soldiers' homes had little to offer men derided as "opium slaves." Each time Bowser managed to gain admission into one of the NHDVS branches, even when he "came . . . to try and break off the morphine habit," he was promptly shown the door. Finally, Bowser found a soldiers' home official with a sympathetic ear and, in 1905, moved into the Marion, Indiana, branch of the NHDVS for good, although even there, he was treated poorly by staff because of his addiction. Bowser ultimately died from "chronic morphism" at the Marion home in 1915, having battled for decades to claim the entitlements he felt the government owed for his military service.[1]

Opium slavery dominated many facets of life for Bowser and other veterans, chipping away at health, manhood, character, and whiteness and landing many users in asylums and morgues. Yet even there, opium slavery's terrible toll did not end. Fraught interactions between veterans, their loved ones, and military entitlement programs amplified the suffering of addiction. Opiate addiction sharply curtailed veterans' access to military entitlements, even when they could directly trace their addictions to military service, like Bowser. This consequence of addiction stemmed from the negative implications of opium slavery for one's character and manhood. Convinced that addiction was an immoral, emasculating vice, gatekeepers of federal and state military entitlement programs routinely prevented these veterans from claiming pensions or obtaining room, board, and medical care at soldiers' homes, the most significant entitlement programs of the nineteenth century. This gatekeeping even extended to veterans' widows and dependents. Fissures in this stonewalling eventually formed in the 1890s, as veterans, their widows, and sympathetic medical practitioners increasingly objected to exclusion from entitlements. Even before that, a few users managed to slip through the cracks of the Pension Bureau and secure payouts. Activists finally made real headway at the NHDVS and some soldiers' homes in Northern states during the 1890s. But for the vast majority of addicted veterans like Bowser, this sympathy was too little, too late.

Investigating conflicts between opiate-addicted Civil War veterans and military entitlement programs illuminates how the state sought to police drug addiction in the nineteenth century. Since the first wave of "drug history" studies appeared in the 1970s, scholars have fruitfully investigated the often-hostile interactions between state police apparatus and drug users. This scholarly project has aimed to uncover the historical roots of America's twentieth-century War on Drugs. Its hallmark criminalization first emerged on a national scale through the Harrison Narcotics Tax Act of 1914, but several studies have located the origins of state policing in the Gilded Age.[2] Incorporating Civil War entitlements into this story helps scholars better explain the origins of policing.

Civil War military entitlements helped spawn the heavy-handed policing of drugs. Addicted Civil War veterans felt the state's police power through pensions and soldiers' homes, although drug historians have largely overlooked these institutions, which were the largest social welfare programs of the nineteenth century. While these programs served pragmatic purposes—feeding, clothing, and caring for ailing veterans, as well as doling out patronage to loyal voters—military entitlements also served the interests of the Gilded Age state during a period of rapid state formation and development. Several historians have convincingly argued that pensions and soldiers' homes were used by federal and state officials and bureaucrats to enforce bourgeois notions of morality, domesticity, and manhood.[3] Historians also recognize Gilded Age hospitals and state welfare programs as emergent manifestations of the state's power to enumerate and uphold social and moral regulations perceived to be in the public interest.[4] Thus by curtailing the access of addicted veterans and their families to pensions and soldiers' homes, postwar military entitlements served as an indirect method of policing and punishing drug addiction among a wide swath of the American population, long before laws were enacted that formally criminalized drugs. Framing the history of criminalization in light of the antecedent policing that occurred in Civil War–era military entitlements underscores how the Progressive Era antidrug measures like the Harrison Act drew on decades of precedent.

Pensions

Opiate-addicted Civil War veterans faced sharply restricted access to pensions, the most symbolically, politically, and economically important entitlement programs of the nineteenth century. Although most Union veterans and many former Confederates ended up getting pensions at some point in their postwar lives, such awards were by no means guaranteed just because a man had served in the Civil War and become disabled. Pension applications were judged by subjective criteria as much as formal guidelines. Awards were not contingent solely on the nature of one's disability but also on the value judgments of the bureaucrats and doctors who processed pension claims or the witnesses who were often asked to weigh in. The appearance of good character and manliness mattered. Just because a disabled veteran met the medical criteria for receiving a pension—for example, losing an arm during the Civil War, preventing him from earning income as a farmer later in life—did not automatically mean that he would secure a pension when he applied. The same went for widows' and dependents' pensions, awarded after the death of a veteran to support his family. The US Pension Bureau interrogated Union veterans' lives, searching for evidence of moral or masculine failings when considering pension applications. Less resourced state pension programs for former Confederate soldiers followed similar investigatory practices, although perhaps relying even more on community input about applicants' honor and reputation. Because of the long-standing, and increasingly salient, stigmas surrounding opium slavery, any physical sign or even rumor of opium eating branded applicants as morally unworthy of receiving pensions, and the same rule applied to his dependents for good measure.

Scholars have long recognized that Civil War pension programs considered both medicalized criteria—missing arms, legs, fingers, and toes—and cultural mores to evaluate applicants. As historian Sarah Handley-Cousins observes, the US Pension Bureau used "gendered moral grounds to separate worthy veterans from the unworthy. . . . Men who exhibited bad moral fiber, seemed like whiners, or failed to bear their pain with appropriate stoicism could all be relegated to the ranks of the unworthy."[5] Although a veteran might appear unambiguously disabled in a medical exam and present substantiating evidence that his disability was the result of Civil War service, those factors alone were not what mattered. Veterans also had to manifest a suitable degree of manliness to persuade the agents who read pension applications to issue an award. Pension agents were liable to deny claims from men who seemed unmanly. Indeed, Handley-Cousins explains, "a disability could be entirely erased if it seemed that a veteran failed to meet standards of genteel manhood."[6] Applications from morally "unworthy" veterans were usually denied as well. The Pension Bureau often rejected the applications of Union veterans deemed morally unworthy because of intemperance.[7] Considering the stigma of the "opium habit" and its close links to drunkenness, opiate-addicted veterans unambiguously fell into this category.

Contemporary ideas about charity also informed gatekeepers' decisions about who was worthy of receiving pension awards. The prevailing understanding of charity in the Gilded Age posited that too much financial assistance could backfire by making men overly dependent on the state, thereby undermining manhood, contingent as it was on independence. Gatekeepers feared that doling out too much charity to individual veterans, no matter how pitiable the case, might actually do more harm than good. That belief is why, in the Civil War's wake, when hundreds of thousands of disabled, indigent veterans clambered for aid, bureaucrats became increasingly stingy with financial assistance, dispensing payouts to only the most severely debilitated men. Moderately disabled veterans, as James Marten argues, were expected to rise above their poor health rather than rely on state assistance, even if their ill fortunes were the direct result of military service to the state.[8] Macabre spectacles—for example, the left-handed penmanship contests that former army surgeon and temperance man William Oland Bourne sponsored in 1865–67 for Union veterans missing their right arms—celebrated gritty disabled men who put on a good show for observers. Little did they know that some of those left-handed veterans "could not have endured" their pain without benumbing, intoxicating morphine.[9] Until sweeping pension reforms late in the Gilded Age, only veterans with the most severe disabilities qualified for public pensions or private charity. Humiliated white men "enchained and enslaved" to opium did not fit these stringent criteria. They simply made too many Americans uncomfortable to receive public aid.

The medical classification of opiate addiction in the nineteenth century also contributed to the stonewalling of addicted veterans from pension programs. Most Civil War–era doctors classified opiate addiction alongside drunkenness as a variety of intemperance, with negative implications for moral character and mental health. "Both of these disorders," opium eating and drunkenness, "are rapidly interchangeable," explained the physician T. D. Crothers in 1892.[10] Intemperance entailed dependency; lack of volition, willpower, and self-control; and recklessness, characteristics that signaled lost manhood and immorality.[11]

Because opiate addiction was considered akin to drunkenness, the criticisms leveled at drunks naturally carried over to "opium slaves."

A perfect storm of late nineteenth-century ideas about manhood, morality, charity, and temperance circumscribed opiate-addicted veterans' access to pensions. It follows that out of nearly 150,000 Union veterans listed on the 1883 pension roll, not one was recorded as receiving a pension for opiate addiction.[12] Yet Civil War pension programs expanded and evolved dramatically in the late nineteenth century, opening up cracks that addicted veterans could attempt to exploit. In its first two decades, the program was conceived as a way for the government to compensate veterans with the most severe disabilities for their inability to support themselves owing to severe war wounds. In contrast, during the 1890s, the US Pension Bureau transformed into a proto-welfare system, generously doling out the federal government's largesse to a much wider swath of Union veterans or their widows.[13] This reform opened the floodgates to a deluge of pension applications from infirm Union veterans and financially dependent widows. Pensions essentially transformed into old-age and survivors' benefits, with much less stringent criteria for receiving an award than were earlier payouts intended to compensate veterans for war wounds. Yet despite the broad liberalization and expansion of the US pension program in the 1890s, opiate-addicted veterans continued to face rejection when they applied for pensions.

The 1890 Dependent Pension Act vastly expanded the pool of veterans and their dependents eligible for pensions, ostensibly creating more opportunities for even addicted veterans to obtain pensions. The act stipulated that all honorably discharged Union veterans who had served at least ninety days and were permanently disabled to the point that they were unable to perform manual labor could apply for a pension, even if their disabilities were not the direct results of wounds, injuries, or sickness acquired during their time in the military. Even "mental disability," ever stigmatized in American society, was pensionable. Soon, old age also became a pensionable disability.[14] Thus, after 1890, nearly any man who had worn Union blues during the war could apply for a pension, and although the application review process remained subjective, disabled veterans now stood a much better chance of securing pensions than under earlier iterations of the program.[15] The Grand Army of the Republic (GAR), which had furiously lobbied for the bill, cheered the 1890 pension act as "the most liberal pension measure ever passed by any legislative body in the world." The veterans lobbying group encouraged its members to apply for the hard-won pension benefits.[16] And they did.

The 1890 pension reform unleashed "an avalanche of claims," according to the Pension Bureau's commissioner. From the 104,044 applications filed between July 1, 1889, and June 30, 1890, the number spiked to an unprecedented 363,799

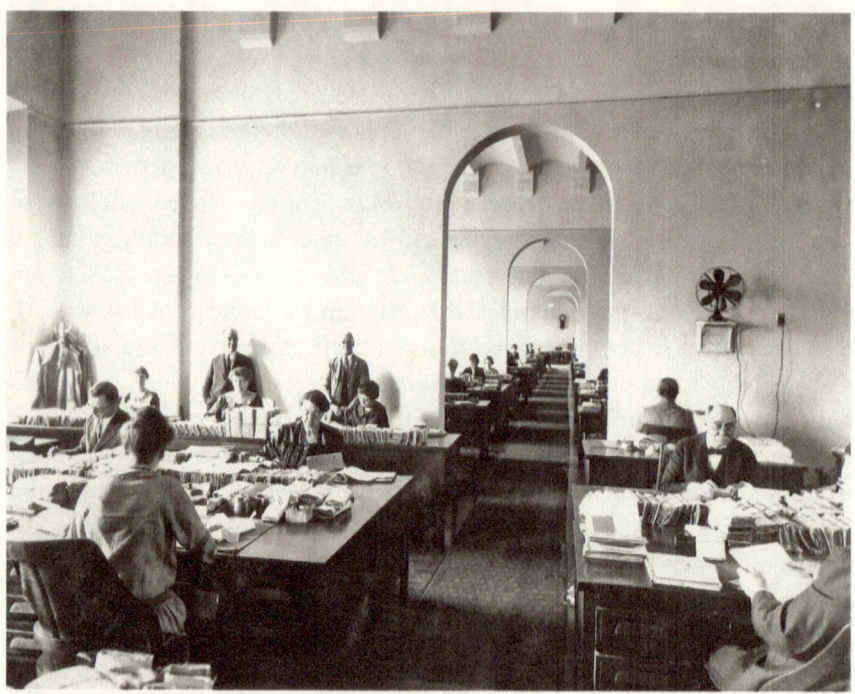

Figure 6.1 Examiners of the pension office preparing claims for action. Undated. Courtesy of National Archives and Records Administration, Washington, DC.

claims in 1890–91, followed by an additional 317,706 applications between 1891 and 1893. Pension agents worked feverishly to keep up, processing fifty claims a day on average (fig. 6.1). Consequently, after the 1890 law's enactment, the pension rate among Union veterans skyrocketed, climbing from just under 40 percent of surviving Union veterans in 1891 to over 90 percent in 1910. By 1893, just two years after the Dependent Pension Act became law, the federal government was spending an astounding 41.5 percent of its annual revenue on pensions for Civil War veterans and their dependents.[17] But by 1894, as the flow of new applications dwindled to a mere 40,148 that year, pension agents, relieved of an extremely high volume of applications, were freed up to spend more time investigating applications. Greater scrutiny and more careful review of individual applications after 1894 increasingly exposed veterans who failed to measure up to the moral requirements of the 1890 law.[18] Among these applicants were veterans with the so-called vicious habit of opiate addiction.

The liberal 1890 pension law singled out for disentitlement any veteran whose disability was "the result of their own vicious habits" or, in other words, habits that the Pension Bureau deemed immoral or unmanly.[19] Simply put, men whose disability could be attributed to "vicious habits" were not to be granted pensions. This restriction was a holdover from previous iterations of the Civil War pension program. Before 1890, surgeons conducting pension examinations had been required to attest that pensioners' disabilities were not the result of vicious habits. However, during the 1870s and early 1880s, the bureau had a flexible understanding of vicious habits, so pension agents largely operated under the notion that they knew them when they saw them. Oftentimes when they encountered questionable cases, examining surgeons and pension agents tended to err on the side of the disabled soldiers. During the toxic political battles of the late 1880s, which pitted pension reform activists like the GAR against antipension politicians like Grover Cleveland, the issue of vicious habits took on new importance. As pensions became ever more politicized, the Pension Bureau developed a renewed interest in exposing veterans who, critics like Cleveland charged, were defrauding the public by illegitimately applying for and drawing pensions. During the late 1880s and 1890s, conservative politicians and media "drew a sharper line between good and bad soldiers" applying for pensions, as Sarah Handley-Cousins observes.[20] Many bureau agents and examining doctors now began ruling against veterans with vicious habits, a trend that continued after the 1890 law came into effect.

These decisions elaborated a more concrete definition of "vicious habits." The phrase was sometimes used in newspapers to describe opium abuse, and perhaps this usage encouraged Pension Bureau officials to firm up their own definition.[21] Within five years of the 1890 Dependent Pension Act, a series of rulings on appealed pension cases defined the excessive use of substances, including opiates, as "vicious habits," along with several other forms of alleged immorality. In an 1894 ruling, the bureau stated that "the use of the word 'vicious' in the act indicated, undoubtedly meant such habits as led to a diseased condition in a claimant where such condition could be avoided by refraining from the habits which led to such condition." "Undoubtedly" meant that vicious habits "are recognized (1) as unnecessary and inadvisable; (2) as harmful to his [the applicant's] physical system." The bureau refused to award pensions to veterans whose "vicious habits" brought on disability, as "Congress never contemplated rewarding or compensating a soldier for physical impairment due to his own indiscretions."[22] In an 1895 ruling clarifying the burden of proof for documenting that disabilities were not the result of vicious habits, a bureau official stated that a veteran with vicious habits was the opposite of "a man of good habits." Veterans with "good habits" were "sober."[23] Men with vicious habits were intemperate. In another case, a bureau official described vicious habits as something that one was "addicted to," implying alcohol and drug abuse.[24] Three years later, the bureau codified its definition of vicious habits in a handbook providing guidance for the processing agents. According to the handbook, veterans with "vicious habits" were the opposite of those men with "good habits and good repute."[25] Considering that opiate addiction had long been referred to as the "opium habit" in many quarters and was widely seen by unsympathetic observers as the product of one's poor choices, immorality, and unmanliness, it naturally fell under the umbrella of vicious habits. Thus, even after the liberalization of US pensions in the 1890s, the vicious habits clause effectively disqualified opiate-addicted veterans from receiving pensions.

To be sure, many opiate-addicted Union veterans applied for pensions under the 1890 law, vicious habits clause notwithstanding. But the bureau tended to reject the applications of Union veterans whose opiate addictions were exposed during the application process. Applying for a pension entailed submitting oneself to a medical exam. Even after securing a pension award, keeping one's pension often entailed being subjected to periodic medical inspections. These examinations were invariably intrusive and, for many men, humiliating. Some veterans were even forced to strip naked and expose their intimate wounds to a board of skeptical doctors. During the poking and prodding that followed, sharp-eyed physicians easily spotted the often-pronounced physical symptoms of opiate addiction: gaunt faces and bodies, constipation, impotence, and abscesses on the skin from hypodermic injections.[26] When confronted by suspicious doctors, addicted veterans sometimes had no choice but to admit that they suffered from the opium habit. Joseph A. Lazelle, a veteran of the 1st Connecticut Volunteer Cavalry, applied for a pension in 1894, claiming that he suffered from piles, rheumatism, and heart disease. But the examining doctor reported to the Pension Bureau that Lazelle "says he has taken 120 grains of opium a day since he was liberated from Andersonville prison in 1865. No evidence of vicious habits[,] except the use of opium[,] and no other disease found." Predictably, this report raised the suspicions of Pension Bureau agents processing Lazelle's application, triggering a follow-up medical investigation. The Bureau medical referee directed the examining doctors to determine: "Has he [Lazelle] the appearance of an habitual user of opium?" Lazelle sensed that he had been unmasked. Realizing that if doctors inquired further into his vicious habit the bureau would deny his pension application, Lazelle refused to submit to another humiliating medical examination. He abandoned his claim, which the bureau formally rejected in 1900 on the grounds of vicious habits.[27]

Like Lazelle, Perry Bowser was unmasked as a morphine user after he applied for a pension increase under the 1890 act. Bowser was previously awarded a pittance of a pension for chronic diarrhea in the early 1870s. At that time, sympathetic doctors had observed traces of opium addiction during a pension medical examination. But they stressed to the bureau that "we did not feel justified in remanding that he be dropped from the rolls" on account of vicious habits because Bowser took opiates to self-medicate for severe diarrhea contracted in the service. In his old age, Bowser found that his paltry eight-dollar-a-month pension was not nearly enough to live on. After the Dependent Pension Act opened an opportunity to apply for a pension increase, Bowser jumped at the chance, like thousands of other Union pensioners. He explained in an affidavit that he suffered from "chronic diarrhea all the time unless I take medicine. Have had attacks every week with eight or ten stools a day." Coupled with piles, nasal catarrh, and a leg injury, Bowser explained that he "cannot do any manual labor at all."

Considering Bowser's prior documented history of addiction, someone at the Pension Bureau grew suspicious. Now that attitudes about opiate addiction had hardened, a sharp-eyed pension agent with a newfound zeal for policing vicious habits flagged Bowser's application for enhanced review. In a note dated March 18, 1891, a Pension Bureau medical referee observed that "it is stated that he [Bowser] has been, if he is not now, a morphia habitué." They directed a team of examining surgeons to follow up, ordering the doctors to "please strip him and subject him to an extra careful examination and describe fully his present physical condition," including the "degree of emaciation," seen as a telltale sign of addiction. The agent also wanted to know if Bowser had syphilis, for which he had apparently been discharged from the army in 1862 before reenlisting in 1863. Finally, examiners were to try to determine the extent to which morphine addiction had caused or worsened Bowser's disability. The doctors found no evidence of syphilis, but they did conclusively determine that Bowser's "nervous system is impaired by morphia." When they confronted him, Bowser claimed that "he acquired [the] habit of taking morphia by using it for chronic diarrhea, but was in [an] insane hospital in 1889, when [the] habit was cured." After processing the medical examination report, the Pension Bureau swiftly rejected Bowser's application.

Over the next several years, a desperate Bowser wrote the Pension Bureau again and again, claiming he had abandoned the morphine habit, although, in hindsight, a preponderance of evidence in his pension file and NHDVS case records suggests otherwise. Because Bowser had been outed as a "morphia habitué," he switched strategies. He no longer intended his queries to the bureau to disguise his addiction but to evoke sympathy and convince pension agents that he had managed to rid himself of the habit, at great personal cost. In an 1896 letter, Bowser explained to a bureau agent that, having been struck down by chronic diarrhea in the winter of 1864–65, he

> was carried home by comrades, being unable to walk, on account of chronic diarrhea, which has clung to me since, unless I use morphine. Contracted the habit on the boat and cannot live without its use unless with the most terrible suffering, both from asthmatic and bronchial trouble, and a recurrence of the diarrhea. I never put in for pension for

lung trouble or malaria, and am now a wreck from service in the army. I tried a cure of my own, and also the Gold Cure for opium habit and have renounced its use some three times but had to resort again to use. It takes me half my pension alone to supply me with morphine.[28]

Yet Bowser's heartfelt pleas for sympathy on account of his efforts to quit taking morphine fell on deaf ears, and the Pension Bureau denied his appeal. Pension applications by addicted veterans were often flagged for review under the vicious habits clause, resulting in investigations that were prolonged, dramatic, and intrusive—even more so than typical pension claim adjudications.

Samuel M. Martin was just a teenager when he enlisted as a musician in the 18th Indiana Infantry. By his twentieth birthday, he had become addicted to morphine, which Union surgeons prescribed for an extraordinary gunshot wound he sustained at Pea Ridge on March 7, 1862. While he was carrying a wounded comrade back from the front lines, a whizzing Minié ball struck Martin near the heart, tearing a hole in his blue sack coat. But an ambrotype in a sturdy brass case, a token from "his lady love" that Martin kept in his shirt's left breast pocket, pancaked the soft lead bullet, deflecting it downward and out of the left side of Martin's rib cage. His life saved by the ambrotype, Martin was carried by comrades back to the surgeon's tent, where he received a dose of opium for the pain and a discharge from the army. Martin's miraculous survival became an Indiana legend, earning him a monthly pension of four dollars beginning in August 1862. Thirty-one years later, an officer from Martin's unit still recalled the miracle of the ambrotype clearly enough to recount it in detail to a Pension Bureau agent during a deposition.[29]

But there would be no more miracles for Martin after Pea Ridge. The stigma of morphine addiction made his life a living hell. A hinge from the ambrotype case lodged against Martin's spine, leaving the veteran partially paralyzed with a tingling numbness across the left side of his body. Returning home to Greenfield, Indiana, Martin trained as a doctor, where he learned how to inject morphine hypodermically. Soon, he began injecting himself for his war wound. Martin tried to keep his addiction secret, but eventually he became erratic from "morphine mania." Martin's friends and family became convinced that drugs had destroyed the veteran's body and mind. Tired of watching Martin inject huge doses of morphine and cocaine—which he attempted to use as a morphine substitute—the veteran's medical partners apparently forced him out of their joint practice. Destitute and debilitated, Martin turned to the Pension Bureau for relief and applied for an increase in September 1892. Naturally, he made no mention of drug addiction in his application, swearing "that I am suffering from physical disabilities of permanent character," ostensibly his war injury, "not the result of my own vicious habits."[30] But to secure a pension adjustment, Martin had to be examined by a board of doctors. On the day of the examination, March 21, 1894, the doctors discovered his secret and reported to the bureau that "this claimant is a 'morphia eater.'" Shortly thereafter, in 1895, Martin's family had him briefly institutionalized at the Indiana Hospital for the Insane in Indianapolis.

The 1894 medical report triggered a special investigation that lasted until the spring of 1897, nearly four years. The bureau dispatched a dogged special examiner to Martin's hometown of Greenfield, Indiana, who documented every facet of Martin's case in painstaking detail. The investigation entailed multiple medical examinations and depositions of Martin and several affiants. In March 1894, Martin was summoned to an intensive medical exam. As soon as he dropped his pants, it became obvious to this second board of surgeons that the previous doctors' reports were correct. Martin's "skin [is] very marked in both legs," they explained to the bureau. They discovered scars that were "the result of hypodermic needle."[31] These scars, often referred to as abscesses, were common among addicted veterans who used the needle and presented unequivocal physical evidence of Martin's secret morphine use. Even more damning were the affidavits from Martin's close friends and former medical partners. Four out of five men who supplied affidavits or depositions reported that Martin was addicted. One man explained, "The first time I knew the doctor Martin was addicted to the use of morphine was in 1893 when I drove him from home to take the train at Maxwell Indiana to get to Lebanon, Ohio for treatment." During the short trip, Martin "had a hypodermic [injection of morphine] five times in going five miles. After that I heard he had been using it for years. I investigated the matter a little after that and I became convinced that he had used it for a great many years. He probably commenced it soon after the war," the affiant reasoned. Under the glare of the special investigator, Martin himself was forced to admit the truth. "Under what circumstances was the use of morphine commenced?" the investigator demanded in a July 1896 deposition. "I commenced the use of opium immediately after I was wounded in March 1862," Martin confessed. "The [army] doctor gave me ergot and opium on account of the hemorrhage from the wound," and he continued taking opiates, eventually becoming addicted. But, Martin insisted, "I do not believe that the use of morphine aggravated the numbness and paralysis. It always gave me a temporary relief."[32]

Martin's admission that he was a morphine user sealed the fate of his pension application. The special investigator wrote to the commission of the Pension Bureau in February 1897 with his final report, more than four years after the veteran's initial application in 1892. "The case was referred for special examination with a view of determining," among other facts, "the extent to which the opium habit is a factor" in Martin's alleged disability. It assuredly was a

(3—)

☞ Attention is invited to the outlines of the human skeleton and figure upon the back of this certificate, and they should be used whenever it is possible to indicate precisely the location of a disease or injury, the entrance and exit of a missile, an amputation, &c.
The absence of a member from a session of a board and the reason therefor, if known, and the name of the absentee, must be indorsed upon each certificate.

Insert character and number of claim: Increase Pension Claim No. 237 259

Name and rank of claimant: Sam'l M Masten, Rank Musician

Company K **18** **Reg't** 2nd Greenfield, Hancock Co., Ind.

Claimant's post-office address: Greenfield Ind **Date of examination** Jan 4, 1893.

We hereby certify that in compliance with the requirements of the law we have carefully examined this applicant, who states that he is suffering from the following disability, incurred in the service, viz: G. S. W-d of left side of abdomen resulting reflex paralysis of left side

and that he receives a pension of four dollars per month

He makes the following statement upon which he bases his claim for Increase.

At the Battle of Pea Ridge Ark on the 2nd day a Musket ball entered abdomen, and for first 3 days vomited blood, then in 3 weeks afterward had severe hemorrhage. The ball passed through body. At this time has partially paralyzed entire left side, has a partial paralysis of bladder & rectum. At times can not control either bladder or rectum. also has rheumatism + heart trouble

Upon examination we find the following objective conditions: Pulse rate, 90 respiration, 24; temperature, 98.4; height, 5 feet 4 inches; weight, 122 pounds; age, 51 years. In the axillary line of the left side & between the 6th and 7th rib Scar of entrance corrugated depressed not adherent tender on pressure one inch in diameter on the ..

This claimant is a "Morphia Eater"

mark in region of wound. The Sphincters nearer but little control over bowels or bladder. The muscles of entire left side Show great loss of tonicity. The grip of left hand not more than ½ of right. walks lame left side foot dragging. All the above conditions we attribute to the gun shot wound above described for which we rate him Twelve dollars per month. Chest at rest 33 Forced In 34½ Forced Ex 31. Lungs normal. Apex beat felt and seen 2 inches below the left nipple. Center of dullness One and one-fourth inches to right of left nipple and two inches in diameter. There are no murmurs but both sounds equal in He is, in our opinion, entitled to a 12/18 rating for the disability caused by G. S. W. left side 4/18 for that caused by disease of heart, and 18/18 10/18 for that caused by rheumatism

Warren King, Pres. J A Comstock, Sec'y. Chas C Bruner, Treas.

N. B.—Always forward a certificate of examination whether a disability is found to exist or not.

factor, the agent reported. "For years Dr. Martin stood very high as a man and a physician until he became a wreck through his unfortunate habit," and now, "during the last few years he has been like all 'morphine fiends' entirely unreliable." With all facts uncovered, the investigator reported, "I believe that whatever disability the claimant has at this time outside of the gunshot wound is due to the constant and excessive use of morphine and cocaine, which in my opinion cannot be charged to his service in the army. I therefore recommend the rejection of the claim." The commissioner evidently agreed, because Martin's claim was rejected under the vicious habits clause of the Dependent Pension Act in the spring of 1897. Someone in the Pension Bureau office went so far as to paste a note to Martin's 1892 application literally labeling him a "morphia eater," perhaps for future reference in case of an appeal that ultimately never came. Physically, emotionally, and financially broken down, Martin died just a few months later.[33] (See fig. 6.2.)

Presumably, most Union veterans realized that the Pension Bureau would deny their applications on the grounds of vicious habits if their opiate addictions were discovered, thus they tended to disguise addictions when applying for pensions. The Pension Bureau's affidavit forms for examining doctors, a crucial element in pension applications, inquired if veterans' disabilities were due to vicious habits.[34] Veterans knew better than to openly disclose their addictions to doctors during medical examinations, lest the doctor make note of their opium habits in the affidavit. Many addicted applicants appear to have concealed their condition from examining doctors when applying for pensions to avoid the outright denial of their applications. As T. D. Crothers observed in 1893, "Many veterans of the late war have become opium maniacs for the relief of their pains and sufferings, and this is often concealed where it might possibly peril the procuring of a pension." For his part, Crothers urged that the "pension bureau should recognize the use of opium as a natural sequence and entailment following the disease and injury in the service." Indeed, "in Prussia both alcohol and opium inebriety are treated as diseases when occurring in the army or civil service."[35] Occasionally, addicted veterans, like Bowser and Lazelle, were caught in the act of covering their tracks, resulting in the denial

---

Figure 6.2 (opposite) Surgeon's report, January 4, 1893, pertaining to Samuel M. Martin's unsuccessful application for a pension increase. Pension Bureau agents flagged Martin's application for a special investigation under the "vicious habits" clause of the Dependent Pension Act. The surgeon confirmed the bureau's suspicion that Martin was addicted to morphine, resulting in the rejection of his application. The Pension Bureau literally labeled Martin a "morphia eater," pasting a note to that effect into his pension file. Surgeon's Certificate, January 4, 1893, Samuel M. Martin pension file, certificate 237259, National Archives and Records Administration, Washington, DC.

of pensions outright or the refusal of the Pension Bureau to increase existing pensions.

But as Crothers observed, an untold number of veterans likely managed to keep their addiction under wraps and secured pensions. For example, Frank E. Pray, a hardened veteran of the 24th, 88th, and 192nd Ohio Infantry regiments, received a pension for chronic diarrhea, rheumatism, and heart disease in 1886. His pension records make no mention of opiate addiction. But six years earlier, Pray had been admitted to the Dayton, Ohio, branch of the NHDVS while suffering from "chronic diarrhea" and the "opium habit," according to his NHDVS file. At some point during or after the Civil War, Pray developed an opiate addiction, perhaps when he worked as a hospital steward during the war. Union hospital stewards were responsible for doling out medicines, an assignment that gave Pray relatively unrestricted access to opium. Of course, it is also possible that Pray managed to quit the drugs after being admitted to the NHDVS in 1880 but before applying for a pension in 1886. Considering the extreme withdrawal symptoms and cravings that prevented most veterans from ever quitting the drugs, however, it is unlikely that Pray managed to beat the odds and break the chains of opium slavery before applying for a pension. A more likely scenario is that Pray successfully disguised his opium addiction from pension examiners when he applied in 1886, thereby avoiding being flagged under the vicious habits clause and thus securing a pension.[36]

Like Pray, Wirt Morris, a veteran of the 14th West Virginia Infantry, made no mention of his opiate addiction in any of the three pension applications he filed during the 1880s and 1890s. Morris told the Pension Bureau that he had picked up a head catarrh in the army in 1864 and had been suffering from debilitating headaches ever since. The first time he applied for a pension in May 1884, Morris noted that "he had uniformly treated himself for his affliction with almost all the so-called medicines with no permanent relief." In all likelihood, one of these "so-called medicines" contained opiates and was the source of Morris's addiction. His mother, Mary A. Morris, confirmed these symptoms in her affidavit. The veteran had "frequent and violent headaches, almost constant discharge from the nostrils," and "has been using some preparation or remedy for catarrh in the head." But, crucially for Morris's sake, the pension application made no mention of opium. This first application for a pension was denied on technical grounds, but after the 1890 Dependent Pension Act came into effect, Morris applied again. This time, the bureau approved Morris's application, awarding him a pension at twelve dollars a month in 1891 for "mass-pharyngeal catarrh, disease of heart, and injury to [the] left knee." In May 1897, a few months before his death, he applied for a pension rate increase, which the bureau ultimately rejected for want of medical evidence. In this affidavit, Morris claimed that "he has not [been] undergoing any treatment by physicians, but has bought and used all sorts and kinds of medicines" to self-medicate for his catarrh. Again, the veteran made no mention of opium. When the bureau refused to grant him an increase, Morris managed to get himself admitted to the Togus, Maine, branch of the NHDVS in August 1897. But, for reasons unknown, he soon left and made his way to Boston, where he died of "alcoholism," according to the city's coroner, in early December 1897. The city's undertaker found Morris's hard-won pension certificate on his corpse. The case is extraordinary, not because the Pension Bureau denied Morris's 1884 and 1897 applications but because the veteran managed to disguise his addiction and secure a pension in 1891, despite being addicted to opium. Morris's strategy—keeping his addiction out of his pension paperwork at all costs—seems to have been common practice for opiate-addicted Union veterans applying for pensions.[37]

Veterans like Pray and Morris understood well the need to disguise their opiate addictions if they hoped to secure pensions. In fact, the GAR warned veterans to do so, albeit obliquely. Its unofficial mouthpiece, the *National Tribune*, published a manual in 1898 advising Union veterans on how to navigate the labyrinthine pension application process. The manual quoted at length from the Pension Bureau's 1890s appeals rulings that laid out a working definition of "vicious habits," unpacking these cases so that Union veterans gained a concrete understanding of the factors that might disqualify them from pensions under the new law.[38] Addicted veterans who read this section of the *National Tribune*'s pension handbook would have recognized the need to disguise their addictions from bureau agents and the doctors conducting medical examinations on the bureau's behalf. In hindsight, veterans' efforts to disguise their addictions to avoid detection by Pension Bureau agents and doctors undermines historians' ability to gauge the extent of addiction among pension applicants. Given the incentive veterans had to mask their addictions, we can reasonably assume that the strategy was widely adopted by addicted veterans. Although this obfuscation served veterans' pragmatic needs, their secrecy about their addictions makes it impossible to gauge the extent of the problem of opiate addiction among veterans using pension records alone.

For its part, the Pension Bureau realized that addicted veterans usually disguised their addictions, and it endeavored to catch fraudsters with "vicious habits" in the act. Members of the federal government had long argued that deception about one's personal habits should disqualify veterans from pensions. During a heated January 1868 House of Representatives floor debate over a contested pension claim, even a Republican congressman who himself had worn the Union blues admitted that the "willful concealment" of drunkenness and other stigmatized habits should disqualify veterans from pensions.[39] The Pension Bureau agreed. According to the bureau, covering up addiction so as to successfully navigate the pension application process constituted fraud, and suspicious applications underwent extra scrutiny to uncover such deception. In an 1881 manual for agents tasked with conducting these investigations, called "special examiners," the bureau instructed that applicants be screened for "intemperance or vicious habits." If found to be addicted, veterans risked having their pending pension applications rejected. This sort of medical fraud was usually obvious, the manual blithely noted. But just in case, whenever agents discovered vicious habits or intemperance, they should take extra care to document the fraud, ostensibly to ensure that any appeal would not succeed.[40]

Opiate-addicted Confederate veterans also faced restricted access to pensions. Most former Confederate states and border states passed laws awarding pensions to disabled Confederate veterans during the late nineteenth and early twentieth centuries.[41] Like the US Pension Bureau, eight southern states barred opiate-addicted Confederate veterans from receiving pensions. Arkansas's pension law prohibited former Confederates from receiving pensions if their disability was "the result of their own vicious habits."[42] Tennessee, Kentucky, and Louisiana required that applicants truthfully answer the question, "Do you use intoxicants to any extent?" Presumably, the states' pension boards would have rejected any applicants who answered affirmatively. And should addicted veterans try to hide their condition when applying, Tennessee required reputable affiants to confirm that "applicant's habits are good and free from dishonor."[43] States that did not have vicious habits or intoxicant clauses imposed character restrictions instead, implicitly barring addicted veterans from receiving pensions. Alabama's pension application form stated that veterans must be "worthy." Missouri's Confederate applications required that two witnesses attest that the veteran in question was a "man of reliability." Oklahoma requested two "credible witnesses" to attest that the "applicant's habits are good and free from dishonor," and North Carolina required that a witness swear that the veteran in question was "respectable." Although these restrictions were ambiguous, they implied that one's physical disability was not the only grounds that should be considered by pension organizations. Thus, these character clauses could reasonably be interpreted by pension examiners to exclude untrustworthy, immoral, or unmanly Confederate veterans—all characteristics closely associated with opiate addiction.[44] Through the use of vicious habits and intoxicants clauses or restrictive, moralizing language, eight former Confederate and border states explicitly or indirectly barred opiate-addicted Confederate veterans from state pension programs. Of the states that had Confederate pension programs, six—Florida, Georgia, Mississippi, South Carolina, Texas, and Virginia—did not restrict opiate-addicted veterans from receiving pensions. Even in these states, though, addicted Confederate veterans likely struggled to secure pensions because doing so often required applicants to submit character references in their pension applications. Considering the stigma surrounding addiction, veteran opiate users would likely have struggled to obtain positive statements in support of their moral fiber or manliness.[45]

Disqualification from pension benefits also applied to the dependents of opiate-addicted Union veterans. Oftentimes, when veterans died of overdoses, their widows and children sought to obtain dependents' pensions. For example, in 1885, "C. H. W." wrote a letter to the *Vermont Watchman and State Journal*, a newspaper that ran an advice column for Union veterans struggling to navigate the convoluted pension process. A pensioner, C. H. W. explained, had died of a morphine overdose, after being prescribed the drug by a physician to remedy the pain stemming from the pensioned disability, and wanted to know if the dead veteran's children were eligible for a pension. Pondering the merits of the "interesting" case, the *Watchman* advised that the children's guardian should apply for a dependent's pension on their behalf. If the Pension Bureau denied the claim, the children ought to appeal to their congressman, who "would very likely give the pension by a special act" of Congress.[46] Many dependents shared the perspective of the *Watchman*'s columnist, applying for survivor's benefits both through the Pension Bureau's standard process and through the special pensions often awarded by Congress.

However, the bereaved widows of veterans who had died from opiate overdoses faced major hurdles when attempting to secure dependents' pensions. One of those hurdles was President Grover Cleveland, who firmly believed that widows of veterans who had fatally overdosed on opium or morphine did not deserve pensions. During his first term, from 1885 to 1889, Cleveland vetoed at least four special pensions granted by Congress to the widows of Union veterans who had died from overdoses. Cleveland's official position was that such deaths were not strictly the result of service-related health problems and therefore were not pensionable. According to the letter of pre-1890 pension laws, he was correct. However, a close reading of Cleveland's veto messages suggests there is more to the story.

Cleveland's veto messages and his public commentary on pensions reveal that he was deeply influenced by prevailing Gilded Age views on manhood and morality. Throughout his first term in office—a period when the Democratic president was embroiled in a political blood feud with the Republican-aligned GAR over the future of the pension program—Cleveland made it a habit to veto as many special congressional pensions as possible, not just those awarded to the widows of veterans who had died from overdoses. He once explained that "I have endeavored within my sphere of official duty to protect our pension roll and make it what it should be, a roll of honor, containing the names of those disabled in their country's service and worthy of their country's affectionate remembrance." Cleveland's obsession with personally policing pension applications troubled his associates, one of whom recalled that the president "took abnormal pains to prevent the success of a fraudulent application for a pension," sometimes working into the early morning hours.⁴⁷

Convinced that the widows of dishonorable, unmanly veterans did not deserve to partake of government largesse, Cleveland used his veto pen to ensure they did not get it. The language Cleveland employed in his veto messages provides a window into his mindset. They reveal a subtle, but persistent, condemnation of opiate-addicted veterans' manhood, which undergirded the president's decisions to veto the special widows' pensions. Cleveland ostensibly denied the pension awarded to the widow of R. J. McIlwain because the Union veteran died by his own hand and not by causes linked, in the president's opinion, to the Civil War. But in his veto message, Cleveland impugned the veteran for his recklessness and lack of self-control—unmanly characteristics. McIlwain died, Cleveland explained, because he injected an "entire purchase of six grains while under the influence of liquor," even though he had been in the habit of taking morphia and *knew how to use it*."⁴⁸ Instead of proceeding with self-control and carefully measuring out safe doses, on the night of his death, McIlwain bought a month's supply of morphine from a pharmacist, got drunk, and recklessly overindulged by taking the morphine all at once. If he had been a man and controlled his cravings, Cleveland's language implied, McIlwain would not have died.

The widows of overdosed veterans often spent years trying to secure pensions, with little success to show for their efforts. John T. Travers, an apothecary and former hospital steward from the 3rd Michigan Infantry, contracted "some form of lung disease, or disease of the throat," during the war, perhaps tuberculosis which spread rampantly in poorly ventilated hospitals. In "great physical pain" after leaving the army in 1866, he took morphine as a cough suppressant. Over the years, Travers become addicted, and in January 1881 he died of an accidental overdose. Alice Travers, John's wife, applied for a widow's pension in October 1884, explaining that her husband's "death [was] caused by [an] overdose of morphine administered by himself."⁴⁹ Alice hoped the Pension Bureau would be sympathetic, considering that the veteran had contracted a lung disease and ensuing morphine addiction through military service. But the bureau was not, so agents denied Alice's application on the grounds that John's death had not stemmed from a disability incurred during the Civil War. At that point, Alice turned to the House of Representatives, which passed a special bill awarding her a pension in the summer of 1886. Unsurprisingly, President Cleveland vetoed the bill in June 1886. Alice appealed the Pension Bureau's original decision, this time claiming that "the soldier contracted in the service some form of lung disease, or disease of the throat, which caused great physical pain at times, to obtain relief from which, the soldier, a practical druggist, administered morphine—causing death." The bureau did not challenge this sequence of events leading to John's death but refused to admit that his overdose was attributable to a disability stemming from military service. It denied the appeal in April 1887. Cleveland's rationale, disclosed in his veto message, explained why Alice had so much difficulty securing a widow's pension. In Cleveland's view, one shared by the Pension Bureau, John's death was the result of his own poor decision-making, not the fault of the army. Cleveland noted in the veto message that John "was in the habit of taking opiates for relief and sleep" and the overdose that killed him was not from a doctor's hand but his own. Cleveland's use of the term "habit" to describe John's addiction suggests that the president thought John was culpable in his death and therefore undeserving of a pension. Indeed, "he administered himself" the fatal dose, Cleveland emphasized.[50] Because of the stigma of opiate addiction, Cleveland felt that John's widow did not deserve a pension.

The Travers case established a precedent that lasted well beyond Cleveland's days in the White House. Cleveland left the office of president in March 1889, and his successor, Republican Benjamin Harrison, oversaw the rollout of the 1890 Dependent Pension Act. But despite the liberalization of the US pension system, the precedent set by Cleveland and his allies in the US Pension Bureau in the Travers case stood throughout the 1890s. After the Travers case, the bureau continued to reject pension applications from widows whose veteran husbands died from opiate overdoses. These decisions were frequently contested under the rules of the 1890 act, and at least nine cases rose to the level of the bureau's appeals body. Winding their way through the labyrinthine appeals process, these cases generated detailed explanations from the bureau that provide unique insight into pension gatekeepers' mindset about opium slavery. In most of these cases, the bureau refused to concede that fatal overdoses constituted a service-related death, even when the medicines had originally been prescribed by doctors. But, as with Cleveland's veto messages, the tone in these final rulings suggests that officials took into consideration the gendering and stigma of opiate addiction when denying dependents' benefits to the widows of overdose victims.

Not content to merely deny the pensions in question, the bureau often impugned the character and masculinity of addicted veterans who had overdosed to death. The language its agents used when handing down rulings on appealed widow's cases hints at subtle, but pernicious, condemnation of the deceased veterans on the grounds that addiction evidenced weakness and immorality and thus rendered their families unworthy of federal support. Take, for instance, the case of James Ladson Hall, a veteran of the 99th Pennsylvania Infantry and successful Philadelphia tobacco merchant. Hall contracted chronic diarrhea during the war, and on returning home, a physician prescribed opiates, which Hall found to be "the only remedy that would effectually relieve the pain."

Toward the end of his life, Hall kept a bottle of laudanum on top of his desk so that he could swallow the drug "at such times as he wished or believed he needed it," according to the bureau's 1898 ruling on his widow's pension case. Hall became addicted, fatally overdosing in 1870. After the 1890 pension law expanded the criteria for widows' pensions, Hall's widow Laura applied for pension benefits. But the bureau rejected her application, reasoning that the veteran's fatal overdose was his own fault. According to the ruling, Hall had simply been too reckless. The bureau condemned such careless overindulgence in painkillers, which branded Hall as weak-willed, intolerant of pain, and unmanly. Chiding the dead veteran for his apparent lack of self-control, the bureau added that "the soldier must have known" laudanum was dangerous and should have "exercise[d] all the more caution." If only Hall had shown restraint instead of taking laudanum intemperately whenever "he wished" to dull the pain, he would not have died, according to the ruling.[51] Such language suggests that in addition to the technical ruling that Hall's death was not strictly service related, the bureau also took his apparent lack of manhood and moral fiber into consideration when judging the claim. Thus, the long shadow of opium slavery not only unmanned Hall and claimed his life but also stalked the veteran's widow for decades after his death.

The hurdles encountered by Hall's widow were not unique. The Pension Bureau ruled similarly on several cases, establishing a precedent that widows of veterans who were addicted to opiates and fatally overdosed were to be excluded from pensions. Eugene M. Whallon, a Union hospital clerk, became addicted to morphine to manage the pain after a gruesome wartime gunshot to the knee. Jessie, Eugene's widow, applied for widow's benefits after he fatally overdosed in April 1884. But the bureau rejected her application, alleging that Eugene had taken morphine of his own volition, which ultimately caused his addiction and fatal overdose. Eugene's decision to indulge in morphine absolved the government of any responsibility for his own death, the bureau reasoned. Jessie disagreed. She appealed, this time procuring testimony from a physician who swore that he had originally prescribed Eugene morphine. But the bureau remained unmoved, rejecting Jessie's appeal and accusing Eugene of immorality in its final ruling in that he stole morphine during the war to support his habit and lied to cover up the theft.[52] The bureau likewise rejected Mary Warburton's application for a widow's pension because of her husband's opiate addiction. According to the bureau's ruling, he "was very intemperate and addicted to the excessive use of opium and morphine," was deceitful, refused to support his wife, and was "disposed to roam about the country" erratically.[53] In the Warburton case, as in the others, the decision was informed by contemporary notions of manhood and morality. Bureau officials viewed opiate addiction as a personal failing, implying that if the veterans had shown greater willpower and self-control or possessed stronger moral fiber, they could have avoided untimely deaths.

In decades of pension rulings, the Pension Bureau allowed only two known payouts to the widow or dependent of a Civil War veteran who had fatally overdosed. In one case, a Union veteran, Augustus F. Caldecott, became addicted to laudanum after a physician prescribed the cough suppressant for a lung disease contracted in the army and for which Caldecott had previously received a pension. He simply "could not live without" laudanum, lest he cough himself to death. Caldecott eventually developed tolerance to the drug, necessitating an ever-increasing dosage that eventually killed him in 1872. His mother Tamezen Ball applied for a dependent's pension, which was initially denied in 1885. But the bureau grudgingly reversed course in 1889 after Ball obtained a physician's sworn statement that her son had "made no improper use of the drug, but used it in the manner and for the purpose prescribed and with no suicidal intent." The doctor's testimony persuaded the Bureau that Caldecott, in life, had possessed strong enough moral character to make his survivors worthy of a federal pension. But lest the ruling set a precedent for the cases of veterans who were less temperate and upstanding, the bureau cautioned, "This case is to be distinguished from those in which it appears that a person contributed to his own death by the careless and reckless use of a dangerous and poisonous drug, upon his own responsibility."[54] The other payout granted by the bureau to the dependent of a veteran who died of an opiate overdose was awarded to Mary A. Buker, widow of Cyrus F. Buker. The veteran died of a laudanum overdose swallowed during "an aberration of mind" in 1873. The bureau rejected Mary's initial application for widow's benefits on the grounds that Cyrus had died by his own hand, either through a reckless accidental overdose or an intentional act of self-destruction. Either way, the bureau claimed, his death was not the government's financial responsibility. Mary, like Tamezen Ball, was able to sway the bureau to change its mind by enlisting three physicians to attest to the dead veteran's moral character, regardless of the manner of his death. Convinced by this formidable "expert medical testimony," the bureau finally admitted in 1887 that Cyrus's death "was a sequela of the injuries received in the line of duty." This reversal secured Mary's pension and absolved Cyrus of the stigma surrounding his overdose death.[55]

These exceptional cases notwithstanding, opiate-addicted veterans and their dependents faced near-universal exclusion from Civil War pensions. Such exclusions represent an especially conspicuous form of suffering experienced by veterans and their loved ones in view of the massive expansion of federal and state Civil War pension programs during the Gilded Age.[56] Yet this growth of pension systems did not apply equitably to all Americans. According to the US Pension Bureau, President Grover Cleveland, and Southern state pension bodies, veterans who suffered from opiate addiction were unworthy of pensions because of their ostensible immorality and unmanliness. Operating under this calculus, gatekeepers used restrictions on military pensions as a way to discriminate against opiate users and formally penalize addiction.

This penalization is significant not only because it made the lives of addicted veterans and their families even harder but also because of the period in which this policing occurred. The Gilded Age carved out new ways to regulate and punish drug addiction, measures that are especially striking because they preceded formal criminalization of drugs by decades. The policing of opiate users and their dependents that developed in the framework of Civil War entitlement programs represents a previously unknown nineteenth-century antecedent to later criminalization measures. Investigating how drug use affected access to entitlement programs thus helps expose the hidden connection between the Civil War and the later War on Drugs.

Soldiers' Homes

Although pensions were the most contentious form of military entitlements, they were not the only kind of government aid extended to Civil War veterans. During the Gilded Age, nearly 120,000 veterans took up residence in dozens of government-funded soldiers' homes across the United States.[57] Yet these facilities did not welcome opiate-addicted men with open arms. In the South, most state-run Confederate soldiers' homes explicitly or indirectly barred opiate-addicted veterans from admission. In the North, addicted veterans could sometimes gain admission into federal and state soldiers' homes—but they could not stay there long or without coercion. The reasoning behind these restrictions mirrored the calculus established by pension programs. The politicians who created the soldiers' homes and the administrators who ran them viewed addicted veterans as immoral and unmanly and therefore undeserving of the room, board, and medical care provided at these facilities.

Restrictions on soldiers' homes were particularly severe in the South. Fueled by Lost Cause fervor, in the late nineteenth century, several former Confederate states and border states that fielded Confederate regiments created publicly funded Confederate soldiers' homes. These facilities, similar to antebellum almshouses, served as a place of refuge where poor, infirm former Confederates and their families could find sanctuary when they could no longer provide for themselves. However, as with all charity in the nineteenth century, admission came with strict qualifiers. Like their federal counterparts, gatekeepers at Confederate soldiers' homes took moral character and masculinity into consideration when screening applicants for admission, not merely financial need or physical disability. Veterans who did not measure up to idealized standards for morality and manhood were denied admissions or, if already living at the home, kicked to the curb.[58]

Many Southern facilities screened for drug and alcohol use and expressly barred heavy users. Like the state's pension agency, the Tennessee State Soldiers Home asked veterans seeking admission: "Do you use intoxicants to any extent?"[59] South Carolina's Confederate Infirmary required that veterans admitted to the home be "persons of good character and habits." The admissions form inquired if applicants had an "opium, chloral or any other drug habit?" Applicants who answered affirmatively were promptly rejected. No "drunkard or deadbeat or a man of bad character" need apply to Arkansas's Confederate home. Most Southern state soldiers' homes posed similar screening questions in their applications for admission, effectively excluding opiate-addicted Confederate veterans from admission.[60] Those rare soldiers' homes that did not inquire about addiction instead barred "insane" applicants. Sometimes admissions forms inquired about habits and mental health. "INSANE PERSONS AND HABITUAL DRUNKARDS WILL NOT BE ADMITTED UNDER ANY CIRCUMSTANCES," warned the admission form for North Carolina's Confederate soldiers' home, complete with capitalized lettering.[61] Physicians endorsing applications for admission into the Confederate Home of Missouri had to attest that veterans were not "habitual drunkards," nor had they "ever been an inmate of an insane asylum."[62] Such language excluded opiate-addicted men from admission because their condition was often framed as a cause of both insanity and a form of intemperance akin to drunkenness.

Deterrence measures were likely effective in preventing opiate-addicted veterans' access to Confederate soldiers' homes. Extant medical records from the hospitals of southern soldiers' homes are few and far between. But a rare hospital patient register dating from 1908 to 1916 records the various ailments that plagued the ailing older Confederates living at North Carolina's Confederate soldiers' home. The volume records hundreds of diagnoses for conditions ranging from cancer to "softening of the brain," insanity, dysentery, sore legs, tuberculosis, apoplexy, and asthma.[63] But the register does not record a single case of opiate addiction treated among the Confederate veterans living at the home. Like hospital records, disapproved applications for admission into Confederate soldiers' homes are also rare. There was little incentive to keep the records of men who did not gain access to the homes, and these denied applications were usually scrapped in the intervening decades after closure of the homes. But the Missouri state archives managed to hold on to the disapproved admissions applications for its Confederate Soldiers' Home. Of the hundreds of extant applications, not even one would-be resident disclosed an opiate addiction.[64] Considering how common opiate addiction was among Civil War veterans well into the twentieth century, these evidentiary silences speak volumes, suggesting that addicted Confederate veterans tried their hardest to conceal drug use or might not have even bothered to apply for admission into Southern state soldiers' homes.

Union veterans faced restricted access to soldiers' homes as well, although to a lesser degree than that faced by addicted former Confederates. In contrast to Southern state homes and the US pension system, the National Home for Disabled Volunteer Soldiers, the federal government's soldiers' homes for Union veterans, did not expressly bar opiate users. While NHDVS managers did not deem addiction alone, absent an accompanying physical disability like a gunshot wound, to be grounds for taking up residence in the system's branch facilities, the NHDVS was sometimes willing to admit opiate-addicted veterans, if their accompanying disabilities warranted admission. Although the total figure is difficult to quantify, medical records indicate that a large number of addicted veterans ultimately spent time in NHDVS branches during the postwar decades. Hundreds of cases of opiate addiction were treated at soldiers' homes for Union veterans, including NHDVS branches and state-run facilities, during the 1870s, 1880s, and 1890s. An 1896 survey of seven NHDVS branches and twenty-six state-run facilities found that, collectively, 102 cases of the "opium habit" had been treated in the preceding year, evidence that many addicted veterans ultimately managed to gain entry, even if addiction in and of itself did not warrant admission.[65]

The NHDVS's relative willingness to open its doors to opiate-addicted veterans reflected the system's mission. Rather than merely charity, the US government used the NHDVS to teach ailing needy veterans how to behave like proper men. There were strings attached to admission into the soldiers' homes, which constituted a kind of paternalistic aid through which the state sought to inculcate domesticity and bourgeois notions of morality into "inmates."[66] To this end, elderly veterans living at the NHDVS wore military uniforms and were forced to adhere to strict military discipline. Bugles woke them up every morning and ordered them to mealtimes, which lasted a mere fifteen minutes. Room searches, compulsory bathing, and bans on possessing liquor checked perceived misbehaviors among the residents. Veterans who violated these disciplinary codes were subjected to harsh fines, forfeiture of pensions, forced work duties, confinement, and, for repeat offenders, dishonorable discharge.[67] Banning drug users and drunkards from admission outright would have conflicted with the NHDVS's mission to teach veterans how to behave like upstanding men. This charge opened a loophole that enabled some opiate-addicted Union veterans to access federal military entitlements, despite the Pension Bureau's best efforts to restrict access of "opium slaves" to state-funded military entitlements.

Addicted veterans might be admitted to the NHDVS, but once inside the doors, they faced harsh treatment that often resulted in expulsion from the soldiers' homes. Ironically, the very rules that were intended to instill virtue among old soldiers ultimately constrained addicted veterans' access within soldiers' homes, even if some of these facilities were open to opium eaters on paper. When inmates exhibited behaviors that were widely ascribed to addiction—lying, stealing, or irrational or abusive conduct—opiate users ran afoul of the NHDVS's strict moral and disciplinary codes, which resulted in censure. Some men, like George M. Barber, were even subjected to medical experimentation intended to correct their behavior. Barber, a veteran of the 3rd New York Infantry, was shot at Dennis Bluffs in May 1864 and "lay in the rain and was wet for four days after before wound was dressed by a surgeon." He also suffered from gonorrhea, typhoid, and pneumonia during the war, all of which were typically treated by opiates. Consequently, according to Barber's NHDVS medical records, "He was addicted to the use of opium from 1864 to 1882." Barber spent the postwar decades being shuttled in and out of six separate branches, a pattern indicating that he presented a persistent behavioral problem for administrators. Finally, in 1893, the NHDVS transferred him to a special medical facility run by doctors at the Leavenworth, Kansas, branch; they described Barber as "restless, uneasy, mean and impertinent to those around him, using abusive and indecent language in the ward at times, and in fact was a bad man." To correct his misbehavior, the doctors planned to subject Barber to trephination, a medical procedure in which a hole was drilled into one's skull, with the aim of relieving pressure on the brain. But Barber ran away before the doctors could do so, thwarting their plan and earning Barber a dishonorable discharge from the NHDVS.[68]

Expulsion from the NHDVS often befell addicted Union veterans who managed to gain admission into soldiers' homes, especially during the 1870s and 1880s. Officials of the NHDVS frequently labeled opium eaters as insane and had them institutionalized at St. Elizabeths in Washington, DC.[69] John Fisk, formerly a colonel in the 2nd New York Mounted Rifles, entered the Dayton, Ohio, NHDVS branch in June 1879 for "chronic diarrhea and debility result of service." Fisk apparently kept his opiate addiction secret upon admission, but when officials discovered his condition in October 1879, they promptly had Fisk committed to St. Elizabeths. Asylum doctors diagnosed him as suffering from long-standing "chronic dementia" caused by the "opium habit." Fisk was eventually discharged from the asylum as "improved" in June 1890, but he never returned to the NHDVS.[70] In December 1893, George W. Michaels, formerly of the 55th Ohio Infantry, arrived at the asylum from the Leavenworth, Kansas, NHDVS branch. His melancholia was attributed to "morphinism."[71] At least twenty-six veterans living at the NHDVS were sent to St. Elizabeths for opiate addiction from the system's various homes between 1865 and 1900.[72] They represented the most severely debilitated men among the larger population of opiate-addicted Civil War veterans living at the NHDVS and state-run soldiers' homes for Union veterans during the postwar decades.

Despite the risk of institutionalization, some veterans sought admission to the NHDVS for the express purpose of obtaining medical treatment for opiate addiction. They hoped that the medical care provided at soldiers' homes might cure addiction and thereby mitigate its health and social consequences. For example, after the Civil War, Alvah V. Oatman, a veteran of the 27th Massachusetts Infantry, developed locomotor ataxia, a painful, degenerative condition afflicting the spinal cord. Chronic, excruciating pain forced Oatman to self-medicate with morphine, and eventually he became addicted. When Oatman's morphine addiction became overwhelming in the early 1890s, he sought relief for his addiction at the Milwaukee, Wisconsin, branch of the NHDVS. Instead of being expelled from the home and committed to St. Elizabeths, the Milwaukee surgeons had mercy on the addicted veteran and provided medical treatment for his addiction. The doctors tapered down Oatman's morphine dose until, eventually, he was able to leave off the habit. Oatman's case was not unique in the 1890s. Indeed, the final decade of the nineteenth century heralded a softening of attitudes toward opiate-addicted veterans at Northern soldiers' homes. As the NHDVS and Northern state homes began adopting sympathetic stances regarding addiction, veterans like Oatman found opportunities to gain admission. The Michigan Soldiers Home, for example, admitted one veteran, Charles L. Williams, in 1895, even though he openly confessed in his admission application that he was addicted to morphine.[73] That the Michigan home provided space for Williams rather than rejecting his application outright suggests that its administrators had come to view the man's plight, and that of others like him, with sympathy. Such liberal views became widespread among Northern administrators during the 1890s. Not content merely to provide room and board for addicted veterans, in the early 1890s the Connecticut legislature went so far as to earmark funds for "the [medical] treatment of veteran soldiers and sailors addicted to the liquor and narcotic habits" at the Connecticut Soldiers Home.[74] These emergent policies marked a stark about-face on the part of Northern soldiers' homes. Rather than having addicted veterans committed to mental asylums, Northern homes began catering to addicted veterans.

If administrators sought to control addicted veterans within soldiers' homes, the NHDVS nevertheless adopted medically innovative policies toward veteran "inmates" who suffered from substance addiction during the 1890s, treating former soldiers on the government's dime. The NHDVS even opened a "Keeley Center" in 1892 at the Leavenworth, Kansas, branch, where between March 1892 and June 1895, thirty-four morphine-addicted veterans underwent Leslie E. Keeley's Gold Cure—a patent medicine for opiate addiction, discussed at length in chapter 7—alongside more than a thousand veterans suffering from alcohol and tobacco addiction.[75] One of these men, William H. Hughes, a veteran from Ohio, "acquired the morphine habit on account of using the drug for the unbearable pains" of rheumatism, according to an NHDVS surgeon. Instead of simply having Hughes committed, as had been the prior practice, the NHDVS sent Hughes to the Leavenworth Keeley Center in 1893. Hughes's surgeon was thrilled with the results of the Gold Cure treatment, proudly reporting to his superiors that Hughes "has taken the Keeley cure for the morphia habit and has now been without the drug for two weeks."[76] Some Northern state soldiers' homes also adopted similar treatment plans. Using the funds earmarked by the Connecticut state legislature for the purpose of medical care for addicted veterans, administrators at the Connecticut Soldiers' Home purchased the "Thompson cure," a patent medicine akin to the Gold Cure, for seven veterans and sent an additional nine men to a clinic run by the German Remedy Company in Birmingham, Connecticut. Unfortunately, the Connecticut home's administrators were dismayed to find out that these patent medicine "cures" for addiction were less "than fully satisfactory."[77] In contrast, the administrators of the New York State Soldiers and Sailors' Home for Disabled Volunteer Soldiers praised Keeley's Gold Cure, reporting in 1894 that several veterans had become "graduates of the Keeley treatment for the cure of drunkenness and the morphine habit," and much to the administers' delight, these recovered men "exert[ed] a salutary influence on other members of the Home." Good news of the Gold Cure quickly spread. Some veterans even penned queries to the *National Tribune* inquiring about the logistics of taking the Gold Cure at the NHDVS, including the treatment's availability and costs.[78]

Shifting policies on opiate addiction in Northern soldiers' homes can be attributed primarily to three factors. First, a core element of the NHDVS's mission was to reform veterans. In the eyes of NHDVS administrators behind the Keeley Institute program, freeing addicted veterans from opium slavery was a way to restore them to true manhood and good character. Administrators had long been sympathetic in practice toward veterans debilitated by substance addiction, even if official policy did not reflect this compassion until the 1890s. For example, in an 1876 report, William S. Tilton, deputy governor of the NHDVS's Eastern Branch, expressed considerable compassion and leniency toward veterans addicted to whiskey:

> Seven years' experience has taught me to look with charity upon the failings of these poor men, or wrecks of men rather, and I cannot help thinking when my patience is most tried by the deceit and ingratitude of the bad ones I say I cannot help asking how much are they to blame, when I know that they were initiated into the Army upon whiskey, had whiskey forced into them by the surgeons as a "prophylactic" before they

were wounded or taken sick, and finally had whiskey poured into them in hospital, either as a stimulant to quiet pain or as a sedative to keep them quiet otherwise.[79]

Such language suggests that Tilton did not blame alcoholic veterans for their "failings" and implies that he was receptive to measures intended to ease the suffering of veterans with substance use problems, perhaps not just alcohol users but also those who used opiates. Indeed, during the Gilded Age, several NHDVS branch managers implemented policies designed to reduce the harm attendant to drunkenness. Some branches even operated beer halls at their campuses—much to the chagrin of temperance activists—so that veterans living at the homes could drink without having to risk the dangers of traveling off campus: being fleeced out of pension monies by locals or freezing to death on the return trip from saloons.[80] Because many nineteenth-century observers classified alcohol and opiate addiction together under the broader label of intemperance, where sympathy toward alcoholic veterans existed, it sometimes extended to men suffering from opiate addiction as well.

Self-advocacy by addicted veterans is another likely explanation for shifting policies at the NHDVS. This phenomenon is difficult to discern in the historical records generated by soldiers' homes, which were produced by administrators and surgeons, providing mostly a one-dimensional top-down perspective on the NHDVS. Admission records and annual reports from the institutions usually do not speak directly to veterans' motivations for seeking entry to the NHDVS, nor do they record veterans' sides of the two-way medical encounters that occurred within the system's hospital wards. Nor do veterans' letters and diaries typically address opiate addiction, because, as in pension applications, veterans tended to refrain from disclosing their addictions in writing unless forced to do so. Occasionally, however, the records of soldiers' homes bear impressions of brave self-advocacy by addicted veterans.

After Alvah Oatman, the veteran treated for locomotor ataxia and morphine addiction at the Milwaukee NHDVS, successfully recovered from his habit, he told the surgeons "that he had lost all desire for morphine." He emphasized that "it was to obtain relief from this habit," not locomotor ataxia, "that he came to the Home."[81] When Charles L. Williams sought admission to the Michigan Soldiers Home in 1895, he was sure to point out that his opium habit was not his fault but that "during the war" the "drug [was] given by [an] army surgeon."[82] Williams pointedly and strategically blamed army surgeons for his opium addiction to claim his entitled support. Considered in the broader context of the successful Union veterans' movement for pension reform in the 1880s and 1890s, it seems likely that like veterans who lobbied hard for expanded access to federal pensions, some addicted veterans wholeheartedly believed the government owed them medical care for addiction as recompense for Civil War military service.[83] Perhaps veterans like Oatman and Williams reasoned that because military surgeons were culpable in causing addiction during the Civil War, government doctors at soldiers' homes shouldered the responsibility for providing medical assistance decades later.

Any self-advocacy by veterans would have tapped into an emerging current of sympathy for opiate-addicted Union veterans during the 1890s, a period when drug historians have observed a softening of attitudes toward white, middle-class medicinal users. One Northern writer, Henry G. Cole, gave voice to this sympathy in 1895. He singled out addicted veterans as uniquely deserving of compassion and medical assistance, rather than condemnation. During the Civil War, Union soldiers "entered the world's arena to do battle for some great cause of humanity," and by way of the war's "severe toil, anxiety, and weary days and nights without rest" ultimately became addicted to medicinal opiates. These veterans deserved "charity, and pity, and sympathy, and forgiveness," not the censure that for decades had been extended to opium "slaves" by the likes of Grover Cleveland and the US Pension Bureau. However, in contrast to veterans, Cole continued, "There is a large and growing class throughout the world with no laudable excuse" for addiction "except, perhaps, ignorance" and "seeking sensual pleasures." This underclass of opiate users did not deserve the same sympathy as addicted veterans, according to Cole. By distinguishing between the deserving and undeserving, his comments harkened back to the antebellum demarcation of "worthy" and "unworthy" drug users.[84] Considering the sympathetic rhetoric expressed by William S. Tilton, deputy governor of the Eastern Branch of the NHDVS, toward drunkenness as early as 1876, it seems likely that at least some administrators agreed with Cole's sympathy for "worthy" drug users. Empathy may have been an animating force behind the relatively liberal practice of treating opiate addiction implemented at the NHDVS during the 1890s. Yet the few veterans who managed to secure addiction care at soldiers' homes still felt the sting of stigma. Even though he found a home at the Marion, Indiana, branch of the NHDVS toward the end of his life, Perry Bowser nonetheless felt that the staff treated him harshly by withholding what he felt was a stable dose of morphine. Bowser described how, in November and December 1899, NHDVS doctors would supply him with only "4 little powders a day, about 4 grains when I needed 16," to avoid withdrawal. They also forced Bowser to pay for the drug and to surrender two months' of his pension, threatening "immediate expulsion" if he refused.[85]

The final force behind shifting policies toward addiction at Northern soldiers' homes was the patent medicine entrepreneur Leslie E. Keeley, who aggressively lobbied NHDVS officials to provide his Gold Cure to alcohol- and opiate-addicted veterans. To promote his products' supposed efficacy, Keeley first had to convince NHDVS administrators and doctors that addiction was a disease, not a vice. Diseases, Keeley insisted, could be cured through medical care, namely his Gold Cure. The Gold Cure path to recovery offered at the NHDVS proved extremely popular with addicted veterans, at least for a while. But far from universally embraced, Keeley's Gold Cure and similar patent medicines for opiate addiction proved controversial among doctors, setting the stage for a battle over the proper medical responses to mass addiction in the postwar decades.

PART III

Reactions

Chapter 7

Buying and Selling the Cure

Veterans and Patent Medicine Remedies for Addiction

In an 1880 letter to the editors of the relatively obscure *Louisville Medical News*, a physician told a grim story of a Civil War veteran, "Mr. J. T. B.," who had tried to buy back his health. Like countless other veterans, J. T. B. contracted diarrhea during the Civil War; during an especially severe bout in April 1862, he began taking opium pills, a standard Civil War antidiarrheal. Opium's constipating effects did the trick, but relief came at a cost. Soon J. T. B. developed the "opium habit."[1]

For eighteen years, according to the report, J. T. B. resolved to quit opium because of addiction's physical and social consequences. Long-term opium use and lingering chronic diarrhea took a terrible physical toll on his body. He had grown emaciated, impotent, and constipated. He also suffered social stigma, seen by others as weak in body, willpower, and moral fiber. Such characteristics may have been expected from Chinese immigrants, who were increasingly associated with opium addiction, but not of an honorable white veteran. Desperate to mitigate these disastrous consequences of addiction, J. T. B. felt that he needed to escape its yoke. The physician's letter did not specify his previous efforts, but if other veterans' experience is an indicator, he probably tried to quit the opium first through sheer willpower, attempting to endure the symptoms of withdrawal. In any case, by 1880, J. T. B. was desperate and willing to try anything.

One fateful day, he chanced on an advertisement for a patent medicine purported to cure opiate addiction without the pains of withdrawal. Perhaps the ad was a postcard for Samuel B. Collins's Painless Opium Antidote or Leslie E. Keeley's Gold Cure, the era's most prolific opiate addiction cures. J. T. B. and other Americans often received such postcards unsolicited in the mail, a Gilded Age version of direct mail marketing. Perhaps J. T. B. spotted a classified advertisement for the remedy in his local newspaper. One could hardly browse a postwar newspaper without spotting these ubiquitous ads. A local pharmacist may also have introduced the cure, solemnly sliding a medical pamphlet across a wooden pharmacy counter. With hope renewed at the possibility of buying his escape from the manacles of opium, J. T. B. mailed a confidential order form and a check to the patent medicine company.

When the cure arrived in the mail weeks later in a discreet, unmarked package, J. T. B. opened up the box, uncorked the glass vial, and gleefully took his first swig of liquid freedom. But his hopes were dashed, as the concoction failed to eliminate his opium cravings. Still, there were other brands on the market, so J. T. B. tried again and again, ultimately experimenting with a series of patent medicines that failed him one after another. By 1880, when he finally came under the care of an open-minded physician who treated opiate addiction liberally with coca, the source of cocaine, J. T. B. had spent $1,800 on opium and the patent medicines, equivalent to about $56,700 in 2025.[2] This small fortune made the case so shocking that J. T. B.'s story soon attracted media attention.[3]

Jarring as J. T. B.'s story might have been, the fraught use of patent medicines to treat opiate addiction was all too common among Civil War veterans during the Gilded Age. Many opiate-addicted veterans experimented with remedies purporting to cure addiction, hoping they would offer freedom from the "slavery" to opium and reverse its deleterious effects on health, manhood, and moral character. One desperate veteran even claimed to have outspent J. T. B., shelling out $2,500 on "all the so-called 'cures' and 'antidotes,'" but felt "worse than ever" when the remedies failed.[4]

If the Civil War played a major role in fostering opium addiction, it also fostered new demand for patent medicines among the thousands of addicted veterans. Like J. T. B., these men were highly motivated to try unproven and dubious "cures" because of the physical suffering and harsh social repercussions of addiction. In their hopelessness, patent medicine makers spotted a medical bonanza. Recognizing a growing demand among veterans and other Americans for opiate addiction remedies, Gilded Age entrepreneurs, many of whom were themselves veterans, invented myriad patent medicine "cures" and "antidotes" for the opium "habit" and marketed these would-be remedies in newspapers, magazines, and pamphlets. Often, but not always, patent medicine sellers specifically targeted addicted veterans, among other demographics, which underscored the contemporary cultural association of veterans and addiction. Countless former soldiers swapped their hard-earned wages for these medicines, hoping to buy freedom from opium and thereby restore lost health, reputations, and livelihoods.

Investigating this phenomenon illuminates several facets of the veterans' opiate addiction epidemic that are otherwise difficult to discern. First, it highlights surprising financial and commercial outcomes of veterans' military service. Historians recognize that amputations often entailed lost wages for laborers and that prosthetic subsidies did little to offset the cost of amputations. Pension payments and room and board provided by soldiers' homes subsidized hundreds of thousands of soldiers during the late nineteenth and early twentieth centuries. But beyond military entitlements, we lack a clear view of the personal financial toll of Civil War service for many disabled veterans. A related question is the extent to which the war's public health catastrophe heightened medical demand and sparked new commercial opportunities for entrepreneurs.[5]

Exploring the buying and selling of patent medicines by veterans complicates the story of the war's financial legacy. On the one hand, opiate addiction literally cost some veterans dearly. The various monetary expenses of addiction—ranging from money needed to purchase opiates to indirect costs like lost pensions and wages—ultimately proved a severe financial burden for many veterans. On the other hand, the burgeoning addiction epidemic opened up new commercial opportunities for savvy veterans. The inventors of patent medicine addiction cures, often veterans themselves, drew on their soldiering experiences and intimate knowledge of the health problems that plagued veterans. Ultimately, the brisk trade in patent medicine remedies illuminates the capricious financial legacy of military service. Although many soldiers were driven to the brink of poverty by addiction and other war-related disabilities, others became rich off their comrades' suffering. This pattern also seems to have been replicated in other niche industries spawned or stimulated by the Civil War, such as prosthetic limbs, undertaking, and pension law.[6]

The postwar growth of the patent medicine industry also illuminates how practitioners of "alternative" medicine responded to the veterans' opiate addiction epidemic and the Civil War more broadly. Most medical histories of the Civil War have focused more on physicians than other medical practitioners. Yet unorthodox medicine was big business in the Gilded Age. Between the Civil War and the Progressive Era, there were relatively few regulations on medical commodities or the practice of medicine. Patent medicine sellers abounded, and their wares commanded a huge segment of the American medical marketplace. Evaluating how the Civil War affected veterans or American medicine must consider patent medicines, because addicted men were as likely to turn to a patent medicine as to a physician. Poor veterans, who could not readily afford large medical bills for extended home care or patronize costly inebriety clinics, seemed especially likely to opt for patent medicines. Although some former soldiers were left unsatisfied, many consumers swore that addiction remedies worked in a clinical sense, perhaps because some brands secretly contained morphine. Testimonials by satisfied customers often hyperbolized the effectiveness of patent medicines, but some consumers may indeed have found that consuming morphine-laced remedies could prevent withdrawal.

Scrutinizing how patent medicines were marketed reveals the strategies adopted by some clever veterans to mitigate and even reverse the damages of opium addiction. Patent medicines were often marketed through long-form testimonials. These narratives flip the typical doctor-patient script seen in pension records and asylum case histories, which tended to describe the body and narrate the actions of drug users from physicians' (often hostile) perspectives. In contrast, patent medicine testimonials enabled veterans to help tell their addiction stories and to do so with a degree of empathy and agency. Certainly, testimonials tended to be embellished and even sensationalized by the proprietors of the products being hawked. Despite their claims to the contrary, patent medicine sellers often solicited (with and without compensation), altered, and sometimes made up testimonials. We can assume that sellers refrained from publishing customer complaints that would have presented "cures" as ineffective or not worth the expense. After all, the goal was to move merchandise. Rather than seeking to benevolently repair damaged reputations, patent medicine sellers were more interested in using veterans as props to support claims of therapeutic efficacy.

Yet opportunities remained for veterans to contest the social damages of addiction. Patent medicine testimonials, when approached critically, can powerfully illuminate veterans' strategies for allaying the stigma surrounding opiate use. Testimonialists invariably portrayed themselves (with an editor's help) as overcoming addiction, much like the evangelical conversion narratives so popular during the nineteenth century. If one converted to Christianity to overcome sin and save the soul, a man could also take patent medicines to emancipate his body from opium slavery and restore the self.[7] Physicians tended to structure case histories around "failures"—that is, addicted people's alleged moral and physical weakness—whereas patent medicine testimonials took the opposite approach by offering up accounts of redemption. Testimonials printed in nationally circulated newspapers and pamphlets served as public venues for performing one's "delivery" from addiction and reclaiming lost manhood and morality. Ironically, narrating their redemption required testimonialists to repeat and implicitly endorse pernicious stereotypes about "opium slaves," so as to situate one's present recovery against a past life of addiction. Thus, testimonials might have benefited individual veterans, but writ large, these narratives ultimately reinforced negative perceptions about drug users. The entire patent medicine addiction "cure" industry depended on Americans' continued belief that substance use needed to be overcome.[8]

The Patent Medicine Industry in the Civil War Era

Patent medicines were pharmaceutical remedies marketed to Americans as do-it-yourself treatments for all manner of medical ailments. Ironically, the remedies were rarely patented, because to do so required proprietors to disclose their products' secret, often dangerous ingredients. Some of the most popular nineteenth-century brands, like Mrs. Winslow's Soothing Syrup and Dr. M'Munn's Elixir of Opium, contained opiates, a fact that was widely known in the Civil War era. For this reason, patent medicines occasionally came under fire in the press as the culprits behind fatal opiate overdoses.[9] Yet despite their dangers, patent medicines were a popular avenue for self-medication, often standing in for physicians. Because many contained opiates as active ingredients, the remedies often proved efficacious against pain, diarrhea, and coughing, which served to reinforce consumers' confidence in patent medicines and increased sales. The products also allowed for medical care in the privacy and comfort of one's home, as opposed to the care provided in public facilities like mental asylums.

Although the antebellum trade in patent medicine was brisk, the industry reached dizzying new heights after the Civil War. On war's eve in 1859, patent medicine sales in the United States stood at about $3.5 million annually. During the Gilded Age—the golden age of patent medicines—new "specifics" and "nostrums," pejorative terms for patent medicines, flooded the medical marketplace and sales skyrocketed. Little to no regulation of the medical marketplace meant that enterprising patent medicine proprietors could successfully advertise their wares as "cures" for practically any ailment under the sun. By 1900, sick Americans could choose from nearly 6,000 brands, and the patent medicine sector had matured into a $74 million-per-year industry.[10]

Alongside other factors in the mid-nineteenth century—increased commercialization in American health care, the expansion of print media and advertising, and decreased shipping and postal costs—the Civil War's long-lasting health consequences amplified demand for medical commodities. The war also led to an influx of novel ailments, prompting the development of innovative treatments. Products like artificial limbs and patent medicines were popular among disabled veterans as they sought to live up to ablest cultural expectations. This new demand fueled the patent medicine industry's meteoric growth, as new inventors entered the market and existing patent medicine makers expanded their sales, targeting veterans.[11]

Opiate-addicted veterans thus represented a significant niche customer base for novel medical remedies. Indeed, before the Civil War led to increased demand for addiction remedies, patent medicine opiate addiction cures were universal commercial failures. In late 1859, Henry Zell, a New York City butcher who apparently lacked any formal medical credentials, invented Dr. Zell's Temperance Powders, a patent medicine that he claimed could "set drunkards against liquor, opium and other narcotics." Zell's product was the first patent medicine for drug addiction in American history. To cure their husbands' addictions, Zell suggested, long-suffering wives could slip the powders into their unsuspecting husbands' tea. Hoping to rustle up sales for the product, Zell placed at least a dozen advertisements in the *New-York Daily Tribune*, the *New York Herald*, and the *Sun* between October and December 1859. Although antebellum New Yorkers were no strangers to opiate addiction—as evidenced by sporadic reports about opium eating in the city's newspapers or the high number of overdose deaths in coroners' records—Dr. Zell's Temperance Powders soon flopped as a cure for opiate addiction. Insufficient demand and poor marketing explain the product's demise. In the antebellum era, most opiate-addicted Americans were women, but Zell marketed his temperance powders as a cure for men's addictions. Evidently facing lackluster sales, Zell retooled his patent medicine in the winter of 1859–60. He omitted references to opium from advertisements and began marketing the medicine solely as a remedy for alcohol abuse.[12] However, within a decade of Zell's commercial failure, the Civil War helped stimulate enough demand to sustain a legion of addiction remedies like those of Zell.

In the Civil War's wake, patent medicine addiction cures proliferated. The caustically anti-patent medicine physician J. B. Mattison lamented in 1886 that one could measure the spread of addiction "by citing the number of individuals engaged in vending the various nostrums" that purported to be "the one genuine, sovereign cure for this phase of human ill."[13] Similar comments were echoed by various doctors and medical bodies throughout the postwar decades. The Massachusetts Board of Health observed in its 1872 report on the opium habit that "among the most dangerous preparations of morphia are those now prescribed and sold by uneducated or villainous individuals as so-called 'cures' for persons afflicted with the uncontrollable appetite for opium." The "very existence of such nostrums certainly indicates the extent of the disease" and its rapid increase, the board concluded.[14] The cures were so prolifically advertised, "so persistently . . . kept before the public," according to a writer in *Frank Leslie's Popular Monthly*, "that a stranger might seriously ask himself whether the mania for the drug be not as strong in this civilized country as in China."[15] Supposed addiction cures were eventually bought and sold in every corner of the United States by both Union and Confederate veterans. Of course, disabled older soldiers were not the only Gilded Age Americans to suffer from opiate addiction. Patent medicines for addiction had broad appeal among Americans of all demographics, reflecting the wide reach of addiction during the late nineteenth century. Yet veterans represented an especially important market segment, which pointed up the heightened visibility of addiction among veterans. Their plight helped inspire the development of the two most successful Gilded Age patent medicine opiate addiction cures.

The first commercially successful patent medicine for opiate addiction was invented by Samuel B. Collins, a La Porte, Indiana, bricklayer and veteran of the 48th Indiana Infantry regiment. Collins launched his product in the Civil War's immediate aftermath, not long after leaving the army, where he had perhaps witnessed how sick and wounded soldiers were treated with opiates, which sometimes fostered addiction. Collins possessed a shrewd and opportunistic business mind. Sensing a commercial opportunity in the postwar surge in addiction and demand for addiction remedies, he invented—or "discovered," as he often claimed—the Painless Opium Antidote in 1868. It appears to have been the first patent medicine opiate addiction cure brought to market after the Civil War. Not only was the remedy developed by a veteran, but ailing soldiers were also some of the first adopters of the antidote. Their praise for Collins's remedy contributed significantly to the product's early commercial success. Joseph Darrow, formerly of the 4th Michigan Infantry, began taking the antidote in April 1869, a few months after the product hit the market. By November 1869 "he was pronounced cured," according to the local justice of the peace, whose affidavit featured heavily in Collins's early advertisements.[16] Another veteran, Newell Gleason, formerly a colonel of the 87th Indiana Infantry who was promoted to brevet general after a heroic performance at Chattanooga, also endorsed Collins's product early on. Gleason's name appeared in a list of references in an 1872 pamphlet for the Painless Opium Antidote. Gleason and Collins both lived in La Porte, so it is possible that the men knew each other well. Gleason had been given opiates by a Union captain during the war and subsequently became addicted. By publicly backing Collins's product, Gleason not only attested to the remedy's efficacy but also provided the name recognition and goodwill attendant to a war hero's endorsement.[17]

Convinced there could be an even greater demand for his Painless Opium Antidote, Collins embarked on a nationwide advertising blitz during the early 1870s. He placed classified advertisements in scores of newspapers and magazines during the Gilded Age and rounded out his campaign with often-unsolicited postcards and flyers sent through the mail. Collins targeted as many demographics as he could think of: women and men, young and old, and veteran and nonveteran alike. Within a few years, sales of the antidote skyrocketed as suggested by Collins's prolific advertising throughout the 1870s and 1880s. During these decades, one could hardly scan the back pages of any major newspaper or magazine without encountering an advertisement for the antidote. For example, in 1879, Collins placed an advertisement in nearly every issue of *Frank Leslie's Illustrated Newspaper*, forty-nine times altogether (fig. 7.1). Such widespread and long-running advertising suggests that Collins attained a considerable degree of sales for his Painless Opium Antidote, otherwise Collins would likely have rebranded his product, like Henry Zell, or simply given up and ceased advertising altogether. After catching readers' eyes with his various advertisements, Collins invited would-be customers to correspond with him, rewarding their interest with a pamphlet replete with satisfied customers' testimonials for the Painless Opium Antidote, including many by formerly addicted veterans like Joseph Darrow.

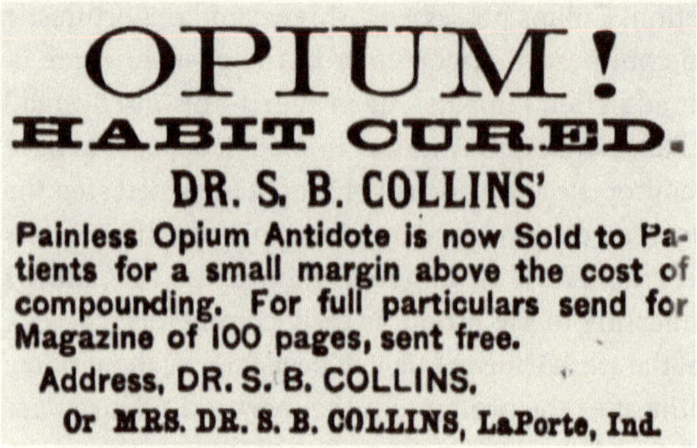

> **OPIUM!**
> **HABIT CURED.**
> **DR. S. B. COLLINS'**
> Painless Opium Antidote is now Sold to Patients for a small margin above the cost of compounding. For full particulars send for Magazine of 100 pages, sent free.
> Address, DR. S. B. COLLINS,
> Or MRS. DR. S. B. COLLINS, LaPorte, Ind.

Figure 7.1 Classified advertisement for Samuel B. Collins's Painless Opium Antidote in *Frank Leslie's Illustrated Newspaper*, August 23, 1879, 419.

Pamphlets were a cornerstone of Collins's commercial success and provide unique insight into the mindset of seller and buyer. In an era before medical regulation or government assurances of product safety, customer testimonials served a vital purpose in the patent medicine industry. Customers had little other recourse for determining a patent medicine's efficacy. Collins, recognizing customers' dependency on testimonials, loaded his pamphlets full of glowing customer references. The sources thus provide a unique window into Collins's business, illustrating both the mechanics of buying, selling, and using the cures and the unique strategies used by Collins to reach various segments of his customer base, such as Civil War veterans. *Theriaki*, Collins's main pamphlet, positively flew off the press, going through several editions with various subtitles during the 1860s, 1870s, and 1880s. The title of the pamphlet was a transliteration of *thériaki*, a French term for opium eaters; the title may also have reminded readers of theriac, a famed medieval panacea comprised of luxury ingredients like opium. Collins's advertisements thus exhibited an air of exoticism, a common advertising technique in Gilded Age America.[18] Collins also used scientific imagery to lend an air of credibility and respectability to the Painless Opium Antidote. Pamphlets included various sections designed to educate would-be customers on the natural history of opium and raise awareness of the alarming health consequences of opium addiction. He also adopted the style and organization of the era's medical journals. Perhaps more impressive to ordinary customers, Collins described his business office in La Porte as a "laboratory" and often styled himself as a "doctor," despite lacking formal medical credentials (a common practice in the Gilded Age).

Theriaki also informed would-be customers how they could go about obtaining and using the Painless Opium Antidote. Collins instructed customers to mail him a letter describing their regular dose of opium, morphine, or laudanum, as well as a detailed description of their symptoms, bodily constitution, and the length of time that they had suffered from addiction. This information supposedly enabled Collins to formulate a dose of the antidote that was tailored specifically to each patient; this strategy reflected the mid-nineteenth-century notion that individuals' unique constitutions required tailored medical remedies, not one-size-fits-all dosing. Collins typically charged about $25 for a month's supply of the Painless Opium Antidote, which was the minimum order. Vials arrived by mail at customers' homes in a specially sealed bottles wrapped in an unmarked package. In return for this steep fee, the antidote would bring about what Collins claimed was "a certain and a perfect cure accomplished without pain and without inconvenience" in the privacy of one's home, therefore avoiding the prying eyes of neighbors.[19]

Collins made a fortune from his patent medicine business. Immediately before the Civil War, he appeared in the 1860 census as a mason possessing no real property.[20] A decade later, after serving in the Union army and founding his nascent patent medicine business, Collins appeared in the 1870 census as a "physician" worth $2,500 dollars—a stunning financial windfall considering he had founded his patent medicine business only two years before.[21] The 1880 census does not enumerate Collins's personal wealth or property, but judging by his standing in his local community, he became very wealthy from his business venture. As Jasper Packard, a local resident, remarked in 1876, "The pecuniary returns of Dr. Collins have been commensurate with the importance of his discovery."[22] To conspicuously display his wealth, Collins purchased or built a massive Victorian mansion, and to house his growing business, Collins erected a striking three-story building with a handsome marble facade in downtown La Porte.[23] The walls bore a billboard hawking the Painless Opium Antidote, and the upper floor housed the laboratory where the product was made. Collins, seemingly with a mind toward enhancing his standing in the community, built up goodwill among his neighbors by donating the lower level of his laboratory building to serve as the town library and by funding local GAR Memorial Day parades. This strategy seemed to pay dividends. As the town chronicler put it in 1876, Collins "spends his means freely among the people where he toiled as a laborer" before the Civil War "and has met and still continues to receive his just reward."[24] There is nothing in the historical record to suggest that Collins achieved his financial success through any enterprise other than the Painless Opium Antidote. Thus, for him, a savvy businessperson with intimate knowledge of veterans' health problems, the Civil War proved to be a rare financial boon—the kind of once-in-a-lifetime windfall that Gilded Age rags-to-riches stories idealized.

The possibility of such spectacular commercial success soon attracted opportunistic competitors. By the mid-1870s, Collins faced stiff competition, as other patent medicine inventors brought a host of similar products to market. The most successful of the lot was Leslie E. Keeley's Double Chloride of Gold, widely known as the Gold Cure, although it contained no gold.[25] Keeley had been a contract surgeon for the Union army. "During the war, and in an active practice since then," Keeley explained in 1881, "I have been favored with many opportunities for successfully observing opium cases." Observation of addicted soldiers convinced Keeley that slavery to opiates and alcohol was, at its core, a disease of the body, rather than simply a personal failing on the part of addicted people. With this medicalized approach to addiction as an intellectual foundation, Keeley concocted the Gold Cure, which, he claimed, treated the physical causes of alcohol and opiate addiction. He achieved unparalleled commercial success selling the Gold Cure during the final two decades of the nineteenth century, even surpassing that of Collins's Painless Opium Antidote. Advertising nationwide in periodicals, pamphlets, and even specially commissioned sheet music, Keeley ultimately sold the Gold Cure to half a million Americans between 1880 and 1920. Many of these customers sought relief for drunkenness, and this element of Keeley's business has been historians' primary interest. But the Gold Cure was widely known in its day as a remedy for the opium habit as well.[26]

Aside from simple demand, the most important reason underpinning Keeley's commercial success was his strategy of developing the use of the Gold Cure into a temperance-style movement. He developed a kind of social club, the "Keeley League," to help drive up use of the Gold Cure and encouragement for customers, and scores of franchised "Keeley Institutes" sprang up around the country, where customers received in-patient treatment with the Gold Cure in conjunction with an early version of group therapy. These Keeley Institutes aped the inebriety clinics that had become increasingly popular since the 1870s, a phenomenon investigated in chapter 8.[27]

Even the military and the GAR embraced Keeley's cause. In 1892, the NHDVS founded a Keeley League to treat opiate- and alcohol-addicted veterans in Leavenworth, Kansas. By 1894, thirty opiate-addicted veterans had received the Gold Cure at the facility on the government's dime, including William H. Hughes, the Union veteran living at the NHDVS during the 1890s whose case appears in chapter 6. Veteran Gold Cure devotees took it upon themselves to found "Keeley Leagues" at several NHDVS branches, receiving praise and support from NHDVS officials. The GAR also endorsed the gospel of Keeley. In fact, "too much praise cannot be given" to soldiers' homes that offered the Gold Cure, one GAR official reported in 1893.[28] For his part, Keeley used these glowing endorsements to boost sales. The NHDVS Keeley Leagues featured prominently in advertising for the Gold Cure. In 1897, for example, an advertisement in the California newspaper *Daily Morning Union* proclaimed in bold print that the "Keeley Cure for Drunkenness[;] The Opium, Morphine and Tobacco habits and Neurasthenia is Indorsed [*sic*] by the US Government and used in the National and State Homes for Disabled Soldiers." To skeptical customers, Keeley reasoned, "What suits Uncle Sam should suit you." His relationship with the NHDVS was a major factor in Keeley's commercial success.[29]

By the 1880s, Americans had only to skim the classifieds in their preferred newspaper to spot advertisements for various brands of patent medicine opiate addiction cures. The *Chicago Tribune*, for example, hawked not only Collins's Painless Opium Antidote and Keeley's Gold Cure but also remedies invented by the city's own Clesson Pratt, H. H. Kane of New York City, W. B. Squire of Indiana, Carlos Bruisard of Cincinnati, and Mark M. Thompson of Chicago, whose Bichloride of Gold blatantly aped Keeley's Gold Cure. Americans could choose among no fewer than thirty brands of opiate addiction cures by 1900. Such widespread advertising suggests that the cures appealed to a great number of people. Indeed, a wide demographic spectrum of Gilded Age Americans suffered from opiate addiction and resorted to patent addiction cures.[30] The mass appeal of such cures underscores how the veterans' addiction epidemic was but one sliver of a larger opioid crisis with diverse causes that extended beyond the Civil War—especially unregulated capitalism that allowed addictive drugs (and their "cures") to circulate widely.

Veterans of the "late war," however, represented one of the most prominent demographics targeted by the proprietors of patent medicine opiate addiction cures. Not only did Collins's and Keeley's Civil War experiences help inspire the two most successful cures, but veterans also provided a key market segment for the products. Many brands explicitly targeted Civil War veterans through advertisements in veterans' periodicals, including the *National Tribune*, the unofficial organ of the GAR. Medical products in high demand among aging and disabled veterans—wheelchairs, prosthetics, and patent remedies for impotence, consumption, and general debility—were some of the *National Tribune*'s most consistently advertised products, and opiate cures were among the most prominent of these. The *Tribune* ran its first advertisement for an opiate addiction cure in May 1883. Dr. F. E. March of Quincy, Michigan, promised to cure veterans of the opium and morphine habits in under a month, with "no pay till cured." His classified advertisement ran alongside others hawking a cure for hemorrhoids, a book of addresses of former army surgeons geared toward pension applicants, and the services of a pension lawyer—all items of equally great interest to soldiers.

Advertisements for opiate addiction cures were staples of veterans' periodicals in the Gilded Age. The *National Tribune* ran hundreds of advertisements for patent opiate addiction cures between 1883 and 1911. A host of proprietors and brands used the periodical to reach out to Union veterans. Advertisers included, among many others, Keeley, M. C. Benham, the Humane Remedy Co., and H. H. Kane, an elite New York City physician who dabbled in patent medicines while simultaneously conducting more mainstream scientific and medical research. Dr. J. Stephens of Lebanon, Ohio, placed at least 120 advertisements for his brand of patent medicine addiction cures during the 1880s and 1890s. Such fierce competition for veteran customers sometimes inspired patent medicine vendors to develop innovative marketing strategies. For example, in 1907, Dr. H. C. Keith of Toledo dared veterans to test the effectiveness of his remedy, offering a handsome payout of $1,000 for any case of opiate addiction he could not cure. In many issues of the *National Tribune*, veterans could spot advertisements for several competing brands on the same page. *Confederate Veteran*, a magazine for former Confederates, also prominently featured advertisements for various opiate addiction cures. In one classified, the Wilson Chemical Company of Dublin, Texas, sought to sway addicted Confederate veterans with endorsements from "physicians, ministers and soldiers."[31]

As the industry expanded during the 1870s and 1880s, several former Confederates launched their own brands of patent medicine cures. One entrepreneurial Southern physician, Basil M. Woolley, formerly a private in the hard-fighting 51st Alabama Partisan Rangers, ironically named his brand the "American Opium Antidote," a testament to sectional reconciliation. Woolley ran his brisk trade in patent medicines out of Atlanta, the quintessential New South city, and his company was exactly the type of innovative commercial operation that boosters hoped to attract so the South could recover from the Civil War's lingering economic damages.[32]

Atlanta also boasted the business operation of John Stith Pemberton, a former Confederate cavalryman–turned-pharmacist who invented the patent medicine Coca-Cola in 1886. It was the precursor to the famed soft drink. Pemberton had been wounded by a saber cut during the war. According to a popular myth, Pemberton became addicted to painkilling morphine and created the cocaine-laced, but alcohol-free, "temperance drink" Coca-Cola to "cure" his addiction. Cocaine was sometimes used to treat opiate addiction, and Pemberton did market Coca-Cola "to the unfortunate who are addicted to the morphine or opium habit." But there is no contemporary evidence to support the notion that Pemberton was himself a morphine user. The allegation that Pemberton was a "drug fiend" first surfaced during a 1916 trial over the ownership of the Coca-Cola brand, decades after Pemberton's death in 1888 from stomach cancer. Regardless, Woolley's and Pemberton's successful businesses illustrate the national reach of the patent medicine industry in the Gilded Age, as well as the broad geographic spread and widespread recognition of the opiate addiction epidemic.[33]

Even Perry Bowser got in on the craze. In 1877, Bowser wrote to President Ulysses Grant seeking assistance in obtaining a pension increase, which the ailing man needed "badly" even decades before being outed as a morphine user by the Pension Bureau in the 1890s. Bowser scrawled his missive on paper bearing the letterhead of "Dr. P. B. Bowser, Proprietor Opium and Liquor Antidote." The paper claimed the remedy was "the ONLY Sure Cure ever discovered for this Terrible Habit," although the product seems to have done Bowser little good, given that he ultimately died from "chronic morphinism" in 1915.[34]

Placing classified advertisements in veterans' periodicals was merely the first step to attracting veteran customers. Most patent medicine proprietors sought to initiate correspondence with addicted veterans, hoping that such communication would culminate in veterans thumbing through full-length advertising pamphlets. These booklets, first introduced by Samuel B. Collins, were replete with testimonials written by Civil War veterans. Such testimonials usually consisted of first-person narratives describing how the veteran author became addicted as well as the great personal toll of opium slavery in his life. The pamphlets also usually included the names and places of residence for the authors of testimonials in case would-be customers wanted to hear about the efficacy of the product in question directly from fellow soldiers.

Anatomy of a Testimonial

Testimonials written on behalf of patent medicine addiction cures provide a unique window into the phenomenon of opiate addiction among Civil War veterans, illuminating veterans' perspectives on opiate addiction and how men sought to contest its consequences. Testimonials hint at what veterans hoped to obtain through the act of consuming patent medicines, as well as how users felt about addiction itself. William H. Chappell, a veteran of the 3rd and 26th Alabama Infantry regiments, furnished Samuel B. Collins with a roughly three-page narrative testimonial in March 1874. Hoping to catch the eye of veterans with experiences similar to Chappell's story, Collins titled the narrative "The Experience of One Redeemed—His Gratitude Expressed" and printed it in an 1874 promotional pamphlet for the Painless Opium Antidote. Chappell's testimonial is representative of the genre, standing in for the numerous stories shared by Civil War veterans on behalf of their preferred brand of patent medicine addiction cures. Many of the elements in Chappell's narrative were mirrored in other veterans' testimonials, including the origin of one's opiate addiction, the dire health and emotional consequences stemming from opium slavery, and, above all, the utility of patent medicines as a tool to heal oneself from addiction and reverse its negative consequences.[35]

Severely wounded at the Battle of Nashville in December 1864, Chappell suffered through a painful amputation of his left leg above the knee. Army surgeons gave the soldier opium to mitigate the pain, the standard of care in many wartime hospitals. "The use of those remedies" during his five-month convalescence at the hospital saved his life, Chappell wrote, but was "followed by the most unhappy results." His amputation did not fully heal but continued to eject "specula of bone" for three years. Suffering from intense chronic pain, Chappell "could get no relief save by using opium." By the time the final bone fragment at last worked its way out of his flesh, as Chappell tortuously described, "my system was completely under the influence of the drug, so that without it, I could not attend to any business." When the wound healed, Chappell attempted to discontinue the opium, believing he no longer needed it to manage the pain. But after years of swallowing some thirty grains of opium and morphine daily, Chappell found himself unable to quit. Each time he attempted to leave off the drugs, his will was overpowered by excruciating withdrawal symptoms, and he was forced to abandon his efforts.[36]

Opium became to Chappell "a tyrant . . . binding me in chains, from which, it seemed to me, no human power could free me." He dreaded his bleak prospects: facing the unbearable pains of withdrawal unaided, which would likely fail again, or continuing to take opiates, but risking a fatal overdose from the ever-increasing dose needed to counteract his body's mounting tolerance of the drugs. Over the next eight years, Chappell tried repeatedly to quit opiates, invariably failing each time, until a chance encounter with a pharmacist in 1874 changed the veteran's fortunes. Out of sympathy for Chappell's condition, so the narrative explained, the pharmacist passed along a copy of Samuel B. Collins's latest pamphlet for the Painless Opium Antidote. "From the moment of reading your magazine, and the numerous testimonials therein," Chappell testified, "I felt the Lord . . . was about to save me from that terrible fate" of fatally overdosing. The Lord and Collins, that is. As Chappell concluded in the narrative's climax: "Deliverance has come, thank God; and to your opium antidote." Chappell purchased a two-month supply of antidote by mail for $50, which cured him "from the thralldom of that enemy which well nigh proved my ruin." Chappell concluded his testimonial by urging other "opium slaves" to waste no time in purchasing Collins's Painless Opium Antidote and, pointedly, expressing his wishes that Collins share his story. For, as Chappell modestly phrased it, "Write this testimony (yea, a more impressive one if possible), in letters of fire and hand it in the heavens for a world to read." Chappell signed his testimonial and listed his residence, a measure intended to assure readers of the story's veracity.[37]

Scores of Civil War veterans shared similar testimonials on behalf of their favorite addiction cures, mirroring the plot and narrative elements of Chappell's account. Naturally, proprietors likely edited testimonials heavily to accentuate claims of clinical efficacy. Collins actively solicited testimonials from veterans and other satisfied customers and swore they were bona fide, even offering a $500 reward payable to any critic who could prove that a testimonial was fraudulent. Yet, because testimonials were created to serve a specific purpose—to sell patent medicines by testifying to their effectiveness in treating opiate addiction—it is hard to imagine that Collins fully resisted the temptation to edit and embellish. The use of these testimonials by historians requires a critical eye, especially concerning claims that patent medicines "cured" addiction. Still, we need not dismiss these sources as unvaluable. Many of the details provided in testimonials can be corroborated in veterans' military service records, lending plausibility to some of the feelings and experiences reported by such veterans as Chappell. For example, Chappell's military record indicates that he spent time as a hospital steward during the Civil War—a position that would likely have given him reliable access to opiates, potentially facilitating addiction, as he described in the narrative published by Collins. The conversion-style script enacted by Chappell also reveals how he and other veterans internalized the stigma of addiction, even as they sought to mitigate its social damage.[38] By filtering out the overt salesmanship injected by Collins into Chappell's story, his and other veterans' testimonials can speak to various facets of addiction absent or obscured from other sources.

Taken together, testimonials emphasize several common elements of opium slavery as experienced by veterans. They illuminate the emotional component of opiate addiction, a theme that comes through less clearly in sources authored by physicians or Pension Bureau agents. Testimonialists also called attention to the various health consequences of addiction, including fatigue, severe weight loss, and impotence, which collectively added up to feelings of hopelessness and despair on the part of addicted men. J. M. Richards, an Illinois veteran, wrote on behalf of Keeley's Gold Cure in 1881 describing his physical suffering when addicted. "I felt that to die and go to hell would involve less torment than that I was suffering every day," Richards reported. "I was emaciated, pallid, weak in body, and my strength of will and energy of mind were all gone." A former Union surgeon, John J. Patterson, suffered a similar experience with addiction, as he testified on behalf of Collins's Painless Opium Antidote. "My wife would get up at all hours of the night and use the syringe on me," Patterson reported. "My health was so poor that I was confined to my room, and at last to my bed. I could not eat until I used the morphine. My nervous system was a total wreck. . . . I was a walking skeleton; no appetite; low spirits."[39] William Chappell's narrative also suggests a sense of hopelessness stemming from the realization that one could not quit taking opium or morphine at will. This realization must have been humbling, and even embarrassing, considering that self-mastery constituted an essential component of manhood in the Civil War era. As Chappell explained, opium dependent men were "like myself . . . fully conscious of the evil effects it will ultimately bring unless abandoned."[40]

Along with an intimate view of the emotional and physical experiences of opiate addiction, a close reading of veterans' testimonials illuminates their reasons for purchasing patent medicines, namely, the cures provided them a relatively straightforward solution for the health and social consequences of opiate addiction. Many users seemed to have wholeheartedly believed that patent medicines could be clinically effective in healing one's body from addiction. Nineteenth-century American medical consumers often retained vestiges of a premodern, "magical" understanding of health that allowed considerable intellectual and spiritual space for secret panaceas to be effective at healing sickness, as historian T. J. Jackson Lears observes.[41] Benjamin F. Sawyer, formerly a lieutenant colonel in the 24th Alabama Infantry, explained after consuming one remedy, "The result was successful—almost magical."[42] Patent medicines did not necessarily seem dubious to all nineteenth-century consumers, although many skeptics rejected exaggerated claims of clinical effectiveness.

Not only could patent medicines potentially cure one's addiction, according to many consumers, but the testimonials central to the marketing of patent medicines also provided veterans with a unique venue for reclaiming manhood and restoring reputations. There was a performative aspect to testimonials, which allowed authors to style themselves as having been redeemed from the ravages of opium slavery. In this sense, testimonials mirrored Christian salvation narratives, in which nineteenth-century authors described their past sins so as to underscore their divine salvation from sin.[43] Veterans who produced testimonials on behalf of Samuel B. Collins, Leslie E. Keeley, or Basil M. Woolley likewise hoped to use advertising pamphlets like *Theriaki* to publicly proclaim that they had renounced the opium habit and had been redeemed to manhood and good character. By confessing their addictions in a testimonial form while also narrating their delivery from opiates, veterans framed addiction as an experience of the past from which they had been delivered. They were enslaved no more but were cured of addiction and thereby restored to health and manhood. In fact, some veterans even used religious imagery to describe their deliverance from opium slavery. William H. Chappell concluded his narrative with a "prayer of deepest gratitude to God for saving me," exclaiming that "deliverance has come, thank God." This language would have resonated with devout readers, especially those who were steeped in temperance literature, which often framed sobriety as a divine transformation. The titles of addiction narratives and patent medicine pamphlets would also have resonated with readers who were familiar with slave narratives like those authored by Frederick Douglass.[44]

The decision to author a public testimonial was not an act that veterans took lightly. Freely admitting one's opiate addiction and thereby exposing one's ostensibly shameful private struggles with drug abuse to public scrutiny stood in marked contrast to the behavior of most opiate users, whose drug dependence remained a closely guarded "concealed practice," as a Gilded Age physician observed.[45] Writing a testimonial was by no means without risks, but veterans braved doing so because providing such on behalf of a respectable patent medicine brand presented a rare opportunity for men to parry criticism of their manhood and moral fiber. Few other means were open to veterans who wished to tell their side of the story, as underscored by addicted Union veterans' fraught struggles to convince the US Pension Bureau to award pensions after evidence of "vicious habits" emerged. Veterans who narrated their stories in testimonials often signed their names, thereby inviting public scrutiny and, potentially, condemnation from critics. Veterans would have put considerable thought into the decision to write public testimonials. Considering the risks involved, the rhetoric espoused by veterans in their addiction narratives should be taken seriously, not overlooked as a mere advertising strategy of patent medicine sellers.

By publicly enacting their redemption from opium slavery, veterans hoped that testimonials would raise their stature among readers. This hope is evident in the exaggerated claims of transformation made by veterans in their narratives. A. W. Henley, a former Confederate surgeon, confessed that in the army he "took Opium, and Opium wound and bound me up with cords that God only knows how often I tried to break, and as many times failed." But Woolley's American Opium Cure changed him, giving him "a new lease on life." The patent medicine enabled him to transform himself by quitting the habit, and "today," Henley wrote, "I am in perfect health, rejoicing in perfect freedom" from opium slavery. A Texas veteran, Byron McKeen, likewise praised Collins's Painless Opium Antidote for allowing for the rejuvenation of his body and manhood. Whereas before taking Collins's antidote, McKeen had been lost, "To-day, I am one week old, and feel like a new human being—no longer a slave to that miserable Opium," he proudly proclaimed. The transformation was dramatic, the veteran explained; he had even gained weight. Joseph Darrow likewise became "addicted" to the condemnable "habit of using Morphine" in 1863, which he deeply regretted. But his self-control was restored by Collins's antidote. Indeed, "since Nov. 15th [1869]," according to Darrow's testimonial, he "has had Morphine at his command, with no necessity or desire to use it." These transformation narratives stressed how veterans had not only been physically cured of opiate addiction but had also redeemed their physical and mental virility, self-control, and, by extension, their manhood and moral fiber.[46]

Testimonials were inherently public facing, meant to be read by potential customers and other curious eyes. Veterans counted on it, hoping their neighbors and colleagues would be swayed by the intensely emotional narratives. Indeed, after freeing themselves from opium slavery by consuming patent medicines, testimonialists often described being positively received in their communities. As George W. Kirk, formerly of the 19th Indiana Infantry, recounted, "I was wounded in 1862, in a skirmish at Lebanon Junction, and ever since have carried in my thigh as a memento of that day, a half ounce of cold lead. To allay in some measure the pain which I suffered, opium was prescribed by the surgeon in charge." Soon, Kirk became addicted, and by "August 1871—I was barely able to walk—not able to set up to exceed two hours a day." But after taking Collins's Painless Opium Antidote, Kirk explained, "I rapidly gained strength—so rapidly that my friends all noticed, and remarked the change."[47] Clearly, some veterans were eager to display their transformation and for friends and neighbors to celebrate their recovery. When testimonials received national circulation, it was all the better, because widely circulated columns offered an expanded public platform for reclaiming one's manhood.

While difficult to determine conclusively, offering their testimonials may have made it easier for opiate-using veterans to secure pensions. Darrow applied for a pension under the Dependent Pension Act, declaring that his chronic rheumatism and general debility were "not due to vicious habits." On medical examination in March 1892, doctors found heart disease, physical weakness, and missing teeth, but no evidence of substance use, so Darrow received a pension of ten dollars a month. According to the public record, the veteran was known to be a former morphine user, but perhaps his testimonial for the Painless Opium Antidote provided persuasive enough evidence that Darrow had quit using morphine for surgeons to feel comfortable signing off. Yet unknown to the Pension Bureau, Darrow was either still using morphine, or he very quickly resumed taking the drug after his medical exam. He was "found dead in bed" from a morphine overdose at the Michigan Soldiers' Home in March 1893. Even if morphine ultimately killed him, Darrow had managed to claim a pension. Addicted veterans who had not so publicly narrated their redemption stories were less fortunate in securing pensions.[48]

Poverty and Opiate Addiction

Veterans' testimonials on behalf of patent medicine addiction cures also seem to have proved effective in drumming up sales, considering the rapid growth of the industry in the postwar decades. Countless veterans ultimately bought the cures during the Gilded Age—and for good reasons. Not only did opium slavery spell disaster for one's manhood, reputation, and physical health, but addiction also presented an extreme financial burden for many veterans, which led to and exacerbated poverty. The monetary costs of addiction, which encompassed direct expenses for medicines as well as indirect costs like lost wages, were unbearable for most addicted veterans. Consequently, the prospect of escaping poverty by freeing oneself from opium proved a powerful motivation for many veterans, who purchased and consumed patent medicine addiction cures to mitigate the financial burdens of addiction.

The financial costs of opiate addiction were immense for most addicted men. A few days' supply of opium, morphine, or laudanum was relatively inexpensive, but the costs added up over years, becoming more burdensome. Many users and observers also claimed that tolerance necessitated increasing the dosage consumed, and thus the amount of drug that was purchased, over time, raising costs. As one New York veteran reported in 1875, "The expense of laudanum to me for the past ten years has been very great." He claimed to have spent ten dollars a month to maintain his addiction, a figure adding up to $1,200 over a decade. Considering that the average New York farmer earned just $36.50 a month in 1875, the cost of laudanum would have likely taken up a large portion of the man's income, squeezing other necessities, such as food, clothing, and shelter, out of the family budget.[49] Pension money did little to ease the financial pressures of addiction. Many veterans' meager pensions failed to cover even basic living expenses, let alone the costs of opiate medicines. In 1889–90, the average Union veteran's pension was a mere $11.16 monthly, and Confederate state pensions were usually even smaller.[50] These payments often did not cover the costs of the opium or morphine that addicted veterans needed to consume to remain functional. Worse still, many veterans were also too physically disabled to work for a living, either from addiction itself or the disability for which opiates had originally been prescribed. Disability and addiction drove these men and their families into grinding, inescapable poverty. As the Virginian Alpheus M. Chappell explained in an 1887, "I have a wife and children to support and can't work." Chappell hoped his correspondent, a former Confederate general in Richmond, might intercede on his behalf and secure a one-time pension payout from the commonwealth. "I can't see General why the auditor don't pay me," Chappell explained, despite several veterans who had served under Chappell's command having already received pensions. Perhaps the stigma of addiction contributed to the denial of the captain's pension. "If you can do me any good General you will confer on me a great and lasting blessing," Chappell added, for "I can never want it worse than at this time." Thus, the various direct expenses of addiction tugged on already threadbare purses, exacerbating poverty among veterans and their families. All things considered, opiate addiction presented "a constant drain on their [users'] purses until the grave closed over them," according to an observer worried about opium eaters' long-term financial prospects.[51] Clearly, addiction presented a huge financial burden in many cases, amplifying the other negative outcomes of addiction.

Patent medicine addiction cures offered the tantalizing prospect of an escape from poverty, although in reality the products usually compounded already severe financial burdens of addiction. The $25 to $30 per month for several months that one needed to hand over when purchasing the cures could cost far more than the monthly cost of opiates needed to avoid withdrawal. Yet even in the face of desperate poverty, men opted to spend what little money they had on patent medicines, hoping and praying that the remedies would provide a quick path to freedom from opium slavery. Recovery meant that one might grow strong enough to work again or even secure a pension, highly attractive prospects for disabled veterans who considered patent medicines as being akin to an investment in one's health—a large expense in the short term, but one that brought the potential of financial solvency in the long term. Thomas Sweeting, a veteran of the 37th Georgia Infantry, described this mindset in an unpublished letter to J. L. Stephens, a former Union army surgeon who founded a patent medicine company in Lebanon, Ohio, in 1879.[52] The 1887 letter, which did not appear as a testimonial, captures Sweeting's raw desperation to be rid of the opium habit because of its harsh financial consequences:

> Dr. Stephens, sir, enclosed you will find $15 for a course of medicine for the cure of the opium habit and I guarantee you to pay you the other $10 dollars so soon as I am cured. Dear Sir, the reason why I did not send [the money] before is my daughter has been sick and to death and it was all together impossible for me to do so. Dear Sir, you can imagine my troubles for you know my state. Sometimes my children don't have a morsel to eat, and if I do get a shilling it has to go for laudanum. Sometimes it almost broke me down to see the wants of my family on account of almost one half of my earnings going for the drug. . . . Dear doctor do your best to get the medicine to me so that I may get on.[53]

Sweeting's despondency over his family's poverty is palpable, as is his willingness to try anything to escape his dire financial straits, which were exacerbated by the cost of laudanum. The budgetary constraints Sweeting described in his desperate letter, as well as his willingness to spend what little money he managed to scrape together on Stephens's remedy, underscores the financial disaster that opiate addiction represented for many veterans.

Customers were often so loyal to their favorite patent medicine brands, or at least the idea of curing oneself with a patent medicine, that they kept on purchasing the dubious remedies, despite overwhelming evidence that the products did not live up to the hype promised in pamphlets. J. T. B., for example, spent $1,800 on opiates and various brands of patent medicine cures for addiction over the course of his eighteen-year struggle. The fact that he experimented with so many different brands suggests that the idea of patent medicines was attractive, even if the individual brands ultimately proved disappointing. Perry B. Bowser, the Union veteran who tried for decades to secure a decent pension and spent his final years living at the NHDVS, protested to the Pension Bureau that "It takes me half my pension alone to supply me with morphine."[54] A New York veteran was admitted to the state's Willard Asylum for the Chronic Insane in September 1884 for melancholia, which the doctors attributed to the man's morphine, chloral, and tobacco habits. Upon entry to the asylum, the veteran "claimed he had several times been cured of his morphine habit by a 'Collins' Remedy' and that he had cured others." Despite the veteran's many relapses, he repeatedly bought and consumed doses of Collins's Painless Opium Antidote and even proselytized on Collins's behalf.[55] Such extreme customer loyalty presented a problem for the physicians who competed with patent medicine sellers in the Gilded Age medical marketplace.

It is possible that veterans' testimonials even swayed some doctors. L. M. Roundtree, a "respectable citizen" and former sergeant of the 59th Georgia Infantry living in eastern Georgia after the Civil War, suffered a gunshot to his thigh at Gettysburg. Roundtree lay in the hot sun on the sweltering battlefield, likely without medical attention, until he was captured on July 5, 1863, by Union soldiers and subsequently confined at Fort McHenry, Maryland. Until the war's end, the soldier remained in federal prisons, where he contracted dysentery, chronic diarrhea, and scurvy, which landed him in the hospital in the fall of 1863 and again in January 1865. Union surgeons would likely have given Roundtree morphine or opium for his many ailments, the standard of care even for captured rebels. Roundtree evidently became addicted to opium, because he turned to Dr. Tanner's Opium and Morphine Cure for help. The patent medicine was sold out of Atlanta for a dollar a bottle. Roundtree was pleased with the results, penning a short testimonial swearing that the patent medicine "cured me of the opium habit after everything, it seemed to me, had failed." The glowing testimonial by a leading member of the community was included in a classified advertisement for Dr. Tanner's Opium and Morphine Cure in local newspapers, where it evidently caught the eye of Charles A. Hentz, a former Confederate surgeon and country doctor practicing in rural postwar North Carolina. Hentz clipped the advertisement for his files in 1887, and eventually the clipping ended up in the Hentz Family Papers in the Southern Historical Collection, a major repository of archival records. Hentz's apparent interest in Dr. Tanner's Opium and Morphine Cure likely stemmed from his prior experience treating opiate-addicted Southerners in the Civil War's aftermath, which the doctor described in his autobiography, part of the same archival collection.[56]

Based on Roundtree's effusive testimonial for Dr. Tanner's Opium and Morphine Cure, perhaps Hentz thought that the patent medicine might be helpful to any addicted patients he might encounter. Sometimes clinicians incorporated patent medicines into their practices, bolstering their therapeutic arsenal.

Hentz's interest in the remedy would not have been abnormal for a doctor of his professional standing. At the very least, the country doctor was curious enough about the patent medicine to save a clipping of Roundtree's testimonial for reference. Patent medicines were even praised at medical society meetings like the February 1896 gathering of the Medical Society of South Carolina, where a doctor told his colleagues that the Keeley Cure was "a benefit to humanity" that "should be recognized by the profession and recommended to patients." Rather than being shouted down, others endorsed these sentiments by chiming in with the positive experiences of patients who had taken the Gold Cure.[57] Coupled with veterans' unbridled expression of faith in patent medicine addiction cures, interest in the remedies among clinicians like Hentz or the Medical Society of South Carolina attracted attention from the era's most powerful and vocal physicians.

The Decline of the Cure

Patent medicine opiate addiction cures were so commercially successful during the Gilded Age that the health craze generated a major backlash among a segment of physicians, who competed with patent medicine sellers for profits and authority in the unregulated, and therefore extraordinarily competitive, medical marketplace. As patent medicine opiate addiction cures proliferated between 1868 and the 1890s, many physicians began attacking the products in earnest, hoping to convince Americans to stop purchasing such remedies. Critics alleged that patent medicines were fraudulent and did not "cure" addiction in a clinical sense. This strategy made sense considering that one of the primary reasons why veterans and other consumers were so willing to spend money on patent medicines was the perception that the products worked. Indeed, evidence suggests that some patent medicines may have been clinically effective in treating addiction—albeit not in the way that proprietors claimed.

Most of these cures for addiction actually contained opiates, although this fact was not widely known until after the turn of the twentieth century. Patent medicine manufacturers refused to disclose the ingredients of their secret formulas, but they insisted that the remedies did not contain opiates. Doctors who were privy to the health effects of opiate addiction knew better, however, and during the 1880s and 1890s, some doctors vocally alleged that the cures were fraudulent, secretly containing opiates, despite the claims of manufacturers like Samuel B. Collins or J. L. Stephens. Therein lay the success of patent medicine addiction cures: for customers to obtain the remedies, vendors required customers to disclose detailed medical information. Collins, for example, required patients to inform him of their exact daily dose and method of consuming opiates, oral or via injection.[58] According to J. B. Mattison, one Gilded

Age addiction expert, nostrum-makers like Collins used this information to manufacture tailored vials of medicine that contained opium or morphine in amounts that were slightly less than customers' usual dosages. Thus, because the cures contained opiates as their secret, active ingredients, the remedies introduced just enough opium or morphine into addicted customers' bodies to stave off withdrawal, without the customers realizing that they were actually taking opiates under the guise of addiction antidotes. Patent medicine sellers essentially tricked customers into thinking they were taking cures for addiction, but consumers were simply ingesting opiates in disguised form. As Mattison explained in an 1886 medical journal article: "The habitué is simply continuing his addiction under a new name."[59] These consumers persisted in taking the remedies over an extended duration of weeks or months. Each time the customer bought another order, the manufacturer put slightly less opium or morphine in the remedy. As one observant doctor reported, "If the patient continues under treatment," gaining a new supply month after month, "the amount of morphia" contained in the patent medicine "is gradually reduced, and he is at last freed of his habit through this deceit."[60]

Chemical analysis of patent medicine opiate addiction cures armed physicians with the evidence they needed to declare open war on the patent medicine industry. One doctor, George F. French of Portland, Maine, performed a chemical analysis on a sample of opium antidote furnished by Samuel B. Collins's former wife and current competitor J. A. Drollinger, who, like Collins, operated her business out of La Porte, Indiana. Although Drollinger insisted that her remedy did not contain opiates, French's analysis contradicted her. Through chemical tests—plus experimentation on a patient he knew to have a "peculiar idiosyncrasy" to morphine—French concluded that the remedy contained morphine. He presented his findings to the local medical society, which hired a firm of New York City chemists to investigate the properties of Drollinger's remedy. They determined that her cure was actually comprised of 1.5 percent morphine, dissolved in glycerin and colored with a splash of red tint to give it a distinctive appearance to customers. For good measure, the committee tested Collins's Painless Opium Antidote as well, which contained twice as much morphine as Drollinger's nostrum. The results were circulated in 1876 in the *Boston Medical and Surgical Journal*, whose editors issued a general call for physicians, especially those in the vicinity of La Porte, Indiana, to "distinguish themselves as guardians of the health of the people" and expose frauds like Drollinger and Collins wherever they might be found.[61]

By the turn of the twentieth century, enraged physicians and skeptical, muckraking journalists became determined to publicly expose patent medicines, especially addiction cures, as frauds, subjecting the industry to scores of medical journal articles, public health reports, and exposés. J. B. Mattison was among the most vocal critic of patent addiction cures. In numerous medical journal articles, he railed against the addiction cures and their proprietors, whom the doctor accused of preying on hapless veterans and other addicted customers. Such men and women deserved assistance from medical experts, Mattison urged. As he explained in 1886, there existed a "mistaken opinion . . . that those who, by force of necessity quite beyond control, have become victims to opium, are simply the slaves of a vicious indulgence, deserving censure rather than charity." Mattison continued: "This feeling, we say, is the main cause of that desire for secrecy on the part of the patient" that was "so essential to the charlatan in this special field, and of which he cunningly takes advantage to his own financial good. In hope of escape the habitué often spends much of both time and treasure to no purpose." Stories like that of J. T. B., of consumers who spent thousands on patent medicine remedies with little to show for it except bankruptcy, supported Mattison's allegations. Critics of patent medicine addiction cures also focused on the fraudulent medical credentials of the many "doctors" peddling these cures. Mattison dismissed Samuel B. Collins as "an illiterate bricklayer in a Western city—who made some presentations to the healing art by virtue of a small stock of herbs stored in a little back apartment—was struck with the shrewd idea that in this peculiar field lay a mine which, perchance, might be worked to no little pecuniary profit."[62] Such ad hominem attacks reflected the animus between regular and alternative medical practitioners in Gilded Age America, as well as frustration on the part of elite physicians, who largely lacked recourse to legally prosecute fraudsters within the patent medicine trade.

Late in the 1890s, the NHDVS's relationship with Leslie E. Keeley also came under fire. In a heated congressional hearing in 1896, a House of Representative member, Republican Richard Whiting Blue of Kansas, accused the manager of the Leavenworth branch of the NHDVS—who doubled as head of the home's Keeley League, drawing a tidy income of $1,200 from this role—of being a drunkard and alleging that the soldiers' home management forced veteran residents to take the Gold Cure against their will, charging them for the cost of the remedy. Some veterans eventually came to resent being treated like medical experiments during the NHDVS's embrace of the Gold Cure. After years of battling over pensions and bouncing around between NHDVS branches, Perry B. Bowser protested to the Pension Bureau in 1900 how much he resented being repeatedly pressured to take the Gold Cure. "I can't live at the Homes on account of the morphine habit, contracted in the service in Oct. '65 for diarrhea," he wrote. Each time he entered the NHDVS facilities, "The Drs. want to practice on me and I am no sooner there than they want me to take some kind of a cure. I have tried that 3 or 4 times and have to resort to it again." If Congress had become skeptical of the Gold Cure, so too had some frustrated veterans.[63]

With the dawning of the Progressive Era, the stalemate between addiction cure peddlers and critics finally broke. During the first decades of the twentieth century, the efforts of anti–patent medicine crusaders eventually turned American legislators and much of the public against "nostrum makers," especially those who peddled fraudulent addiction remedies. Journalist Samuel Hopkins Adams's landmark 1905 *Collier's* series, "The Great American Fraud," helped bring the anti–patent medicine crusade championed by Mattison in the 1870s and 1880s into the mainstream of progressive politics. Adams singled out J. L. Stephens, B. M. Woolley, and other patent medicine makers as "scavengers" and "vampires of the drug addiction school," who cruelly preyed on desperate men by fraudulently lacing so-called cures with morphine.[64] Adams hoped to prod the federal government to regulate the patent medicine industry, and he found willing allies in the physicians who comprised the increasingly powerful American Medical Association. The AMA famously printed and disseminated thousands of copies of Adams's exposé, a strategy that helped marshal political capital against the patent medicine industry. The move paid off, inspiring federal legislation—including the landmark 1906 Pure Food and Drug Act, which required patent medicine sellers to disclose their products' ingredients and imposed purity standards—that finally brought patent medicine proprietors like Samuel B. Collins and Leslie E. Keeley to heel. Although some patent medicine brands persisted for decades, the 1906 law helped usher in the decline of the Gilded Age patent medicine craze and, with it, the opiate addiction cure industry.[65]

Yet for decades after the Civil War, enormous demand for opiate addiction medicines powered a brisk trade in patent medicine addiction cures and their widespread consumption by veterans and other Americans. Desperate to secure freedom from opium slavery and to reverse its physical and social consequences at almost any cost, addicted veterans helped inspire the development of patent medicines purporting to cure drug addiction, and they provided a key customer base for the most successful brands, invented by veterans. The buying and selling of patent medicine opiate addiction remedies by Civil War veterans, particularly the advertisements used to promote the products, reveal how veterans felt about their addictions and the strategies some men pursued to mitigate the worst effects of opium slavery. Above all, the brisk trade in addiction cures in postwar America also serves as an extraordinary window into the financial hardships and, alternately, commercial windfalls prompted by Civil War military service. Of course, patent medicines were not the only forms of addiction treatments available to veterans and other Americans with financial means—far from it. Chapter 8 investigates how physicians reacted to mass addiction in the late nineteenth century, exploring shifting prescribing patterns and the rise of inebriety clinics in Gilded Age America, where countless Americans received medical care for opiate addiction from specialist physicians.

Chapter 8

The Revolt against Opium

Physicians React to Mass Addiction

Joseph Janvier Woodward feared for the American medical profession. Woodward—famous for his work as a Union army surgeon and, later, for tending to President James Garfield after he was shot in 1881 by Charles Guiteau—had good reason for alarm. After decades of warnings by colleagues, including many former Union army surgeons, Woodward had become convinced that physicians were responsible for the ongoing opiate addiction epidemic among Civil War veterans and other Americans. Woodward recognized that the widespread overprescribing of opiates had spread addiction. During the war, surgeons had prescribed opiates "with a freedom which borders on recklessness" for chronic conditions like diarrhea and pain, Woodward observed in 1879 in *The Medical and Surgical History of the War of the Rebellion*, which he coauthored. Woodward fretted about the welfare of drug-using former soldiers and worried that the addiction crisis might blow back on physicians. Throughout the 1860s and 1870s, a cacophony of veterans, patent medicine sellers, and even some doctors had vocally blamed the profession for carelessly prescribing opiates, causing many cases of addiction. These accusations, Woodward feared, threatened to undermine the reputation and authority of the "regular" medical profession in the competitive Gilded Age medical marketplace. Evidence could be seen in the commercial success of patent medicines like Samuel B. Collins's Painless Opium Antidote.

In response, Woodward proposed a radical solution, one that flew in the face of fifty years of mainstream therapeutic practices. Describing the "chronic opium intoxication" that so often stemmed from doctors' prescriptions, Woodward warned, "the more I learn of the behavior of such cases under treatment, the more I am inclined to advise that opiates should be as far as possible avoided." Woodward, chronicler of the US government's official medical history of the Civil War, admitted physicians' culpability in opiate addiction, linked the phenomenon to military medicine, and urged doctors to refrain from overprescribing opiates moving forward.[1]

This chapter investigates how mass opiate addiction shaped Gilded Age medical practices and ideas about addiction. The epidemic challenged physicians' long-standing reliance on prescription opiates to treat all manner of ailments and encouraged doctors to rethink old ideas about the nature of addiction.

Gilded Age physicians faced a deluge of criticism in newspapers, patent medicine advertisements, and medical literature for inadvertently causing opiate addiction through overprescribing. These allegations had the potential to undermine allopathic physicians' position in the extraordinarily competitive Gilded Age medical marketplace, where they competed with sectarian medical practitioners, patent medicine sellers, and even the temperance movement for business and professional authority. Any bad press, especially when it came from or concerned Civil War veterans, made it harder for doctors to stay ahead. Sensitive to criticism of professional malfeasance, some of the nation's leading physicians—including Joseph Woodward and other respected "medical veterans" of the Civil War, to borrow a phrase from Margaret Humphreys—conceded that overprescribing lay at the root of the postwar addiction crisis and called for professional reforms.[2]

Highly motivated to stem the tide of addiction and mitigate its blowback, reform-minded physicians "revolted" against opiates during the 1870s and 1880s, embarking on a mission to radically alter prevailing therapeutic practices and concepts of drug addiction. They began relying less heavily on addictive opiates, prescribing the drugs less frequently while adopting supposedly less addictive substitutes such as chloral hydrate and cocaine. Leading doctors also urged their colleagues to adopt the same practices in widely read medical journals, textbooks, and scientific studies. Considering that for a generation, opiates had been among the most widely prescribed drugs in America, these therapeutic innovations were truly radical measures, signaling an outright rejection of medical orthodoxy. The "revolt" against opium, a phrase coined by former Union navy surgeon J. F. A. Adams, caught on quickly, especially among influential Northeastern physicians. Consequently, clinical records reflect a steep decline in opiate prescribing rates during the 1870s and 1880s.

Physicians who rejected the very concept of opium slavery and presented alternative theories of addiction represented another ambitious element of the revolt against opium. Central to the cultural and medical construction of addiction as "slavery" was the notion that addicted men were culpable for their condition because they failed to uphold conventions of morality or manhood. This victim blaming was terribly harmful for opiate users. Yet as more physicians came to recognize their profession's culpability for the epidemic, many doctors became sympathetic toward addicted people. The growing number of "respectable" white and middle-class Americans who used drugs, including but certainly not limited to Civil War veterans, also challenged the notion that drug users were inherently bad people.[3] A cocktail of sympathy and public criticism prompted a movement to medicalize opiate addiction, that is, redefine it as a physical disease called "inebriety" rather than the personal failings of unmanly or immoral men. Proponents hoped this rethinking of opiate addiction would reduce the stigma surrounding the condition, lead to innovative and effective medical care for addiction, and perhaps even absolve physicians of blame for addiction. To this end, inebriety specialists and some asylum doctors argued that addicted people did not belong in mental asylums and should not purchase patent medicines but instead seek medical care at specialized "inebriety clinics"—among the earliest iterations of drug addiction rehabilitation centers in American history. The medicalization movement also helped supplant older labels for addiction, such as opium slavery, in favor of a disease-oriented vocabulary of addiction.

The late nineteenth-century shift away from prescription opiates and the inebriety movement have been well documented by historians. Yet the connection between this revolt against opium and the Civil War has been largely overlooked. Scholars have long recognized that the therapeutic importance of opiates declined late in the nineteenth century. David Courtwright has shown that the decline in prescribing rates in the 1890s led to a steep decrease in addiction. The introduction of new nonopiate painkillers, advances in medical knowledge and education, and lobbying by physicians and pharmacists to regulate poisons have also been convincingly cited as factors that helped drive this therapeutic shift.[4] Similarly, the inebriety movement has often been described in the historiography of drugs, alcohol, and addiction. The Civil War helped inspire these developments as well. Historians cannot fully explain the origins of the revolt against opium without considering how the Civil War informed the context from which the movement emerged. Key figures like Woodward, Silas Weir Mitchell, and Jacob Mendes Da Costa were deeply troubled by their observations that widespread if well-meant use of opium and morphine in Civil War hospitals and postwar clinics had left many veterans addicted. Equally motivating were allegations against physicians leveled by veterans in public forums. Moreover, a close look at clinical records indicates that the shift away from opiates began shortly after the Civil War in the 1870s, decades before historians have realized and in contrast to rising opiate consumption overall until the 1890s. Ultimately, by recognizing the Civil War's role in the revolt against opium, historians can gain a clearer understanding of the war's place in broader transformations in American medical practice and thought. A closer look at how former Civil War physicians responded to addiction in this era also brings new evidence to light and presents a richer view of therapeutic changes.

"The Doctors Are to Blame"

Medical observers began attributing the rapid growth of opiate addiction to doctors' prescriptions immediately after the Civil War. As one doctor observed in 1868, "The habit has crept upon" most opium eaters "almost unconsciously, during the medicinal use of opiates to soothe pain, to remove sleeplessness, or to arrest protracted bowel-complaint."[5] Alonzo Calkins, an early chronicler of opiate addiction, reported one such case in 1871. A "gentleman . . . suffered much from a diseased ankle" and went to see his physician, who "advised (professionally) to use morphine hypodermically." According to Calkins, "after a habituation for two years, the invalid" became "helplessly delivered over, an abject slave to the habit, enervated in body and enfeebled in mind." His thigh was "literally studded with punctures," a tragic result of the doctor's misguided prescription.[6] Media coverage in the late 1860s and 1870s also attributed the upward trend in opiate addiction to doctors' prescriptions. A Maine newspaper in 1868 counted at least fifty opium eaters in the vicinity around the town of Auburn, and "without doubt the largest part [of them] formed the habit by first using opium as a medical prescription against pain."[7] The author Fitz Hugh Ludlow, in his widely read 1867 *Harper's New Monthly Magazine* story on the opium habit, likewise reported a causative link between prescriptions and the spread of opiate addiction. "The vast majority of Anglo-Saxon opium-eaters" in America, Ludlow explained, "first learned its seductions . . . through a medical prescription."[8]

As the post–Civil War opiate addiction crisis reached a fever pitch in the 1880s and 1890s, observers moved beyond simple attribution and angrily blamed the addiction crisis on doctors. According to the magazine *Banner of Light* in 1874, "There is—and it is fast growing on the people of this country—one curse, if possible, worse than rum, and that is the use of opium, or what is called laudanum. This habit has in part been formed by the ignorant doctors, who first administer the sleep drug as medicine; it is afterward taken by the patient as a soothing balm—the end of which is misery and death."[9] The charge of "ignorance" on the part of physicians signaled the growing opinion that doctors bore much of the blame for opiate addiction. Such rhetoric implied that physicians were at fault because they carelessly prescribed addictive opiates for minor complaints. Doctors wielding hypodermic syringes were no longer simply the vectors of opiate addiction. Now, they shared culpability for the addiction crisis ravaging the nation.

Many veterans joined in this chorus of criticism, in part to deflect accusations of unmanliness and immorality so often leveled against addicted men. Alpheus M. Chappell, the Confederate captain wounded at Pickett's Charge, blamed his addiction on doctors' prescriptions. Explaining his circumstances in an 1886 letter to a benefactor, Chappell was careful to explain that the "Drs. put me on morphine," implicitly denying that he initially contracted the morphine habit of his own volition.[10] When Charles L. Williams, a Michigan veteran, applied for admission to the Michigan Soldiers' Home in March 1895, he claimed he was "totally unable to earn a living" because he had "contracted [the] opium habit during war." Likely sensing that the home's gatekeepers might reject his application on character grounds, Williams was careful to point out that the "drug [was] given by [an] army surgeon" and not originally taken of his own volition.[11] The anonymous Union veteran behind the 1876 addiction narrative *Opium Eating* also laid the blame for his morphine addiction squarely on the doctor who had initially prescribed the drug as a panacea. Surviving captivity at the notorious Andersonville prison and Libby Prison, the young veteran returned home as a gaunt old soldier suffering from lingering gastrointestinal distress. He soon fell under the care of an "ignoramus," a syringe-wielding doctor who "hung about me for six months to allow him to treat my case." The physician secretly began dosing the veteran with hypodermic morphine, launching the young man down a lifelong path of slavery to morphine. The doctor "used every persuasive art within his command to get me to his office, and under his professional care, only for the purpose of giving me bare morphia by way of a syringe!" Viewed in this light, the doctor and his prescription were not merely passive vectors through which the veteran contracted morphine addiction. Instead, the doctor was cast as the agent behind addiction, his actions directly responsible for the veteran's misery. The book was a scathing indictment of the prescribing physician and of mainstream medicine by proxy.[12]

William Rosser Cobbe, a noted Chicago journalist who claimed to have fought in the Civil War, likewise blamed doctors for his opiate addiction. Cobbe's reporting in the *Chicago Tribune* and his 1895 addiction narrative *Doctor Judas: A Portrayal of the Opium Habit* presented a scathing critique of physicians for overprescribing opiates, even to patients whose constitutions made them predisposed to addiction. Cobbe, who survived a lengthy addiction to opium, blamed his condition on the prescriptions of the titular "Doctor Judas" coupled with a constitution that had started off infirm and was broken down further during the Civil War. As a child, Cobbe explained, "I was heir to physical weakness," prone to "sensitiveness to pain" and "nervous disorder." To shore up his constitution and quiet the boy's complaints, the Cobbe family's doctor had prescribed opiate-laced medicines. "Unhappily," Cobbe recalled, "in those days the dicta of physicians were deemed infallible, and they not only gave medicine for every ailment, small or great, but they also prescribed it in heroic doses." Cobbe was reared on laudanum, paregoric, and Godfrey's cordial. "The persistent use of them in early childhood" at the doctors' behest "gave to the physical cells an appetite" for opium "which they never lost." During the Civil War, Cobbe claimed to have suffered "mental strains" and "incarceration in military prisons," followed by postwar failures in business and a hard stint in the navy. Consequently, because of his childhood doctor's prescriptions coupled with the hardships of service, Cobbe developed "a consuming desire for stimulants," namely, "the hell drug, morphine."[13] Physicians whose patients became addicted to opiates, according to Cobbe, ultimately did more harm than good, violating the central aim of medicine. "I warn physicians to exercise greater caution in the use of opium," Cobbe concluded, lest doctors lose their hard-fought standing in the medical marketplace.[14] Cobbe made similar accusations in the *Chicago Tribune*, writing in 1894 that "the army of opium habitués is appalling in size" and that "careful investigation shows that three-fourths of the opium 'fiends' of this country owe their habit directly to the physician." Cobbe too had been like "clay in the hands of the potter" of the "family physician," the doctor Judas who "placed me under my bondage" to morphine.[15]

Addiction narratives that blamed doctors, especially accounts written by Civil War veterans, presented a formidable challenge to physicians' reputations and professional standing. Doctors could not simply dismiss veterans' accusations out of hand. The profession had to take allegations seriously because soldiers held considerable sway over political and public discourse in the Gilded Age. Although opiate addiction afflicted all sorts of Americans, Civil War veterans were a uniquely conspicuous demographic that wielded an unusually effective lobby. When veterans like Cobbe accused physicians of causing opiate addiction, their criticisms carried more weight than allegations by women who comprised a majority among opium users but lacked a comparable public platform. Throughout the Gilded Age, veterans provided sustained and influential commentary on a variety of public issues through periodicals like the *National Tribune* and *Confederate Veteran*, which served as the mouthpieces of the Grand Army of the Republic and the United Confederate Veterans, respectively. Veterans' organizations, especially the GAR, successfully lobbied Congress on issues pertaining to veterans' welfare, namely, the expansion and liberalization of the federal pension system during the 1880s and 1890s.[16] As the influence wielded by Civil War veterans grew during the 1880s and 1890s, particularly after the expansion of pension programs and through popular mediums such as soldier memoirs, veterans gained considerable social and political capital. This cult of the soldier, living and fallen, made it impossible for physicians to dismiss veterans' criticisms out of hand.[17]

Although veterans' organizations did not formally address the epidemic of opiate addiction among veterans, individual veterans frequently broached the topic, influencing public discourse about opiate addiction. The reception of veterans' addiction narratives illustrates how much influence older soldiers could bring to bear on public discourse about addiction. *Opium Eating*, published in 1876 by the anonymous survivor of Andersonville, generated positive reviews in the popular press but heated backlash among doctors. Whereas *Penn Monthly*, a literary magazine, judged *Opium Eating* a success that "should serve the good purpose its author has in view," the veterans' narrative was "trash," according to the erudite doctor who reviewed the book for the *Boston Medical and Surgical Journal.*[18] William Rosser Cobbe's book *Doctor Judas* also generated much attention upon publication in 1895, with glowing reviews in *Chicago Tribune* and the *Arena*. According to the latter, Cobbe's riveting account of the "fantastic nightmare" of opium slavery, including his depiction of doctors' culpability in the ongoing addiction crisis, put his book on par with De Quincey's *Confessions of an English Opium-Eater*. From then on, "he who speaks of De Quincey will feel compelled to mention Cobbe," high praise indeed. According to the *Chicago Tribune*, "its [*Doctor Judas*'s] influence must be for incalculable good," because the narrative raised awareness about the prevalence of opiate addiction and highlighted physicians' role in the crisis.[19]

The numerous testimonials written by veterans on behalf of patent medicine addiction remedies also made it impossible for physicians to dismiss allegations of their culpability for addiction. Samuel B. Collins, Leslie E. Keeley, and other entrepreneurial patent medicine proprietors seized on veterans' complaints, reprinting them as advertisements in newspapers and pamphlets while casting themselves as anti-physicians who could undo doctors' malfeasance. "Physicians are responsible for nineteen-twentieths of" addiction "and all the misery, the wasted life, the early death, lies at the doors of our profession," claimed Collins, who referred to himself as a doctor even as he undercut the position of physicians in the medical marketplace.[20] Keeley likewise alleged in the *Chicago Tribune* that "74 percent of all the patients [treated for opiate addiction at Keeley Institutes] claimed the drug was first given by physicians, and in many cases continued without their knowledge till they had formed the habit. . . . The medical fraternity is responsible to a large extent for the terrible indulgence in narcotics."[21] Keeley even reprinted William Rosser Cobbe's account of opium slavery in a pamphlet advertising the Gold Cure.[22] Accusations of culpability leveled by patent medicine purveyors struck a nerve among physicians, both because these criticisms drew on long-standing critiques of allopathic medicine and because the extreme competition of the Gilded Age medical marketplace meant that physicians risked hard-won professional legitimacy. Physician Frederick Heman Hubbard acknowledged that morphine "now counts its victims by thousands," yet "the medical profession has been strangely apathetic with respect to the increase of this vice." Doctors needed to act, and fast, to prevent further reputational damage from "unprincipled quacks" like Collins and Keeley.[23] Investigations by public health officials and journalists during the 1880s added credence to the accusations leveled by veterans and patent medicine proprietors, while underscoring how much ground patent medicine sellers had gained. As J. M. Hull, a member of the Iowa State Board of Health, explained in 1885: "The way these poor victims are fleeced by advertising quacks is pitiable, indeed. No better proof can be given of the rapid increase of this evil than the number of advertisers who claim to cure the habit. So common are they that one or more may be seen in nearly all the papers and journals of the country."[24]

Gilded Age journalists loudly blamed physicians for the addiction epidemic. "It is said," one reporter observed in 1891, "that many physicians lend their hands too willingly and are ready with the injecting needle to check a pain that could easily be borne" without drugs. Physicians who were too willing to administer hypodermic morphine "encourage[d] effeminacy" by "plant[ing] the germ of the morphine habit" among their patients.[25] Muckraker Virgil E. Eaton's 1888 exposé in *Popular Science Monthly* attracted considerable attention and provoked a backlash among physicians. Eaton claimed to have meticulously studied opium addiction in Boston for over a year, consulting druggists and surveying pharmacy logbooks that detailed physicians' prescriptions. His grim findings confirmed the allegations against doctors leveled by Civil War veterans and patent medicine vendors. A meticulous investigator, Eaton reviewed "10,200 recipes [prescriptions] taken in thirty-four drug-stores" across the Boston area, finding that about 14 percent of prescriptions contained opiates. "I found them [opiates] prescribed for every ailment which flesh is heir to," Eaton reported, from neuralgia, rheumatism, and headache to sore throat, gallstones, and chest complaints like tuberculosis, pneumonia, and bronchitis. The frequency of refills proved even more alarming than the high opiate prescribing rate. Forty-two percent of prescriptions were refilled twice, and 23 percent of these refills included opiates. Of prescriptions refilled three times or more, between 61 and 78 percent contained opiates. Such a high rate of opiate prescriptions and refills, Eaton concluded, proved that "the parties who are responsible for the increase of the habit are the physicians who give the prescriptions." The widespread overprescribing of opiates by doctors was a terrible injustice of which "the result is to convert their patients into opium-slaves."[26] Eaton's *Popular Science Monthly* exposé culminated in a call to action. "The doctors are to blame," Eaton argued, "and they are the men who need reforming." Laws were badly needed to restrict patients from refilling opiate prescriptions, a measure that Eaton hoped would make doctors "more guarded" in doling out opiates "for trivial ailments." Lazy practitioners who persisted in overprescribing the drugs for minor complaints could be fined. Finally, Eaton urged American medical consumers to pressure physicians by taking their business elsewhere. "They should forsake medicine, and patronize the gymnasium" instead, a novel form of preventative health care in vogue during the late nineteenth century.[27] Eaton represented a growing chorus of observers who believed doctors were to blame for the Civil War–era opiate addiction crisis.

Eaton's 1888 exposé ignited a firestorm in the medical press, and many doctors roundly rejected such criticisms from laypeople. The AMA, in particular, was hypervigilant about countering bad press, which stood to undermine physicians' precarious standing in the Gilded Age medical marketplace. A few weeks after Eaton's piece appeared in *Popular Science Monthly*, the AMA responded with an aggressive rebuttal in the *Journal of the American Medical Association*. Resorting to ad hominem attacks, the journal insulted Eaton as an "unscientific and unthinking man" peddling "arrant nonsense." Dismissing Eaton's evidence out of hand, the AMA insisted that "physicians are not responsible for the increase of the opium-habit."[28] This hostile response to mounting evidence illustrates how some physicians could not bring themselves to admit their profession was to blame for the addiction epidemic. Such an acknowledgment would amount to an admission that a prized therapeutic innovation, hypodermic morphine, might do more harm than good.

Yet in the face of overwhelming evidence, many physicians came to concede that the profession, to some degree, was at fault. One professor of medicine, describing how to effectively treat opiate addiction in the *Richmond Medical Journal* in 1868, expressed sympathy for patients who had been exposed to opiates by their doctors' orders. "In many instances," he explained, "the sufferers are more objects of pity than of blame. For . . . in not a few the habit has crept upon them almost unconsciously, during the medicinal use of opiates to soothe pain, to remove sleeplessness, or to arrest protracted bowel-complaint." The professor urged that "the risk of this evil should therefore be carefully borne in mind, for life-long misery has often been caused by undue laxity in the prescribing of opiates."[29] The next year, Roberts Bartholow, the former Union army surgeon and a leading authority on the use of hypodermic syringes, noted in his influential handbook on hypodermic medicine that "when morphia is administered for a lengthened period . . . the brain and nervous system become accustomed to the influence, and demand its repetition." The habituated patient "fidgets" unless morphine injections are regularly administered, followed by "wakefulness, a suicidal tendency, hallucinations, and decided mental alienation" if the drug was long withheld.[30] Such warnings were crucial because during the late 1860s, some doctors, perhaps with willful ignorance, considered hypodermic morphine to be less addictive than orally administered opium or laudanum. This was nonsense, according to an exasperated physician writing in the *BMSJ* in 1870, who rejected the dangerous notion that hypodermic morphine "avoided" the "danger of the habit of opium-eating." This was not the case, to which the doctor could personally attest from several cases. When practitioners carelessly administered hypodermic morphine, wishfully hoping that it was not addictive, the drug ultimately did more harm than good, and patients ended up becoming "confirmed slave[s] to the degrading habit of opium-taking."[31]

In the 1860s, such admissions of culpability for the addiction epidemic were few and far between. But during the 1870s, the link between opiate prescriptions and opiate addiction grew increasingly obvious to anyone willing to see it. Bartholow, the pioneer of hypodermic medicine, began openly questioning the benefit of his expertise because of the hypodermic syringe's predilection for spreading addiction when employed by careless doctors.[32] By that point, the myth that hypodermic morphine was less addictive had been shattered. George Miller Beard, the eminent medical and racial theorist who developed the disease concept of neurasthenia, admitted in 1870 that "there is, I think ... truth in the charge that opium eating is caused by opium prescribing."[33] In 1872, the Massachusetts Board of Health's investigation of opiate addiction found most cases of addiction originated in "the injudicious and often unnecessary prescription of opium by the physician." The opium habit was "on the increase, because doctors prescribe it [opium] more indiscriminately now than formerly, thus establishing the habit with the patients," according to one druggist consulted by the board. Another druggist added that he "thinks that physicians are not sufficiently careful in regulating and restricting the use of opium before it becomes a habit." The board was alarmed, concluding that this was "so grave a statement, and one so generally endorsed," that it "should not be allowed to pass unnoticed by those who, as guardians of the public health, are in no small measure responsible for the moral, as well as physical, welfare of their patients."[34]

By the late 1870s, physicians were hotly debating their profession's culpability for the addiction crisis in medical journals and at professional conferences. It was no coincidence that Joseph Woodward expressed grave concerns about "chronic opium intoxication" in the 1879 volume of *The Medical and Surgical History of the War of the Rebellion*, urging doctors to avoid prescribing opiates needlessly.[35] Such commentary had become mainstream in medical circles, reflecting a growing consensus among physicians. The same year, a frustrated Bartholow added that "no matter how much the original [morphine] prescription may have been justified in the condition of the patient, and how conscientious the physician in his efforts to prevent abuse, if the habit be formed, the mental and moral degradation which ensues will always be referred to as the blunder or the crime of Dr. So-and-so," rather than the patient's fault.[36] Another doctor, E. M. Sell, angrily lectured an audience of well-to-do New York Medical Society members in 1883, charging that "there is an awful responsibility resting upon those [practitioners] who have been aiding and abetting in constituting and establishing a large army of miserable wretches, who are enslaved soul and body by this direful opium habit."[37] Sell's frustration and alarm at the toll of the addiction crisis on the medical profession's standing was palpable.

Physicians like Woodward, Bartholow, and Sell pointed to bad actors within physicians' ranks as a major part of the problem. Despite the widespread recognition that addiction often had iatrogenic origins, some clinicians still bragged about the enormous doses of opiates they prescribed over long durations. Anyone who doubted doctors' culpability in the addiction crisis, critics charged, need only flip through the pages of the day's medical journals. In the *Pacific Medical and Surgical Journal*, one doctor, George E. Jones of Cincinnati, described how he administered over 2,300 injections of morphine to a single pain patient over the course of just twenty months in the late 1870s. "Commencing with half a grain subcutaneously," Jones recalled, "the morphia had to be increased in amount until... the daily dose was thirty grains; fifteen in the morning, the balance in the evening. This was continued twenty-one consecutive days" before the doctor attempted to gradually lower the patient's daily dose. Although Jones did not record the patient's subsequent medical history, it must have been hard for the journal's experienced readers to imagine that the protracted administration of hypodermic morphine in such enormous doses did not result in addiction. Yet, astonishingly, Jones insisted that none of his patients had ever developed opiate addictions.[38] Another doctor, Richard J. Noble of North Carolina, described administering between 2,500 and 3,000 morphine injections to one patient in eighteen months. But "so far," Noble insisted in 1880, "I see no signs of the opium habit."[39] The actions of such stubborn physicians as Jones and Noble reflected poorly on the profession as a whole.

By the late 1880s, what began as a minority opinion among doctors morphed into a cacophony of self-criticism within the profession, putting the likes of Jones and Noble increasingly out of step with their colleagues. "We all know how the opium habit is formed," quipped Frank Woodbury, a fellow of the prestigious College of Physicians of Philadelphia in 1886.[40] The Philadelphia physician J. C. Wilson lectured an audience of doctors at the American Academy of Medicine's 1889 annual meeting that "it is an unfortunate fact," not merely an opinion, "that the greater number of the victims of habitual vicious narcotism become so through the prolonged abuse of narcotics originally prescribed for the relief of pain."[41] The eminent neurologist Silas Weir Mitchell agreed. "Often, in my experience," Mitchell explained in 1888, "the opium habit is learned during an illness of limited duration, and for the consequences of which there is always someone to be blamed." Ever the elitist, Mitchell blamed poorly trained doctors who were "weak, or too tender, or too prone to escape trouble by the easy help of some pain-lulling agent" when badgering patients came calling.[42] "It is pleasanter," chided another physician, "to give a hypodermic injection than to refuse it to a suffering and unreasonable patient."[43] This shift in doctors' thinking about addiction and their role causing it was consistently reflected in American medical literature throughout the 1880s and 1890s. An 1889 article in the *BMSJ* synthesized the medical knowledge known about "morphiomania" by describing a typical patient's cycle of addiction: "A patient shall be suffering from frequent attacks of angina pectoris, sciatica, hectic colic, or some other very painful affection, for which his physician has resorted to subcutaneous injections of morphine." This was the first step to addiction. Next, finding that "the relief has been speedy and magical" but "the painful disease persisting, the hypodermic injections are continued, but larger and still larger doses are soon required to reduce the effect which small doses at first produced." Finally, as tolerance builds up, "the patient obtains a hypodermic syringe of his physician or some druggist, and a quantity of morphine." Soon, "he is now on a downward road; he has become a morphiomaniac."[44]

"The Therapeutics Need Revising"

Recognizing professional culpability in the opiate addiction epidemic was the first step. Forward-thinking physicians also believed there was an urgent need to alter the ways in which they prescribed opiates if doctors were going to stop the spread of addiction and mitigate its impact on the profession's standing. The addiction crisis thus sparked a reevaluation of opiates' medical benefits in relation to the danger of addiction, which ultimately led to radical changes in opiate prescribing practices during the Gilded Age. Leading American physicians, especially influential former Union army surgeons, openly revolted against opiates by bucking the profession's historical reliance on them. Instead, they sharply curtailed opiate prescriptions and began substituting supposedly less addictive alternatives like cocaine and chloral hydrate, while urging other doctors to do the same. "The [opium] habit is wide-spread, prevailing and increasing," as one doctor put it, so "physicians must attempt to stay its disastrous progress. The therapeutics need revising."[45] Indeed, "the honor, interest and respectability of the profession" were at stake unless doctors took "action to prevent the abuse of opium."[46]

Yet shifting away from prescription opiates was a radical proposition. Opiates had long been considered the "magnum Dei donum" of the materia medica and remained among the most commonly prescribed medicines in the nation—used to treat hundreds of ailments. American doctors had been trained to rely on opiates, and experience during the Civil War only reinforced doctors' impulse to reach for opiates when treating symptoms like pain and diarrhea. Many doctors could not imagine a world in which opiates were not essential medicines. Even those physicians who recognized the early warning signs of the nascent addiction epidemic nonetheless struggled to envision a world without opiates. As a group of former Union army surgeons and US Sanitary Commission leaders explained in 1869, "Opium and alcohol are more largely used in medicine than any other drugs, and it cannot be denied that the effects of the abuse of these two wonderful products are most pernicious and destructive." But the profession was caught in a difficult position. Opiates "cannot be abandoned as remedies," the committee members reasoned, simply because "they are too essential and too potent to be overlooked."[47]

Resistance to change was staunch in some quarters, especially among older practitioners trained before the Civil War. Boston physician William Mason Cornell, renowned for his work on epilepsy, relied heavily on prescription opiates during the 1840s and 1850s. Cornell had become so reliant on opium in his practice that he refused to give it up, flatly rejecting any talk of therapeutic reforms. "Are we to relinquish a remedy indicated in a certain disease, and which we have found by experience to be useful, because unprofessional men abuse it, or because some physicians ride it as a hobby, and prescribe it for all diseases," he asked with exasperation in 1867. "Suppose we were to subject opium or quinine to this test, would the profession be willing to do it? There are thousands who get intoxicated every day by opium." But "must our profession, therefore, cease to prescribe opium as a medicine?"[48] During the late 1860s and 1870s, many practitioners like Cornell continued to rely heavily on prescription opiates, despite mounting evidence in medical journals and newspapers that the overprescribing of the drugs was fueling the opiate addiction epidemic among Civil War veterans and others. Overall, opiate consumption rates remained high until declining in the 1890s.

Yet calls to "revise the therapeutics" seemed to resonate among a cadre of reform-minded former Union army surgeons, including Silas Weir Mitchell and Jacob Mendes Da Costa. Their appetite for therapeutic change differed sharply from that of physicians like Cornell, more than two decades senior. By the 1870s, Mitchell and Da Costa were already at the cutting edge of American medicine and renowned for their pioneering Civil War research.[49] Crucially, they had witnessed the spread of iatrogenic opiate addiction among soldiers during and after the war. Age and experience help explain why these doctors were more receptive to calls to move away from prescription opiates. Long before developing his infamous rest cure or identifying phantom limb, Mitchell had cultivated a reputation for innovation during the Civil War, when he worked as a contract physician at Turner's Lane Hospital, the Union army facility in Philadelphia that specialized in nerve injuries. Mitchell's wartime medical research quickly catapulted him to the heights of the American medical profession. In 1875, at a relatively young forty-six years old, the president of the Smithsonian Institution described Mitchell as "an eminent physician and physiologist of Philadelphia."[50] Such lofty praise attests to his influence among American physicians in the Civil War era. When Mitchell spoke out about an issue in medicine, his colleagues listened.

Mitchell was particularly concerned with the well-being of injured Civil War veterans. In an 1890 letter to the superintendent of the Hampton, Virginia, branch of the NHDVS, Mitchell wrote that he was "anxious" to "find out the later history of these men."⁵¹ The fate of Civil War veterans was an animating theme throughout much of Mitchell's postwar medical research and his prolific literary career. He penned several works of fiction after the Civil War, as was common among elite American physicians of the day. In "The Case of George Dedlow," a short story published in 1866 in *Atlantic Monthly*, Mitchell depicted a fictional Union veteran quadruple amputee who struggled to cope with pain and reintegrate into civilian life. Mitchell's depiction of veteranhood and its many traumas was so vivid and realistic that the story prompted donations from readers moved by the plight of Dedlow, for they did not realize the heart-wrenching tale was fictional.⁵² During the postwar decades, Mitchell's concern for veterans' well-being, coupled with his commitment to scientific medical research, motivated him to turn his powerful pen toward the issue of opiate addiction.

Mitchell initially learned about opiate addiction while working at Turner's Lane Hospital, where he conducted some of the Civil War's most innovative medical research. Mitchell and his colleagues William Keen and George Morehouse specialized in treating complex nerve injuries. This work was challenging, for nerve wounds were tremendously painful for soldiers and poorly understood by physicians. To help wounded soldiers cope with intractable nerve pain, Mitchell and his colleagues administered hypodermic morphine injections "incessantly." In a study on morphine he published in August 1865, Mitchell described his experimental use of hypodermic morphine to treat nerve wounds, noting that he and his colleagues administered on average twenty to thirty morphine injections a day collectively among their patients. They gave one man nearly 400 shots of morphine during his hospitalization.⁵³

The addictive potential of hypodermic morphine had not been lost on the young surgeon. Mitchell described several cases of addiction in his landmark 1872 study *Injuries of Nerves and Their Consequences*, compiled from research at Turner's Lane. One troubling case was that of A. F. Swann, the Pennsylvania captain who developed shocking "abscesses" from his reliance on hypodermic morphine to ease his painful war wound. At the height of his addiction, Swann injected himself twenty times a day, imperiling health and manhood, even in the eyes of sympathetic physicians like Mitchell.⁵⁴ The doctor was deeply concerned about the fate of veteran patients, and he authored several longitudinal studies documenting their poor outcomes in the postwar decades. In 1891, Mitchell wrote to a fellow ex-army surgeon inquiring about Swann's postwar health. The correspondent replied that Swann had died in 1878, adding, "I would ask for your private ear that his death was mainly due to bad habits," namely, morphine addiction. Swann's recklessness had, according to the surgeon's point of view, cost the veteran his life. Considering his concern over Swann's fate, Mitchell would have likely believed the veteran's overdose death was a tragedy, and an avoidable one at that.⁵⁵

Mitchell's concern about opiate addiction among Civil War veterans influenced his postwar prescribing practices. Well aware that opiate prescriptions for painful war wounds had resulted in addiction among his former patients, Mitchell was receptive to calls in medical journals and at conferences urging doctors to prescribe fewer opiates. The clinical records of the Philadelphia Orthopaedic Hospital and Infirmary for Nervous Diseases, where Mitchell held a clinic every Friday for decades, indicate that he largely abandoned opiates after the Civil War. Like the wartime facility at Turner's Lane, Mitchell's postwar Philadelphia Orthopaedic Hospital and Infirmary for Nervous Diseases was a pioneering center of neurology in the Gilded Age, the sort of place where doctors did not cling to antebellum therapies but instead embraced therapeutic revisionism.[56] Patients, including some veterans, traveled from across the city and the nation to receive care for burning nerve pain, intractable headaches, and various neuralgias from the eminent Mitchell (fig. 8.1). During the previous decades, most of the hospital's patients would have been treated with opium, morphine, or laudanum. Although Mitchell had prescribed opiates heavily at Turner's Lane during the Civil War, by the 1880s he had reversed course and abandoned prescription opiates. Mitchell's postwar casebook reveals that he did not prescribe opiates to any of the sixty-two individuals for whom he recorded clinical notes between 1887 and 1900.[57] Mitchell's rejection of opiates represented a major departure from the norms of Civil War–era American medicine, a truly radical medical reform that reflected his personal experiences with opiate-addicted veterans and sensitivity to postwar calls to prescribe fewer opiates.

Mitchell's Philadelphia colleague, Jacob Mendes Da Costa, also largely abandoned prescription opiates in the postwar decades. Like Mitchell, Da Costa had treated Union soldiers and became renowned among American doctors for the wartime research he conducted in Union general hospital wards. Da Costa's most influential study identified a condition he named "irritable heart" among Civil War veterans. Some historians suggest that Da Costa's irritable heart was perhaps the earliest clinical observation of war-related psychological trauma among soldiers—a precursor to modern post-traumatic stress disorder (PTSD).[58] "On Irritable Heart" appeared in the influential *American Journal of Medical Sciences* in 1871. In it, Da Costa explicitly warned that opiates were addictive when prescribed for chronic pain, an observation he reached after giving opium to a veteran suffering from irritable heart. Opiates should be avoided, the doctor explained, because "in the long continuance of the treatment required" to remedy chronic pain there was "great risk of making the patient an opium eater."[59]

Shortly after the Civil War, Da Costa accepted an appointment as professor of theory and practice of medicine at Philadelphia's Jefferson Medical College.

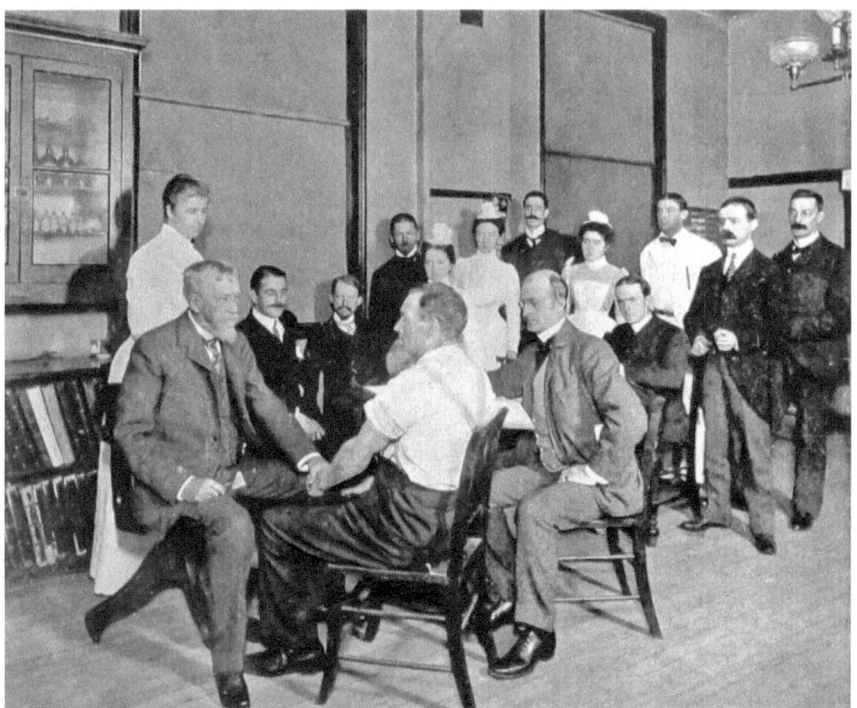

Figure 8.1 Silas Weir Mitchell examines a Civil War veteran, Philadelphia Orthopaedic Hospital and Infirmary for Nervous Diseases, 1902. From *International Clinics*, 12th ser., vol. 1 (Philadelphia: J. B. Lippincott, 1902), frontispiece.

In this capacity, Da Costa directed the college's medical clinic, where he practiced medicine and supervised a team of medical students. The clinic filled a unique niche in postwar Philadelphia's medical landscape. Unlike Mitchell's nerve hospital, Da Costa's clinic served the city's urban poor. Unable to afford the services of private physicians, impoverished patients obtained free medical care for all manner of ailments at the Jefferson Medical College clinic. It doubled as a training facility for Jefferson medical students, who acquired invaluable hands-on practice under the direction of Da Costa. Few nineteenth-century general hospital records are extant, but those generated by Da Costa's clinic dating from October 1870 to October 1875 were preserved. These rare clinical records provide an unparalleled window into Da Costa's prescribing practices around the time that he published his 1871 warning about prescription opiate addiction.

The Jefferson Medical College clinic records show that Da Costa heeded his warnings about prescription opiate addiction. In 1,945 cases between 1870 and 1875, only about 19 percent, or 371 patients, received prescriptions for opiates. By comparison, just over 42 percent of cases treated at a comparable public hospital in Boston during the 1870s contained opiates. In the Civil War's wake, Da Costa and his medical students were far less likely to prescribe opiates than other physicians who treated similar patients in comparable clinical settings. Da Costa's personal experience treating Civil War soldiers, through which he came to realize that opiates were addictive, convinced him of the need to refrain from prescribing opiates lest his patients become addicted. Consequently, he implemented this new treatment practice at the Jefferson Medical College clinic during the 1870s.[60] Da Costa also disseminated his stance on prescription opiates in an influential textbook on diagnostic techniques. In the book, which went through nine editions and taught a generation of American doctors how to diagnose patients' ailments, Da Costa reiterated his reservations about prescription opiates. Doctors should proceed cautiously when prescribing opiates, Da Costa warned, as "the employment of morphine hypodermically has become an alarmingly frequent form of the opium habit."[61]

Da Costa's stance on opiates left an indelible mark on his subordinates. J. C. Wilson, Da Costa's chief lieutenant at the Jefferson Medical College clinic, soon became a vocal proponent of the anti-prescription opiate movement. Like his supervisor and mentor, Wilson had also served as a Union army surgeon. The two men worked closely together at the Jefferson College clinic during the 1870s, where they would have exchanged views about the therapeutic use and merits of opiates. A decade later, at an 1888 meeting of American Academy of Medicine, Wilson presented a paper on opiate addiction, explaining to his audience that "it is an unfortunate fact that the greater number of the victims of habitual vicious narcotism become so through the prolonged abuse of narcotics originally prescribed for the relief of pain." With this fact in mind, Wilson reasoned, the solution to the problem of opiate addiction was "the exercise of every possible precaution on the part of physicians in prescribing narcotics." Doctors should refrain from prescribing opiates whenever possible, resorting to the drugs only as therapies of last resort. "Under no circumstances," Wilson warned, "except in the final stages of hopelessly incurable painful affections, should the hypodermic syringe be placed in the hands of the patient" because possessing the instrument was likely to lead to addiction. If opiates must be administered, Wilson concluded, then patients should be kept "in ignorance" about the ingredients of doctors' prescriptions. If patients did not know that relief was brought about by opiates, Wilson's thinking went, then they would not seek out the drugs at pharmacies. This rhetoric mirrored Da Costa's 1871 warning about prescription opiate addiction and his prescribing practices at the Jefferson Medical College clinic, which suggests that Da Costa's cautionary warnings about prescription opiates had influenced Wilson to join the anti-opium camp.[62]

Cocaine, Chloral Hydrate, and Drug Substitution

If physicians were to reduce their reliance on opiates, they would have to develop alternative painkillers and antidiarrheals. Thus, as physicians decreased their reliance on opiates, they also sought to replace opium and morphine with seemingly safer substitutes. In the *Boston Medical and Surgical Journal* in 1889, James Forster Alleyne (J. F. A.) Adams, a physician who during the Civil War was a Union army medical cadet and navy surgeon, made a radical "argument in favor of restricting the use of opiates to a greater degree than has hitherto been the prevailing custom." He explained that "opium is the most conspicuous article in the pharmacopeia," and "its extraordinary efficacy in relieving pain, the versatility of its powers, and its reliability in emergencies, give it a preeminent standing." "In acute cases the use of opium is comparatively safe," Adams noted, because it did not require prolonged administration. The same could be said of morphine "in the last stage of incurable diseases," such as cancer or tuberculosis. "But in chronic cases opium needs to be used with the greatest caution." Adams had learned about opium's "remarkable ... power for harm" through observing "slaves of opium" firsthand, perhaps Civil War veterans. Indeed, "there are probably few physicians who are not cognizant of some such cases," he added. Like most observers of the opium habit, Adams recognized that the widespread medicinal use of opiates, their "unrestricted sale" and "unlimited renewal of the prescriptions," as well as the "multitude of proprietary nostrums containing opium," including "alleged 'cures for the opium-habit,'" all contributed to the crisis.[63] Each of these evils could be solved by substituting alternative medicines for opiates. This was a radical proposition, considering that opium was "generally recognized by the medical profession as the most indispensable of drugs." Nevertheless, "there are times when the dangers and disadvantages of this most brilliant of drugs seem wholly out of proportion to its benefits." The time had come to replace opiates as the central drugs of American medicine.[64]

The "recent discoveries" of Gilded Age science provided substitutes in the form of "several safer remedies which are capable of being used as substitutes." By the late 1880s, Adams began to replace opiates with other drugs in his own practice. He believed these "new analgesics," which included acetanilide, the precursor to acetaminophen, as well as antipyrine, phenacetin, sodium salicylate, and cocaine, promised to replace the traditional use of opiates in the treatment of many painful ailments. These medicines' "power for relieving pain is extraordinary," and "in many cases," they were "superior to opium." Indeed, several of these drugs ultimately became widely prescribed anti-inflammatory analgesics in the twentieth century. The drugs also had the "advantage over opium" of "not leading to any enslaving habit." Chronic diarrhea was a case in point. "Among the veterans of the war, a very large number are still suffering from this disease," Adams observed, and "as might be expected, some have become opium-eaters." Instead of addictive opiates, Adams prescribed sodium salicylate for chronic diarrhea. One of Adams's patients, a fifty-four-year-old Civil War veteran called "J. C.," suffered from debilitating chronic diarrhea, having "from four to seven stools daily, containing mucus and blood." Adams treated J. C. with ten grains of sodium salicylate four times daily, and within a few weeks, the veteran's bowels had resumed their normal function. The key to reducing opiate addiction, Adams concluded, was drug substitution. Summing up his position, Adams urged his fellow physicians to "revolt against opium."[65]

American physicians embarked on a flurry of experiments during the 1870s and 1880s in search of effective, less addictive substitutions for opiates. Doctors tried out scores of potential alternatives in hospitals, clinics, and private practices, some drugs safer than others. One doctor, W. C. Blalock, recommended hydrocyanic acid—cyanide and water—three times daily, "as an efficient substitute for opium and morphia, in the treatment of the opium habit." "No patient," Blalock insisted, "could not quit morphia while under the influence" of the remedy, which was highly toxic, unbeknownst to Blalock or his unfortunate patients.[66] Cyanide aside, most doctors eventually settled on two main substitutes for opiates, chloral hydrate and cocaine, which became popular medicines during the 1870s and 1880s. By 1890, the centrality of opium, morphine, and laudanum to physicians' therapeutic practices had greatly diminished. As the Massachusetts Board of Health surmised in 1888, "Chloral, [and] cocaine . . . were taking the place of opium."[67]

Chloral hydrate was the most promising substitute for opiates. The drug, introduced to the United States in its modern form in 1869, had been known since the 1830s and was a component in chloroform. Chloral hydrate was the first fully synthetic psychotropic drug used in Western mental health care. Often referred to simply as chloral, the drug was a liquid comprised of equal parts chloral and water. It was usually injected subcutaneously with hypodermic syringes. Not merely a substitute for opiates, chloral represents, according to one recent study, "the start of modern psychopharmacology"—meaning that chloral was intimately tied to the emergence of scientific medicine in the Western medical world. Elite reform-minded American doctors thus embraced chloral with gusto as an example of how scientific research could benefit the therapeutic practice of medicine, particularly chloral hydrate's utility as a substitute for opiates. Chloral was initially thought to be as potent a sedative and painkiller as morphine, but far less addictive. This made chloral a natural substitute for morphine amid the postwar opiate addiction crisis. A powerful sedative, chloral hydrate also helped doctors mitigate the effects of overcrowding in mental asylums by keeping patients calm and quiet.[68]

Physicians raced to adopt chloral hydrate after its introduction in 1869. In June 1870, Edward Hammond Clarke, professor of materia medica at Harvard Medical School and a correspondent of William A. Hammond, Silas Weir Mitchell, and Jacob Mendes Da Costa, published an article in the *BMSJ* praising chloral and recommending it for delirium tremens, hysteria, insomnia, and tuberculosis. Perhaps with Mitchell's commentary on opiate-addicted Civil War veterans in mind, Clarke even posited that chloral was a promising treatment for morphine addiction.[69] Chloral was superior to opiates because the new drug did not cause "congestion of the brain as morphia does."[70] Another doctor preferred chloral over opiates for treating neuralgia pain, namely, because "the patient does not acquire a habit for it."[71] According to a writer in the *Journal of Insanity*, "In many cases it is not desirable to use opium or any of its preparations." In opium's place, "we resort to chloral, because it has none of the subsequent bad effects of opiates, it is more reliable, it is convenient, palatable and reliable."[72] Such high praise for chloral appeared consistently in medical publications throughout the 1870s, 1880s, and 1890s, which illustrates how the drug was supplanting the therapeutic grip of opium and morphine.

Chloral was adopted widely during the Gilded Age to manage mental asylum patients, a role formerly filled by opiates. The May 1874 annual meeting of the Association of Medical Superintendents, the professional organization of mental asylum doctors, included a robust discussion about the merits of chloral as a substitute for opiates. "The most popular remedy, at present, in a large majority of hospitals for the insane, I doubt not, is chloral hydrate," noted one asylum doctor. The drug's main benefit was that it could calm excited patients and procure sleep. But like morphine, chloral hydrate could be dangerous, as some doctors quickly realized. The drug suppressed breathing and led to "intoxication," facial swelling, rashes on patients' skin, and even fatal overdoses on occasion. Most alarming of all was the realization that chloral hydrate was addictive. One doctor warned the audience, "It seems to me, brethren, that some of us can have but very little knowledge of the rapid spread of chloral drunkenness in our large cities, and among females. It is a notorious fact, beyond all question, that women in our large cities, are using chloral to-day to a most alarming degree, and solely because of the almost criminal carelessness with which physicians recommend its use."[73]

Thus, chloral hydrate was no panacea. Not long after its introduction, observant physicians realized that chloral was a poor substitute for opiates. "The bromides, chloral, ether and alcohol are all bad, and tend to do much damage by causing headaches and unpleasant reactions," J. M. Hull warned the Iowa Board of Health in 1885.[74] "Since the introduction of chloral hydrate into the practice of medicine it has rapidly grown in favor with the majority of the medical profession, until it has come into almost universal use," explained a New Hampshire doctor in 1872. Such reports had focused on the chloral's "bright side," quipped the doctor, who wrote to warn his colleagues about the dangers hiding behind "the curtain of silence," including overdose. The doctor recounted a case in which he had left a bottle of chloral hydrate and a hypodermic syringe with a woman suffering from facial pain. Following his orders, she injected ten grains of the chloral, only to find that her hands and feet grew numb, followed by difficulty breathing, hysteria, and, finally, unconsciousness. She narrowly survived the overdose, and shocked by her case, the doctor publicized her brush with death "to put every careful practitioner upon his guard."[75]

By the 1880s, Civil War veterans were dying from chloral hydrate overdoses. Less common than opium eating, chloral use nonetheless became stigmatized and often resulted in similar outcomes. Chloral could cost veterans their pensions and their lives and sometimes even landed them in mental asylums. John J. Wright, an Indiana veteran, died of a suspected overdose of chloral or "some other narcotic." When his widow, Laura, applied for a pension in 1888, her application and subsequent appeal were both denied. In the appeals decision, the US Pension Bureau denounced Wright as intemperate because of hard drinking and chloral use.[76] Willis B. Pomeroy, a veteran of 24th New York Cavalry, likewise died from a chloral overdose in 1899, which he had been "in the habit" of taking to relieve insomnia and lingering wartime sickness.[77] After observing cases of chloral addiction, some doctors came to believe that long-term chloral use could actually drive one insane—ironic, because chloral was used so widely in asylums to sedate institutionalized people. Edward Andrew Brown, a Confederate veteran and express agent from New Hanover, North Carolina, was admitted to the Dorothea Dix Hospital in Raleigh, North Carolina, on January 10, 1888, for mania caused by "excessive use of bromidia & chloral," the former being a popular patent medicine. Brown suffered from hallucinations, could barely draw a breath, and struggled to walk in a straight line without tottering over, which the doctors attributed to drug abuse. The asylum doctors promptly withdrew Brown from the chloral and bromidia, and after the hallucinations subsided and he gained strength, the veteran was released on April 2, 1888.[78]

Some physicians preferred cocaine, introduced to the United States with much acclaim in 1884, as a substitute for opium and morphine. Da Costa became an early and influential advocate for cocaine.[79] Shortly after identifying the risk of opiate addiction in Civil War veterans treated for chronic pain, Da Costa made up his mind to identify substitutes for opiates. Through a process of experimentation—injecting patients with hypodermic cocaine and observing the results—Da Costa concluded that the drug was a promising treatment for a variety of ailments for which opiates had been formerly indicated, including "diseases of the eye, ear, throat, tongue, nose, and rectum," as well as heart disease and as a local anesthetic.[80] During the 1880s, American physicians increasingly turned to cocaine as a substitute for opiates. Samuel M. Martin, the Civil War veteran whose "vicious habits" triggered a lengthy special investigation into his pension claim in 1896, tried cocaine as a substitute for morphine, which he felt was destroying his body and manhood. Martin, a physician by trade, had heard about cocaine's wonders. Soon, he "got to using cocaine," alongside his daily injections of morphine, perhaps "excessively" so, according to witnesses.[81] Other physicians began administering cocaine as a treatment for opiate addiction, especially as a stimulant to aid patients during withdrawal.[82]

Observant doctors thus quickly realized that cocaine, like chloral, was dangerous in its own right. "The use of cocaine in the alcoholic and opium inebriates is not satisfactory; while it is a more or less perfect substitute," one physician warned in 1886, "its use is attended with greater danger than alcohol and opium."[83] At the annual meeting of the American Association for the Study and Cure of Inebriety (AASCI) in November 1886, a paper on cocaine inebriety presented by T. D. Crothers sparked a lively discussion about the merits of cocaine as a substitute for opiates. Crothers reported treating several cases of cocaine inebriety, including among Civil War veterans. One man "was a neurotic dating from wounds in the army" who became addicted to cocaine after suffering "a severe army experience" punctuated by "attacks of malaria and typhoid fever." Cocaine was a dangerous drug, Crothers warned, and "it cannot be used as a substitute for any other narcotic, or as an antidote or remedy" for addiction. After Crothers read his paper, several of the nation's leading inebriety experts, who were in the audience, added that they too had treated cases of cocaine inebriety. J. B. Mattison had seen ten patients so afflicted. "All took it [cocaine] hypodermically, and nearly all had begun it in the hope of freeing themselves from opium, to which they were more or less addicted." Their hope was misguided, Mattison explained, for "none succeeded in the effort at self-cure, and all but one forged another link in their chains." Mattison urged his colleagues to administer cocaine with "caution," as "cases of its habitual use" were even "more disastrous, and less hopeful" than cases of morphine addiction. Another doctor in the audience, J. A. Blanchard, added that he treated a cocaine user who had been forced by cravings to use the drug every fifteen minutes, resulting in "brain delusions and hallucinations." It was "impossible," Blanchard warned, "for anyone to use this drug" in large doses daily "without becoming insane." Albert Day agreed, having recently treated more than a dozen cocaine inebriates in his Boston Washingtonian Home. Most had been substituting cocaine for opium or alcohol, and all had developed "pronounced and delirious mania." "I should never use cocaine for its narcotic properties," Day solemnly warned, for "it is too dangerous and uncertain." Joseph Parrish, an AASCI founder, beseeched his colleagues to study cocaine inebriety and report back any additional evidence of the drug's addictiveness and other dangers. Lewis D. Mason, a Brooklyn doctor, also in the audience, went a step further, concluding that "it was the duty of physicians to warn others of its [cocaine's] dangerous effects," just as it had been the profession's duty to revolt against opium. Cocaine ultimately did not turn out to be the safe or effective substitute for opiates that some doctors had hoped, a lesson that many inebriates and doctors learned the hard way.[84] Indeed, cocaine addiction became a serious problem among younger Americans during the Gilded Age, as has been well documented by historians.[85]

By the 1880s, the idea that physicians should prescribe fewer opiates and substitute them with supposedly less addictive alternatives became embedded into mainstream medical thought and practice, even if chloral hydrate and cocaine did not exactly live up to the nonaddictive hype. Joseph Woodward's warning about opiate addiction and his calls for doctors to avoid prescribing the addictive medicines in the 1879 volume of *The Medical and Surgical History of the War of the Rebellion* attest to the success of the revolt against opium, which was even incorporated into the US government's official medical account of the war.

Yet it is difficult to gauge how the therapeutic reforms advocated by well-heeled elite doctors affected the day-to-day practices of more ordinary American doctors. Unlike the famed Mitchell and Da Costa, most nineteenth-century doctors' prescription records were not preserved in historical medical archives.[86] Pharmacy and hospital records, however, can help fill this evidentiary gap, as they reveal impressions of changing therapeutic practices among ordinary American doctors, many of whom began prescribing fewer opiates from the 1880s onward than at any previous period in the nineteenth century. Following the lead of Mitchell, Hammond, and Da Costa, elite Northeastern physicians soon began prescribing opiates less frequently. Historian John Harley Warner, analyzing the records of two nineteenth-century American hospitals, has found that the percentage of prescriptions containing opiates declined beginning in the 1870s. Out of a sample of 274 prescriptions by doctors at Boston's Massachusetts General Hospital in the 1860s, 50.4 percent of prescriptions contained opiates. Of 341 prescriptions dating from the 1870s, only 42.2 percent contained opiates, and just 34.7 percent of the 222 prescriptions from the 1880s contained opiates. Doctors at the Commercial Hospital of Cincinnati also prescribed opiates less frequently during the 1870s and 1880s. They included opiates in 41.2 percent of 243 prescriptions Warner sampled from the 1860s, 24.4 percent of 700 prescriptions from the 1870s, and 24.8 percent of the 109 prescriptions dating from the 1880s. During the same thirty-year window, the average dosage of opiate prescribed at the Cincinnati hospital was also significantly higher than that of the Boston hospital, ranging from nearly three times higher in the 1860s to about 50 percent higher in the 1880s.[87] No such records from Southern hospitals are extant for direct comparison, but of 100 prescriptions sampled from a New Orleans pharmacy's prescription logs dating from 1886 to 1889, which would have been ordered by perhaps several dozen local doctors, 30 percent contained opiates.[88]

Although based on limited data, these statistics indicate two trends. First, the frequency and potency of opiate prescriptions began to markedly decline in several regions as early as the 1870s, keeping pace with growing allegations that physicians were culpable for the addiction crisis. Second, the influential voices of physicians like Mitchell and Da Costa mattered. The Northeastern physicians who worked at the Boston hospital—well-trained, elite practitioners who practiced in the same professional circles as Mitchell and Da Costa and thus would likely have been the most aware of the revolt against opium—prescribed opiates even less frequently than Midwestern or Southern doctors. There was always a degree of regional differences in nineteenth-century American medicine, although these distinctions softened during the Gilded Age. Regional distinctiveness, along with any number of additional factors, could have informed the disparity between Northeastern, Midwestern, and Southern opiate prescribing rates. Boston, home of the *BMSJ* and the Massachusetts Board of Health, had also been the site of much discussion of opium eating, dating back to the 1830s. But in all likelihood, an important factor in the Boston doctors' comparatively low opiate prescribing rate was their exposure to the warnings about opiate addiction frequently voiced by the nation's leading physicians, including Mitchell, Hammond, and Da Costa.[89]

Perhaps physicians at Massachusetts General Hospital took their cues from Silas Weir Mitchell, who, in 1882, corresponded with Edward Cowles, superintendent of the hospital's associated mental asylum. Cowles adored Mitchell, effusively praising his medical wisdom and clinical prowess. Cowles even described Mitchell's rest cure as "one of the most important contributions to the healing art in modern times."[90] Cowles's colleagues at the hospital may have likewise embraced Mitchell's advice about prescription opiates and responded by reducing their reliance on opiates there. Certainly, the writings of Mitchell and like-minded proponents of the revolt against opium were not the only factor driving the decline in its prescribing rates during the Gilded Age.[91] But the influence of these prominent former Civil War surgeons who warned about prescription opiate addiction early, often, and in important venues was an important factor in the decline of prescription opiate use in nineteenth-century American medicine.

Medicalization and Inebriety Clinics

Scientifically minded physicians also responded to the addiction epidemic with an effort to medicalize opiate addiction by redefining opium slavery as a physical disease called "inebriety." This change, proponents hoped, would reduce the stigma surrounding the condition; lead to innovative, effective medical care for addiction; and elevate the professional status of physicians who specialized in addiction medicine. To this end, doctors formulated complex theories about the pathology of inebriety and advocated for the treatment of the disease at inebriety clinics, early iterations of drug addiction rehabilitation centers. Although it would ultimately collapse in the early twentieth century, the inebriety model of addiction presaged later concepts of drug addiction as a substance use "disorder" and provided a template for modern addiction treatment centers. The inebriety movement thus helped push "opium slavery" to the margins of drug discourse, at least for a time, and bring more medicalized understandings of addiction to the forefront.

Gilded Age physicians who adopted a medicalized understanding of opiate addiction were responding both to criticisms of the profession as culpable for addiction and to calls for sympathy voiced by a growing number of opiate-addicted Americans. In 1867, the popular author Fitz Hugh Ludlow published a widely read *Harper's New Monthly Magazine* story on opium addiction. Ludlow was already famous for his 1857 narrative of cannabis use, or "hasheesh eating," but he also experimented with opium. He advocated for a radically medicalized understanding of addiction, describing opium eating "as purely physical as ... small-pox." "When this truth," Ludlow hoped, "is widely understood among the laity as it is known by physicians, some progress may be made in staying the frightful ravages of opium among the present generation."[92] Perhaps overestimating the degree to which most physicians agreed with him, Ludlow nevertheless found receptive audiences in some quarters, especially elite Northeastern physicians who had served in the Civil War. They had witnessed firsthand how the war's health conditions and medical practices facilitated opiate addiction among veterans.

In June 1868, the influential Medical Society of the State of Pennsylvania formed the Committee on Intemperance as a Disease to investigate the apparent increase in alcohol and opium intemperance.[93] Several of the committee's members had been involved in wartime medical and relief work. Joseph Parrish, who had initially pitched the idea for the committee, was already one of the nation's foremost experts on drug and alcohol addiction. During the Civil War, he served as inspector for the US Sanitary Commission and editor of its *Sanitary Commission Bulletin*. In these capacities, Parrish visited gargantuan military hospitals and dirty, disease-ridden army camps. Parrish's extensive observations meant that he understood the medical and health landscape of Civil War America. Like Silas Weir Mitchell at Turner's Lane Hospital, Parrish would have likely observed how veterans seemed prone to abusing substances like alcohol and morphine.[94] Around the time he joined the committee, Parrish also opened a sanitarium for drunkards and opium eaters near Philadelphia.[95] James King, another committee member, had been medical chief of Pennsylvania's Camp Curtain before assuming the medical directorship of the Pennsylvania reserves and, from late 1862 through August 1864, serving as the surgeon general of Pennsylvania. In 1866, as recently discharged, ailing, impoverished Union veterans flooded the streets of Philadelphia, Pittsburgh, and other Pennsylvania cities, King assumed the presidency of the Medical Society of the State of Pennsylvania.[96] In this capacity, King would likely have witnessed the plague of drug and alcohol addiction among soldiers. William Biddle Atkinson, a noted obstetrician and the longtime secretary of the AMA and the Medical Society of the State of Pennsylvania, spent the Civil War serving as an acting assistant surgeon in Philadelphia, where he would have dedicated much time to attending sick and wounded Union troops in Philadelphia's labyrinth of general hospitals.[97]

Primed to understand veterans' health needs and the urgency of addressing this issue, the committee completed its task quickly. Its June 1868 report generated much attention and was widely reprinted and circulated in the medical press.[98] The committee's findings on opiate addiction were bleak. First, they warned, "the opinion that the opium habit is greatly on the increase in nearly all communities seems to be gaining strength," demanding a concerted response by the medical profession.[99] The danger of addiction for patients should alarm every physician "when we consider the damaging influence of the opium habit, especially, how it degenerates nervous force, demoralizes manhood, and paralyzes labor—how it holds its victim a bondman, with no intermission of freedom and no promise of escape."[100] The committee singled out the hardships of army life, such as fatigue and hunger, to help explain why opiate addiction, drunkenness, and tobacco use were on the rise. "Soldiers, during our late war, frequently and cheerfully sacrificed a ration for" tobacco and opium, the root of the growing substance abuse crisis among veterans.[101]

In addition to uncovering the causes of substance abuse, the committee was also charged with determining if "those who are addicted to alcoholic and opium excess" were physically diseased, as Ludlow had argued, or merely depraved.[102] This question was of the utmost importance because it would dictate the proper response by physicians to the growing addiction crisis. If opium eaters were insane, then medical resources and professional energy should be channeled into states' existing public mental asylums. If opiate addiction was a disorder "as purely physical as one of small-pox," then a concerted medical solution would be warranted. A medicalized understanding would also "modif[y] the relation of the subject to morals and law," excusing opium eaters from culpability in their condition and the ensuing consequences, such as lost pensions for addicted veterans.[103]

The committee ultimately concluded that opiate addiction stemmed from a physical pathology. "Medical observation and diagnosis have, we think, distinctly proved that the diseased portion of the mind in such cases is chiefly of the will, not the intellect." This impairment of the will, the committee reasoned, must have its origin in some physical disorder of the brain. Opium made users "captives" whose "will yields to the insatiable demand of physical unrest and depression, or moral infirmity." But "when it [intoxication] is over, they are stung with the bitterest remorse, and sink into the deepest penitence and sorrow. Such, however, are not the fruits of insanity."[104] After all, how could an insane or depraved man feel remorse? Consequently, those who were addicted to opium deserved "sympathy and assistance" from physicians and from American society, not "arrest and fine, or imprisonment."[105] This finding directly contradicted accepted wisdom about opium slavery. For decades, most Americans had believed that addiction was a kind of intemperance or an expression of immorality, effeminacy, or insanity. This view would persist in many quarters well into the twentieth century, especially among proponents of the temperance movement, who vocally opposed the medicalization of addiction.[106] But the Committee on Intemperance as a Disease was nonetheless significant as the earliest organized effort by physicians to challenge the status quo by medicalizing opiate addiction.

A cadre of physicians took up the committee's call to action, forming the AASCI in November 1870.[107] Joseph Parrish, fresh from his work with the committee, together with physician Willard Parker, spearheaded the AASCI.[108] Parrish, Parker, and like-minded doctors who joined the organization rejected the temperance approach to addiction, which placed much moral culpability on the inebriate. The AASCI, they insisted, was "not a temperance, but a scientific gathering" seeking medical solutions for inebriety. The organization never fielded more than 500 members, but it would play an outsized role in the discourse of drug addiction in the Gilded Age and the Progressive Era. Many members were prominent Northeastern and Midwestern physicians, who were influential beyond their small numbers because their works were voraciously read by other doctors.[109] The first AASCI meeting was held at a Manhattan Young Men's Christian Association in November 1870, an ironic location considering the latter organization's close ties to the temperance movement.[110] The AASCI quickly emerged as the vanguard of the movement to medicalize opiate addiction in late nineteenth-century America, spearheading a fifty-year campaign to redefine addiction as a disease.

At its first meeting, the AASCI adopted a guiding principle that "intemperance is a disease" called "inebriety," which was "curable in the same sense that other diseases are."[111] One of the organization's prominent theorists, Edward Mann, elaborated that inebriety was "a disease of certain parts of the brain, resulting from some morbid irritation of the cortical sensory centers of the brain or from special molecular changes in the centers, perverting brain function." Inebriety "evidences outwardly by great nervous irritability or restlessness, unnatural sensations, and uncontrollable desire for" intoxicants such as alcohol and opium.[112] Thomas Davison "T. D." Crothers, the organization's longtime secretary and a leading inebriety theorist and clinician, defined inebriety as "a cerebro-psychal disorder manifest in cravings for fluids" that intoxicate, like morphine and whiskey.[113] These medicalized definitions rationalized addicted people's troubling behavior while offering up the prospect of a medical solution. Although "the inebriate loses his manhood, his self-respect," they were deserving of medical intervention and might even be cured when cared for under the right conditions, according to a speaker at the AASCI's 1871 annual meeting.[114] Although the term "inebriety" had been in limited use prior to its adoption by the AASCI, the organization popularized it.[115] The AASCI's stance presaged the model of addiction hawked by Leslie E. Keeley, who repackaged the organization's rhetoric to sell his Gold Cure, ultimately achieving more buy-in for a medicalized understanding of opiate addiction from the American public and the government than the AASCI ever would. But the organization did make some headway among elite doctors and state legislatures during the Gilded Age, before the inebriety movement came crashing down against the surging tide of prohibition in the 1910s and 1920s.

Advocates of the inebriety model of addiction developed a complicated array of views about the causes and nature of inebriety. Reflecting a broader scientific obsession with it, many theorists argued that heredity was the root of the disease. Some distant physical or mental infirmity handed down from parent to child grew worse with each successive generation until finally manifesting in the predilection for drunkenness or opium eating.[116] Once an inebriate appeared in a family line, unless he was cured, the disease doomed all descendants. Further, some doctors suggested that inebriety might stem not only from "progressive degeneration [that] often dates back to ancestors" but also "to defects of growth, retarded development and early physical and psychic injuries" in childhood.[117] A third theory suggested that excessively high doses of alcohol or opium damaged the brain, leaving it with a "diathesis," or craving, for the substances. Diathesis might lay dormant until activated when the inebriate received a swig of opium or alcohol later in life. Most AASCI members thus recognized that exposure to opiates through medical prescriptions increased the likelihood that patients would become addicted to opiates later in life. As Crothers explained, "Opium in any of its forms, given for any length of time... predisposes it [the nervous system] to functional and organic diseases marked by a craving for drugs and other narcotics."[118] After exposure to addictive substances, the sufferer's brain deteriorated until, finally, "both structural and functional degenerations are usually present."[119] Other doctors argued that physical "traumatism," or injury, could damage a healthy brain, leaving it susceptible to developing inebriety when exposed to intoxicants later in life.[120] Telltale proof of inebriety could be found in lesions and infirmities that seemed to appear on the brains of inebriates in postmortem autopsies, much like the needle marks that could be observed on the skin of hypodermic morphine users. Lesions helped explain the inebriate's erratic, immoral, unmanly actions.[121] According to Crothers, the "want of veracity," the "indiscriminate slandering and lying," the apparent "moral prostration, or paralysis of the will," the "unwonted risks" in business "or displays [of] trickery" to conceal opium use were simply manifestations of a lesion-riddled brain.[122]

Inebriety's theorists were heavily influenced by George Miller Beard, who had argued that neurasthenic "brain-workers," or desk-bound white-collar workers, were more liable to becoming inebriates than previous generations of American men, who had mostly worked with their hands outdoors. Beard joined the AASCI soon after its founding in 1870. The next year, he published a book on stimulants and narcotics in which he claimed that opiate addiction was on the rise in the United States, which counted at least 150,000 opium eaters. "All druggists know that in every community there are more or less" many users "who buy their opiates as regularly as others buy their tobacco," Beard warned. Although at times Beard utilized language describing opium addiction as "slavery," he often characterized addiction in medicalized language, explaining that "opio-mania is sometimes as truly a disease as dipsomania." Addiction was "partly a vice and partly a disease," Beard added, but "in either case the drunkard is to be pitied more than blamed." He concluded that "I would rather risk my life by jumping off Niagara Falls, than by forming the habit of opium-eating."[123] Doctors affiliated with AASCI built on the foundation provided by Beard's neurasthenia thesis to explain the kinds of people who became addicted to opiates. White-collar workers, especially doctors, were liable to addiction, argued the physician J. B. Mattison, because working long hours at mentally strenuous activities left such workers vulnerable to neurasthenia.[124]

Proponents of medicalization argued that, like any other disease, inebriety was curable with proper medical intervention. The AASCI thus echoed earlier calls for medicalization. The organization's members considered themselves to be true scientists, being distinguished from the temperance movement by a rejection of moral suasion, prayer, and contrition, as the proper solution for inebriety. However, inebriety theorists did not yet possess effective medical interventions for inebriety in 1870. It would take considerable scientific inquiry to discover effective and humane treatments for inebriety, especially through direct observation of those afflicted and clinical experimentation with various remedies. The AASCI advocated for scientific research to develop theoretical knowledge and clinical solutions for a burgeoning epidemic. The AASCI founded an influential specialty medical journal, the *Quarterly Journal of Inebriety* (*QJI*), to disseminate research and elevate the treatment of inebriety as a medical specialty during a time of intense specialization in American medicine.[125] Between the first issue in December 1876 and the last in 1914, the journal published more than 2,000 articles on the pathology and treatment of inebriety as well as its social and legal dimensions.[126] By 1891, the journal boasted over 2,000 subscribers in the United States and abroad.[127] The need for *QJI* was great amid the growing epidemic of inebriety. According to Albert Day, "The many forms of neuroses which arise from the action of these toxic agents are increasing and becoming more complex, requiring special study, and, as yet, are comparatively unknown to the profession."[128] Some of the most prominent American doctors of the Gilded Age published articles on various facets of inebriety in *QJI*, including Silas Weir Mitchell and George Miller Beard.

Efforts to monopolize the clinical spaces where inebriates received treatment was crucial to the development of inebriety medicine. During the Civil War, many AASCI members had seen how a glut of sick bodies under the direct control of physicians could generate a rapid development in scientific knowledge and medical interventions. To that end, inebriety specialists proposed the creation of residential clinics where inebriates could receive expert care, while also providing inebriety doctors with more data about the disease. As one advocate for inebriety clinics explained, the "rational data collection and analysis in the 'lab-oratory' of the inebriate asylum would unlock the secrets" of inebriety, which "moral and penal authorities had failed to cure."[129] Doctors had long recognized that opiates could be poisonous, but exactly how they damaged the body remained unclear. "Notwithstanding the numerous researches and observations which have been made on the influence of opium," one doctor explained, the "conditions have not yet been precisely laid down under which it [opium] may act beneficially or mischievously."[130] The inebriety clinic, with its large supply of opium users, thus provided a unique opportunity to investigate how opium affected the body and impaired the mind. Antebellum opportunities for drug addiction research had been rare, limited to private practices or to unsafe public asylums with poor cure rates. Instead, a "sick" inebriate "must seek the hospital and the physician, and not moral treatment, if he would be cured, as his disease depends upon physical conditions that have to be remedied."[131]

Channeling inebriates to dedicated clinics would not only benefit patients and the doctors who treated them but society as well. Most inebriety theorists considered the disease to be essentially contagious—not through contact with miasmas or infected bodies but through social or hereditary contact with inebriates. Clinics could thus provide opportunities for the study and treatment of inebriety while also quarantining inebriates, who "should be no more permitted to go at large" and spread sickness "than the man deprived of reason from any other source."[132] Deteriorating conditions at public mental asylums also worked in favor of the nascent inebriety clinic movement. As large state-funded mental asylums grew increasingly crowded with patients during the late nineteenth century, many pragmatist asylum doctors came to believe that treating inebriates in asylums was a waste of scarce resources that were better directed toward other patients. A vocal cohort of asylum superintendents argued that inebriates, who had only temporarily lost their wits while intoxicated, recovered their sanity quickly. Inebriates did not belong among the chronically insane, who recovered slowly over years and decades, if at all. For their part, many inebriates, feeling out of place among those deemed insane, balked at asylum rules and proved difficult to manage. In 1889, the superintendent of the Connecticut Hospital for the Insane aired his frustrations at the constant misbehavior exhibited by alcohol, opium, and cocaine inebriates. The presence of inebriates in the asylum undermined the precarious balance of power between the few attendants tasked with maintaining order and the many patients to be managed. "As soon as they rally from the toxic effects of the drug which inspired them," the superintendent explained in 1887, "and seriously reflect upon their situation, [inebriates] begin to chafe under the restrictions which govern the insane [in the asylum]." Such patients "protest against associations with lunatics," "are not usually disposed to engage in any useful occupation," and "are often prone to plot mischief."[133] Thus, shunting inebriates into dedicated inebriety clinics proved an attractive measure for asylum doctors seeking to alleviate the problems of scarce funding, overcrowding, and patient misbehavior.

Scores of inebriety clinics were founded during the late nineteenth and early twentieth century in all corners of the United States. The clinics treated inebriety in all its forms. Rather than opium users, the majority of patients at most clinics were alcohol inebriates. Historians recognize the clinics as pivotal in the movement to medicalize drunkenness as "alcoholism," although their importance to the history of narcotics has been less studied.[134] Inebriety clinics gained traction during the 1870s and 1880s, although there were a few earlier iterations.[135] J. Edward Turner, an early advocate of inebriate clinics and a member of the AASCI, founded the nation's first public and most influential inebriate asylum at Binghamton, New York, in 1859.[136] Operations were delayed by the Civil War, but New York State Inebriate Asylum accepted its first patients in 1864. By December 1867, the asylum had admitted eighty men.[137] Private patients were sometimes admitted to the asylum on their own volition at ten to twenty dollars per week, but more often, inebriates were committed to the Binghamton asylum against their will. "More than half" of the inmates, according to an *Atlantic Monthly* reporter, were "officers of the army or navy during the late war, and lost control of themselves then" by abusing alcohol and opiates.[138] Turner left the asylum shortly after its founding, replaced in 1867 by Albert Day, the noted inebriety expert, who had previously practiced for a decade at Boston's Washingtonian Home for drunkards. Like Turner, Day had previously been a temperance activist. But in Binghamton, Day adopted the inebriety model, learning to treat the disease through a combination of medical intervention and moral suasion.[139]

Day claimed in 1868 that fully half of the patients treated at the Binghamton asylum had been discharged, their inebriety ostensibly improved or cured by Day's unique therapeutic regimen. The premise that inebriety eroded one's manhood and moral character, despite absolving one of moral culpability, was central to this treatment plan. Inebriates "had been deeply degraded and steeped in all the vices indulgent to a dissipated life," but innovative medical care at the asylum promised to transform inebriates into "truly regenerated men."[140] Despite the idea that inebriates were distinct from the insane, the system of care at Binghamton included hallmarks of nineteenth-century psychiatry: rest, nutritious food, and outdoor labor. Equally crucial in the restorative regimen was the notion that inebriates must be separated from the poisons of alcohol and opiates, thus allowing one's body, brain, and, by extension, manhood to be restored. Naturally, many inebriates resisted abstinence, but the asylum's charter allowed for patients to be involuntarily committed by judges, just as insane patients could be legally committed to New York's public mental asylums.[141] Patients were immediately withdrawn from stimulants at admission and, during the agonizing process, might be sedated with bromides. Amid the agony of withdrawal, many patients lost control of themselves. Staff at the Binghamton asylum thus sometimes resorted to physical restraints to control patients, a flash point of controversy in nineteenth-century psychiatry. Once withdrawal pains faded and physical restraints came off, Day prescribed cricket, billiards, and copious reading to occupy and stimulate inmates' recovering brains after withdrawal. To that end, Harriet Beecher Stowe visited the asylum around 1867, where she performed a reading from her book *Uncle Tom's Cabin*, supposedly using a tattered copy of the book supplied by a self-emancipated, formerly enslaved man who, in freedom, worked at the asylum. Stowe's son, Frederick, a Union army veteran wounded at Gettysburg, was a patient at the asylum during the late 1860s, where he received Day's treatment for alcoholic inebriety.[142]

The asylum's managers claimed unprecedented success at curing inebriety through this system of care. While the facility's medical records are no longer extant, Willard Parker, president of the asylum's board of directors, quoted from former patients' letters in an 1867 report. According to Parker, their outcomes evidenced the asylum's success at curing inebriety. "I am living quietly and steadily . . . as I think becomes a man," wrote one newly sober patient. "I have entirely abstained from touching the accursed thing [intoxicants]," added another man, "and trust I may be kept from it forever."[143] For many addicted men, the inebriety clinics represented an opportunity to be rid of addiction and restored to manhood, much like addiction "antidotes" peddled by Samuel B. Collins and other patent medicine sellers. Yet, despite its great promise, the pioneering New York State Inebriate Asylum was short-lived. Turner's tenure during the 1860s was marred by accusations of mismanagement, fraud, and arson, a controversy that cast a pall over the asylum's public standing. The notion that inebriates were not morally culpable for their condition remained deeply controversial, further animating hostility toward the institution. Citing allegations of mismanagement as well as overcrowding at the state's public mental asylums, New York State assumed control over the Binghamton asylum in 1879, opening the institution's doors to the insane, not just inebriates.[144]

Yet despite its brief existence, the Binghamton asylum catalyzed the growth of the inebriety movement. The sheer spectacle of the asylum garnered considerable media attention, amplifying inebriety activists' message. After visiting the asylum in 1868 for an *Atlantic Monthly* story, a journalist predicted that "there will, perhaps, one day be in every state an asylum for incurable drunkards, wherein they will be permanently detained, and compelled to live temperately."[145] While there was a trace of sarcasm in this prediction, it nonetheless buoyed the confidence of inebriety activists. Citing the Binghamton asylum, the Committee on Intemperance as a Disease, likewise highlighted the urgent need for inebriety clinics in the Civil War's wake: "What experience have we to justify the establishment of institutions for the care and treatment of persons who are addicted to alcoholic and opium excess? Our answer is that the experiment has been successfully tried in Massachusetts and New York, under the patronage of these States, and, for the last two years, at Media, Pennsylvania, by a private corporation" and led by Joseph Parrish.[146] Optimistic observers believed the cure rates claimed by inebriate clinic doctors were convincing enough to warrant more such facilities, where some "90 percent, of opium cases are curable, under institution treatment."[147]

The experiment at Binghamton set the tone for the founding of some 100 public and private clinics by 1910, the peak of the inebriety movement.[148] The AASCI's organizational charter made the establishment of inebriate asylums a priority, calling for "every large city" in the United States to found a "local or temporary home for inebriates, and every state, one or more asylums for the treatment and care of such persons." Furthermore, the organization insisted that "the law should recognize intemperance as a disease, and provide other means for its management, than fines, stationhouses and jails."[149] Responding in part to the AASCI's call for action and in part to growing demand for treatments for addiction, enterprising physicians founded scores of inebriate homes around the United States during the Gilded Age.

Inebriety clinics came in two varieties: public inebriate "asylums" and small, private inebriate "homes." Public inebriate asylums were generally modeled after the Binghamton asylum. They were large, publicly funded institutions where inebriates could be subjected legally to coercive treatment. In many states, inebriates might find themselves involuntarily committed by families or judges to such facilities.[150] In Brooklyn, New York, inebriates who were arrested for disorderly behavior oftentimes wound up in the Kings County Inebriate Asylum, also known as Fort Hamilton. It was founded in 1867 with the pragmatic aim of relieving overcrowding at the local Kings County jails, which were inundated with inebriates.[151] Like the Binghamton asylum, Fort Hamilton admitted many Civil War veteran inebriates, at least in its early years. According to the 1871 annual report of its superintendent, "Of the 105 male patients treated in the home during the past year, thirty-five were returned soldiers, who had fought and conquered in our late civil war." Like many institutions that targeted veterans in the late 1860s–70s, commitment to Fort Hamilton was sometimes pitched as a way of protecting veteran inebriates who had fallen on hard times. As the superintendent explained in 1871, "Most of their [veteran inebriates] number had, since that time [the Civil War], been constantly immured in prisons, sharing the companionship, and suffering all the penal afflictions of the felon," having been jailed for disorderly or deviant behavior stemming from addiction.[152] Indeed, opiate-addicted veterans occasionally landed in Gilded Age jails, despite the absence of criminal laws against opiate use or possession. In 1874, the warden of the United States Jail in Washington, DC, reported that his institution held several prisoners with opiate addictions. When encountered with such prisoners, his "usual treatment" was immediate withdrawal from opiates. The warden's phrasing implied that the jail had seen such cases previously.[153]

Under the leadership of J. B. Mattison, Fort Hamilton became nationally famous for treating opiate inebriates. It admitted public patients from Kings County jails and elsewhere in the state, as well as private-pay patients. According to Mattison, most opiate inebriates were middle-class men with professional occupations, especially doctors, who could afford to stay at the clinic at the rate of five to thirty-five dollars a week, payable in three-month increments. The "seclusion and repose" of the facilities were especially conducive to "the treatment of the victims of the Opium Habit," according to one advertisement for Fort Hamilton.[154] The conditions for admission were strict. To secure entry, voluntary patients had to humble themselves, admitting to "indulging" in the use of opiates "until such practice has become a confirmed habit, which I cannot control, and which I feel powerless to overcome without assistance." Patients also had to consent to stay for as long as the medical staff deemed necessary, up to six months, as well as submit to the use of restraints during withdrawal or whenever the staff deemed such measures necessary. Inebriates who refused to enter the asylum voluntarily could be committed by state or county courts, at the request of their families, for up to a year.[155]

Armed with the conviction that addiction was a curable physical disease, Mattison's work at Fort Hamilton earned him a reputation as one of the nation's foremost experts on the treatment of opium inebriety. His asylum attracted patients and inquiries from all corners of the United States. An Alabama doctor, who apparently had been addicted to opium for a decade, wrote to Mattison in 1883. "Opiomania" is "a subject in which I am deeply interested," the doctor explained. "Do you think it can be cured?" he inquired. "If so," he added, "advise me what course to pursue in order to attain the important privilege of being rationally treated." "Most emphatically—Yes," Mattison replied. The Alabama doctor should not "hopelessly resign himself to a bondage for life," because even long-standing cases can "undoubtedly" be cured with proper care. "Opium addiction" is "a functional disorder" of the body, Mattison insisted. "Opium addiction," like other diseases of the body, "is curable in the sense that other diseases are."[156] Mattison recommended gradual withdrawal and cited several cases under his or his colleagues' care as clinical examples. Mattison typically withdrew his patients from opiates gradually over the course of a week. In case histories of seven doctors whom he treated for opiate addiction in the 1880s, Mattison described how he reduced the patient's dose every day while administering sedatives and hot baths to mitigate withdrawal symptoms. The recovered patients were released from the clinic about a month after admission.[157]

Several states considered opening public inebriate asylums like those in Binghamton and Brooklyn during the postwar decades, although only a handful of long-lasting inebriate asylums materialized.[158] In 1868, the Massachusetts legislature's Joint Special Committee on Inebriation as a Disease concluded that "opium eating is rapidly on the increase in this country, as every physician can testify." "There is little hope for such patients outside of an inebriate asylum," but the problem could be contained if the state established an inebriate asylum for the cure of drunkards and opium eaters. The state was already home to Boston's Washingtonian Home, but more must be done, the committee declared. "Beyond all question the legislature ought to make the same provisions of persons who have lost self-control through habitual inebriation" as it had made for mental asylums. Little ultimately came of the report, which was followed by subsequent State Board of Health investigations on the subject in

1872 and 1888. But the 1868 committee's report illustrates the increasing alarm over opiate addiction in the Civil War's aftermath, as well as the impetus for physicians to act to tackle the problem.[159] In 1872, the legislature of Kentucky passed a bill "in order to check the practice of opium eating, which is greatly on the increase." It allowed for the voluntary or involuntary commitment of those found to be addicted to opiates, "as is in the case of habitual drunkards."[160] In March, the legislature passed an act incorporating the "Central Kentucky Inebriate Asylum," although a dedicated facility never came to fruition.[161]

Despite the initial optimism surrounding public inebriate asylums, during the late 1870s, the movement for such facilities largely collapsed. Several factors were responsible. First, the Panic of 1873 forced most states' budgets into the red. Northeastern states, where inebriety asylum proponents had made most headway among state legislatures, were hit especially hard. In the ensuing depression, funding for inebriate asylums simply evaporated. The Pennsylvania Sanitarium, a short-lived public inebriate asylum founded in 1868, was denied state funding during the Panic of 1873, and the facility shuttered its doors the next year. The depression that cemented the Northern "retreat from Reconstruction," to quote Eric Foner, also killed the AASCI's vision of a nationwide system of public inebriate asylums.[162] When funding dried up, the bottom simply fell out of proposed asylums, and several existing asylums converted to private facilities. Additionally, despite the AASCI's passionate appeals for sympathy toward inebriates, the idea of inebriate asylums remained controversial in many quarters, especially as the temperance movement surged during the Gilded Age. Many Americans could not stomach the idea that drunkenness and opium slavery were diseases, instead of condemnable failures of manhood or morality. It was thus difficult to secure funding for the controversial asylums, especially after 1873. The use of coercive restraints against inebriates in asylums like Binghamton also proved controversial, working against the movement to found public inebriate asylums. The practice disturbed many observers, who questioned the effectiveness of forcing drunkards to receive treatment in inebriate asylums against their will. Finally, the presence of large and growing state mental asylum systems made specialty inebriate asylums seem superfluous. Most state legislatures simply did not see a need for inebriate asylums because inebriates could be funneled into existing mental asylums. In fact, inebriates would continue to be committed to mental asylums well into the twentieth century.[163]

Frustrated by the collapse of public asylums, inebriety specialists increasingly turned to private practice from the mid-1870s onward. In contrast to public inebriate asylums, private inebriate "homes" tended to have fewer than fifty beds and admitted patients voluntarily and selectively. In 1878, J. B. Mattison, superintendent of Brooklyn's Fort Hamilton, left the public asylum and opened a private inebriety clinic in Brooklyn called Parrish Hall. Mattison exclusively treated opiate inebriates at the new private clinic. He billed the institution as a "private medical home for opium habituates," the "only one of its kind in existence."[164] Like Fort Hamilton, Mattison's private clinic became a mecca for opiate-addicted patients with the means to afford travel and care costs. "Dr. Mattison of Brooklyn, N.Y., the veteran specialist of opium inebriety, has his home constantly crowded with patients," reported *QJI* in 1889, which advertised his clinic.[165] By 1909, when just three state inebriate hospitals remained, scores of private inebriety clinics like Mattison's were scattered around the nation.[166] Several clinics were run by former Union army surgeons who had treated addicted veterans.

T. D. Crothers, longtime secretary of the AASCI and editor of *QJI*, directed Walnut Hill Asylum, another prominent clinic in Hartford, Connecticut. During the Civil War, Crothers had served as a medical cadet at the US General Hospital in Albany, New York. No account exists of his time at the hospital, but Crothers would almost certainly have administered opiates to ailing soldiers. Perhaps the Albany hospital is where he first recognized that long-term exposure to opiates could lead to addiction. Crothers became a proponent of inebriety clinics during his time as assistant physician in the New York State Inebriate Asylum at Binghamton, where he arrived around 1875 and where he would have treated Civil War veteran inebriates.[167] According to Crothers, all the inebriate needed "to recover" was the "restraint and quiet of hospitals."[168] The collapse of the asylum at Binghamton seems to have prompted Crothers to strike out on his own, and he soon became the superintendent of the Walnut Lodge Hospital in Hartford, Connecticut, where he remained for decades.[169] From Walnut Lodge, Crothers meticulously studied inebriates, experimenting with various medical treatments and observing the pathology of the disease in hundreds of patients. Through his ambitious research agenda, at the time of his death in 1918, Crothers had become the nation's most prominent authority on opiate addiction.

Among the scores of papers Crothers published on inebriety, including at least seventy-one papers in *QJI* alone, were numerous studies on opiate addiction based on observations and clinical experiments conducted at Walnut Lodge.[170] Crothers described treating Civil War veterans, recalling one notable case in 1900. A merchant recovering from influenza "was given a small quantity of opium daily for two weeks" and could not muster the self-control to quit taking the drug after recovering. At first, ashamed of his habit, the man "secretly" consumed the drug. But soon he "threw off all restraint," abandoning any bourgeois attachment to self-control, "and used it boldly in large quantities" in plain view. "Coming under my care," Crothers investigated the man's case, hoping to identify the event that had generated the man's diathesis.

Upon interrogating the patient, the doctor "found that opium had been used twenty years before for chronic diarrhea following a term for service in the Civil War."[171] Crothers came to believe that addiction to opiates and other narcotics, which he named "narcomania," ultimately left opium users out of touch with their physical and moral senses. Consequently, narcomaniacs became unaware of their surroundings and actions. A sophisticated elaboration of inebriety theory, Crothers's narcomania model rejected the prevailing sentiment that opium slavery eroded morality and manhood, explaining that the narcomaniacs' sensual deprivation excused them from culpability for any crimes and immoral actions they committed while under the influence. Crothers's narcomania model of opiate addiction thus represented the apex of the movement to medicalize opiate addiction. But it was far too radical of a proposition for most observers to accept. Most Americans ultimately rejected narcomania, clinging to the belief that drug users were culpable when they developed the "habit."[172]

The Postwar Temperance Movement

In contrast to the broader American public, during the final decades of the nineteenth century, the medicalization of opiate addiction gained significant traction among elite American physicians, especially those who, like Hammond and Crothers, had served as surgeons during the Civil War. As they adopted the medicalized perspective on addiction, these physicians increasingly considered inebriety clinics as promising avenues for restoring opium eaters and other inebriates. Indeed, "the only reliable means of escape" from slavery to opium, concluded an 1877 editorial in *Medical and Surgical Reporter*, "is by the patient wholly and willingly resigning himself to the care and supervision of a physician in an institution especially adapted for that purpose." In particular, the article lauded Mattison's Brooklyn clinic and Crothers's Walnut Hill as successful models.[173] Eventually, the AASCI even managed to get major medical organizations to endorse the inebriety clinic model and, by extension, the medicalization of opiate addiction. The Association of Medical Superintendents of American Institutions for the Insane, the nineteenth-century precursor to the modern American Psychiatric Association, endorsed public inebriate asylums in 1875, although many superintendents maintained the older view that opiate addiction was a cause of insanity.[174] The AMA sponsored a session on alcoholic and narcotic inebriety at its 1891 annual meeting.[175] When Albert Day, president of the New York State Inebriate Asylum at Binghamton during the late 1860s and among the founders of the AASCI, died in 1894, obituaries appeared in several leading medical journals lauding Day's medical work. Such attention illustrates the notoriety achieved by the medicalization movement during the Gilded Age.[176]

Throughout the post–Civil War decades, however, there remained considerable popular opposition to the inebriety model. Ultimately, despite the best efforts of inebriety doctors, most Americans did not adopt a medicalized concept of opiate addiction. Temperance proponents, some mental asylum superintendents, and public officials like Grover Cleveland maintained that addiction was a condemnable "habit," not an uncontrollable compulsion stemming from a diseased constitution. The medicalization of addiction cut against many decades of medical-moral dogma, and these headwinds proved too strong to overcome. Moreover, many observers were troubled by the implications of the inebriety model's medicalized take on addiction for men's willpower. According to inebriety doctors like Crothers, the inebriate had no self-control. But the notion that the user was entirely beholden to the drug absolved him of the actions he committed when intoxicated. Most Americans were not intellectually or emotionally prepared to dismiss the existence of volition out of hand, as the inebriety theorists seemed comfortable doing. Many people thus rejected the inebriety model on moralistic grounds, insisting that the drunk and the opium slave were culpable for their sins.

The postwar temperance movement was a case in point. Temperance proponents had denounced opium, with its addictive and intoxicating properties, for decades. With addiction surging in the Gilded Age, increasingly powerful temperance organizations such as the Woman's Christian Temperance Union (WCTU) doubled down on the notion that addiction was a moral failing, not a disease. With Frances Willard at the helm, the organization's narcotics division set about "fighting the devil in the morphine bottle," as one observer put it, around 1885. Much of this campaign involved teaming up with British and American missionaries to lobby for the end of the international opium traffic, which scholars have argued amounted to little in the short term. Less studied is the WCTU's effort to combat opiate addiction at home. Considering the organization's stated goals of improving women's lives by way of prohibition, it is not surprising that much of its domestic anti-opium campaign focused on saving "white-souled women of exquisite culture and natural mental qualities" by publicizing the growing addiction problem and calling for opiate bans. Chinese opium smokers in places like San Francisco presented a special menace to the virtue of white women, Willard argued, finding common ground with anti-immigration and pro-segregation politicians.[177]

The WCTU also found natural male allies in patent medicine sellers, who had a vested interest in increasing business. In the 1890s, the Anti Opium Department of the WCTU officially endorsed Samuel B. Collins's Painless Opium Antidote. The department's superintendent, Jessie A. Ackerman, lived in Chicago, where Collins had moved his bustling laboratory earlier in the decade. It seems plausible that the two met to discuss their common cause. Concerned about race suicide and opium slavery, Ackerman praised Collins's antidote as a "boon to the race" for freeing so many whites from "the slavery of these drugs." Collins milked this resounding endorsement for all it was worth, churning out flyers emblazoned with Ackerman's praise.[178] Columns praising the WCTU's anti-opium crusade ran side-by-side in newspapers with stories praising Leslie E. Keeley's Gold Cure.[179] Shared ground between Collins, Keeley, and the WCTU might seem puzzling at first glance, considering that patent medicines represented an expression of medicalization, not far removed from inebriety clinics. After all, Collins and Keeley needed their customers to envision opium slavery as a disease so they would buy the remedies. Yet this apparent contradiction between moralizing and medicalization did not prevent an alliance between patent medicine sellers and the temperance movement. Businesspeople like Collins and Keeley were committed chiefly to profit at the end of the day. If the WCTU's moralizing would guilt men into purchasing the Painless Opium Antidote or the Gold Cure, so much the better.

Not all inebriety doctors, either, saw their movement as being at odds with temperance. After all, both wanted the same goal: the emancipation of "opium slaves." But temperance proponents and their patent medicine allies had no room for scientific rhetoric about the moral neutrality of addiction. Throughout the country, temperance speakers, writers, and activists loudly condemned the "sin" of opium "abuse" and urged users to turn to God for forgiveness. Newspapers printed temperance sermons alongside advertisements for addiction "cures." In one sermon about hell, a doom-and-gloom preacher railed that the opium eater "has no fear of an angry God" in his soul.[180] Some preachers even claimed that "faith alone" could cure opium eating, rejecting medicine altogether. One inveterate opium eater of forty years was healed during a prayer session. When she came away praising the "blessings of the Holy Spirit," her church endorsed the faith healing by holding a revival, and the *New-York Times* echoed the story to excited readers around the nation.[181] In the Gilded Age competition over how to define addiction, the temperance movement's cacophony—with its potent mix of moral suasion, fear mongering, and faith healing—drowned out the logic and intellectual appeals of the inebriety movement.

Beyond the ranks of the WCTU, many ordinary Americans continued to subscribe to the view that addiction represented a form of intemperance, with moral implications for the opium eater. Opium was condemned from the pulpit at temperance meetings, as it had been before the Civil War. Drawing on the rhetoric of opium slavery, one St. Louis preacher shocked revival goers in 1880 with his claim that there were "at least 10,000 persons who were addicted to the habitual use of opium, and who were surely becoming victims to its galling chains, or had already become so." In that wicked city, opium was "sold here by the dram, ounce or pound" when "physicians only used it by the grain." Too many people "were perfect slaves to it." Opium was "detrimental of health and moral character," and if allowed to go unchecked, the preacher warned, it would imperil souls and ruin the nation. With the audience already on the edge of their seats, the preacher then "created something of a stir" by a confession: *He* had been a "slave" to opium for years, reforming after he joined the Methodist church. Mimicking antebellum drunkard narratives, the preacher's "intensely interesting" story of redemption "filled his audience with deepest sympathy." Finally, a local doctor with experience at treating opium eaters materialized on stage. He sent the enraptured audience home with a solemn warning to "run away from the drug."[182]

The persistence of the older, moralistic model of opiate addiction helped stifle the medicalization movement and its inebriety clinics, which largely died out by the 1920s. Also important was the growing number of non-white opiate users in an era of explosive immigration to the United States. Immigrants were often crammed into the poorest neighborhoods and vice districts of America's growing metropolises. When urban non-white immigrants used opiates, it made drug use seem less sympathetic and helped spur heavy-handed policing. The same rationale also worked against morphine maintenance clinics in the 1920s.[183] Equally significant, historians also attribute the decline of the inebriety movement to the inability of specialists to develop effective therapeutic measures for addiction. "As institutions failed to realize this utopian promise" of curing inebriety with medicine, one scholar concludes, "the theory that inebriety was a curable medical condition suffered."[184] Unable to clinically check the spread of drunkenness and narcotic addiction, inebriety specialists had little ammunition to oppose the resurgent Progressive Era movement to ban alcohol. Prohibition finally killed off the AASCI's movement to medicalize addiction. Despite its early promise to cure the evils of addiction, the organization's medicalization efforts were eventually eclipsed by prohibitionist laws like the Harrison Narcotics Tax Act and the Eighteenth Amendment.[185]

The AASCI's efforts to medicalize opiate addiction ultimately proved unsuccessful. The cadre of scientifically minded physicians, many of them former Union surgeons, succeeded at changing the discourse around drug and alcohol addiction from "opium slavery" to "inebriety" in some corners of the American medical profession during the Gilded Age. But the proponents of medicalization failed to change popular discourse about opiate addiction or to convince most Americans that opiate addiction was a disease, not a form of insanity or a failure of manhood or morality. As the AASCI's signature inebriety clinics shuttered, the bottom fell out of the medicalization movement.

Oblivion

Even if medicalization largely failed as a solution to opiate addiction, the broader revolt against opium profoundly altered American medicine. Before the revolt, doctors had leaned heavily on prescription opiates for most of the nineteenth century. But during the 1870s and 1880s, some American doctors began relying less heavily on opiates, shifting to supposedly nonaddictive substitutes that offered solutions for the addiction crisis. This shift was especially true of former Civil War surgeons and the postwar generation of physicians, like J. C. Wilson, Da Costa's medical mentee during the 1870s who later trumpeted the revolt against opium at the American Academy of Medicine in the 1880s. By the turn of the twentieth century, American doctors had sharply curtailed opiate overprescribing. Younger, better trained American physicians relied less on prescription opiates, once widely prescribed and heralded as the "magnum Dei donum" of the materia medica. When doctors prescribed opiates less frequently, fewer patients became addicted, which decreased the extent of physician-caused opiate addiction. As David T. Courtwright observed on the centenary of the Harrison Act, "progressive physicians and pharmacists" by 1914 had "managed to contain the first major US epidemic of iatrogenic opiate addiction." "They had succeeded through primary prevention," that is, "creating fewer new addicts as existing addicts began quitting or died of old age, chronic disease, or overdose."[186]

As the years passed, aging morphine-addicted Civil War veterans were simply eclipsed in number and in the public eye by other, usually derogatory stereotypes—the Chinese opium smoker, the fallen white prostitute, the Black cocaine user, the immigrant urban heroin user, or, ironically, the invalid World War I "doughboy." The next generation of American drug users often became addicted not through doctors' prescriptions but through substance use outside of formal medical bounds, in part because access to medicinal opiates grew increasingly restricted. Prescription opiates became the purview of middle-class whites.[187] Historian Charles E. Rosenberg observes that "epidemics ordinarily end with a whimper, not a bang. Susceptible individuals flee, die, or recover, and incidence of the disease gradually declines."[188] This pattern held true during the early twentieth century for addiction among Civil War veterans. As they slowly faded away with a metaphorical whimper, they were overshadowed by a more worrisome cohort of narcotic users.

In the end, the revolt against opium ultimately came too little, too late for many opiate-addicted Civil War veterans. Some men managed to find emotional solace in patent medicines, although many consumers found only poverty. Some former soldiers found help at inebriety clinics, although this avenue was restricted to the wealthy. For most Civil War veterans who used opiates, addiction ended up lasting a lifetime. By the time the revolt against opium yielded mainstream therapeutic reforms, countless veterans, like Francis C. Clewell or James Ladson Hall, had already died of drug overdoses years beforehand, leaving behind grieving families. Many old soldiers, such as Robert B. Andrews and Charles Y. Sturgeon, wasted away in gloomy mental asylums, having been institutionalized by families who hated to see their loved ones go but had no other recourse for managing their addictions at home. Some aging users, like Perry B. Bowser and John T. Goolrick, soldiered on into the twentieth century. Ostracized and frustrated, with little hope for a cure, they kept on swallowing opium pills or injecting morphine day after day to get by until succumbing to complications, comorbidities, or old age. Ironically, the revolt against opium, which hastened the overall decline of iatrogenic opiate addiction in nineteenth-century America, did little to help most addicted veterans break the chains of opium slavery. The Civil War's addiction epidemic only ended when addicted veterans themselves faded into oblivion.

Epilogue

The Army Disease

Remembering Addicted Veterans in the Twentieth- and Twenty-First-Century United States

> The United States has a unique history with opioids. . . . And it starts with the US Civil War.
>
> —Rep. Alexandria Ocasio-Cortez (D-NY), 2019

The last opiate-addicted Civil War veterans died off during the early twentieth century, but their memory lived on through depictions of the "army disease." For more than a century, references to the so-called army disease (sometimes styled as the "soldier's disease") have appeared in drug policy debates, medical studies, pop culture, and histories of the Civil War. If many Americans today remember traces of the addiction epidemic among Civil War veterans, it is largely because Progressive Era drug warriors wanted us to. When these veterans departed, they left behind a politically useful legacy for those who sought to further police and criminalize drug addiction in the early twentieth century. The use of morphine by veterans was widely cited during discussions and debates over the prohibitionist regime that formed around the Harrison Act of 1914. If the addicted veteran proved problematic in life, after death, his memory helped drug warriors convince lawmakers that narcotics should be brought under the federal government's heel. Even today, as the United States grapples with its worst opioid crisis to date, the memory of drug use among Civil War soldiers and veterans remains useful as politicians, doctors, and the American public reckon with the ongoing opioid epidemic.

Reflecting in hindsight on the state of medical practice during the Civil War, Progressive Era medical experts and social scientists spilled much ink describing opiate addiction among veterans of "the late war," which remained within living memory. These drug warriors coined the label "army disease" and the like, which have remained popular for a century, although such terms were anachronisms that were totally unfamiliar to the Civil War generation.[1] The army disease narrative emerged as the earliest scholarly interpretation of opiate addiction among Civil War veterans, and it proved deeply influential. The army disease model posited that the careless overprescribing of medicinal opiates, especially hypodermic morphine, by military surgeons triggered a surge of iatrogenic addiction in the postwar decades among former soldiers, who emerged as the first cohort of opiate-addicted Americans. Certainly, there is a nucleus of truth to this narrative, as we have seen. Yet the army disease model was deeply flawed in that it pinned the entirety of the late nineteenth-century addiction epidemic solely on the Civil War, overlooking the myriad other causes of addiction. The use of "army disease" as a shorthand for addiction also framed Civil War veterans as the only demographic of drug-addicted Americans at that time, leaving unnoticed the women and civilian men who were the majority of users. The army disease narrative also ignored the lived experiences of addicted people in favor of a more cut-and-dried narrative about causation, leaving veterans' suffering unacknowledged and scholars' understanding of addiction in the nineteenth century limited.

The first tellers of the army disease narrative obsessed over the use of hypodermic morphine by Civil War surgeons, which was framed as the exclusive vector of opiate addiction, even though many users preferred other preparations. Implicit in this story was the critique of Civil War surgeons for overzealously, carelessly administering hypodermic morphine injections. Jeannette Marks, an anti-narcotics crusader and English professor at Mount Holyoke College, was influential in spreading the army disease narrative during the 1910s. In a 1913 novel, Marks warned that drug use had become the "great leviathan" of American life. "In this country" drug addiction "came in the first place through the horrors of the Civil War," she claimed. Disremembering the long, prewar history of opiate use and addiction, as well as the fact that most nineteenth-century drug users were not veterans, Marks selectively claimed that "there was no opium question before then [the Civil War]."[2] She hoped that raising the specter of the army disease would drive home her broader message—that narcotics were inherently immoral, dangerous, and should be regulated—and might generate support for the Harrison Narcotics Tax Act, which hastened the criminalization of addiction nationwide after it was enacted in 1914.

Of course, Marks found that the Harrison Act did not resolve the "problem" of narcotic use and addiction. In reality, historians recognize that the law and its enforcement mechanism segmented drug users into white and black markets, criminalizing the latter while legitimizing the former.[3] Not content with the Harrison Act, Marks continued to wage a personal war on drugs. Calling herself "a bugler sounding a reveille," in 1914 she told an audience of physicians and public health workers that "there is practically no old American family of Civil War reputation which has not had its addicts." "Did you know that it was called 'the army disease' because of its prevalence?" she asked.[4] As the United States mobilized for World War I, Marks predicted a resurgence of drug addiction among a new generation of American veterans. Writing in the *North American Review* in December 1917, she again claimed that the United States' "narcotic problem took its rise on the battlefields of the Civil War." Yet despite "the lesson we have learned from our own Civil War battlefields," a new addiction crisis loomed unless urgent preventative measures were taken.[5] Military leaders were warned that some 500,000 drug users might volunteer or be drafted, overwhelming the army's psychiatric services and disciplinary systems. Only 3,284 men were flagged and rejected for drug use, but the Great War generated new examples of drug-using veterans.[6] Morphine was a useful palliative for painful gas attacks, war wounds, and shell shock, and some "doughboys" returned home addicted.[7]

During the 1920s, a decade defined by prohibitionist anti-alcohol and anti-narcotic regimes, the army disease continued to provide a useful frame of reference for reformers and politicians. Prohibition raised complex questions about what to do with addicted people. As Congress considered the fate of morphine maintenance clinics and the prospect of opening federal "narcotics farms" to police addiction, Civil War veterans became a valuable foil to the "drug fiend" stereotype that emerged in the early twentieth century. During a 1928 congressional hearing on the narcotics farms, one congressman explained that "I recall an old man who was wounded in the Civil War and became an addict and lived to a ripe old age. He was not the menace to society that the heroin or cocaine addict is." The former, once derided as an "opium slave," was now venerable and stood in stark contrast to the "menace to society that the heroin or cocaine addict is."[8] Conveniently overlooking the victim blaming and policing leveled at "opium slaves" during their lives allowed policymakers to sanitize addicted Civil War veterans' memory, who could serve as sympathetic foils to the "drug fiends" of the 1920s. After addicted veterans died, their memory became a political weapon to wield against younger generations of drug users.

The addicted Civil War veteran remained a powerful metaphor in drug policy debates throughout the twentieth century. Charles E. Terry and Mildred Pellens, social hygienists and drug addiction experts, claimed in 1928 that American doctors of the Civil War generation had been too slow to recognize the addictiveness of hypodermic morphine. "Medical journals of the day," they argued, "were full of enthusiastic descriptions" of "the hypodermic use of morphin[e]" and naively overlooked the obvious potential for addiction among veterans. The ignorance of syringe-wielding Civil War surgeons, Terry and Pellens chided, meant that "following the Civil War the increase in opiate use was so marked among ex-soldiers as to give rise to the term 'army disease' and today in more than one old soldiers' home are cases of chronic opium intoxication which date from this period."[9] Misguided "enthusiasm" for addictive narcotics and the absence of regulation, Terry and Pellens implied, helped spark the first opioid epidemic in the United States. Their reductionist take overlooked and obscured much—Marks, Terry and Pellens were uninterested in the suffering endured by addicted veterans, in their self-advocacy, or in taking a more comprehensive view of the causes of addiction during the previous generation. History took a back seat to politics and policy.

Yet the army disease model, as articulated by Marks, Terry, and Pellens, stuck around because it continued to be useful for drug warriors. During the 1970s, the US National Commission on Marihuana and Drug Abuse, tasked by President Richard Nixon with recommending updates to US drug policy, recalled Terry and Pellens's Progressive Era commentary on the army disease. Sketching the historical origins of the "drug problem" in America, the commission's 1973 report explained that hypodermic morphine "was used indiscriminately during the Civil War for the wholesale relief of pain and, most significantly, to treat common gastrointestinal ailments. After the War, morphine was widely used in medical practice and was easily available outside the medical system in proprietary medicines. Within a few years, 'morphinomania (or the 'army' disease) became a recognizable medical entity."[10] Nixon found it politically expedient to "other" and demonize drug users, especially Black Americans.[11] But even the US Army found the idea of the Civil War–era army disease to be a useful foil. In 1972, during the heroin scare of the Vietnam War, the army circulated a handbook to warn commanders about drug use in the ranks. It included a photo of wounded Civil War soldiers along with the claim that "vast numbers of soldiers . . . returned to civilian life addicted to morphine. A term prevalent at the time, 'Soldier's Illness,' actually meant narcotic addiction."[12]

The army disease bled over into pop culture and was even discussed within families. A 1976 episode of the popular television show *Little House on the Prairie* narrated the moral decline and overdose death of a fictional Civil War veteran, Granville Whipple.[13] The show's unusually dark episode took inspiration from the army disease as well as contemporary depictions of heroin use among Vietnam veterans. When musician James Taylor began using heroin, his father warned about the drug's dangers by recalling the addiction epidemic among Civil War veterans a century prior.[14] In 1982, during President Ronald Reagan's revival of the War on Drugs, the National Institute on Drug Abuse explained in a glossary of drug terms that "because only [Civil War] soldiers were so widely affected" by morphine addiction before the twentieth century, "the addiction became known as the army disease."[15] Throughout the twentieth century, the army disease remained an essential concept in the discourse of drugs and drug policy, and the narrative provided a useful origin story for those who sought to frame drug use as a "problem."

Drug policy debates did much to keep the army disease model alive, but medical literature also carried this narrative forward into the mid-twentieth century. A 1962 medical textbook on addiction, coauthored by a former senior doctor at the federal "narcotics farm" in Lexington, Kentucky, claimed matter-of-factly, "The Civil War in America provided the first opportunity for the widespread use of morphine administered hypodermically, and the Pension Bureau had difficulties well into the twentieth century as a result of the large numbers of Civil War veterans who became addicts to morphine and other opiates, euphemistically referred to as suffering from the 'army disease.'"[16] The ominous passage reminded medical students of the 1960s to carefully avoid ostensible mistakes made by Civil War surgeons a century prior. Numerous contemporary studies on drug addiction echoed these warnings, keeping the army disease at the forefront of addiction studies in the mid-twentieth century.[17]

The army disease also helped frame Civil War medicine within the context of dizzyingly rapid late nineteenth- and early twentieth-century medical advances, including the discovery of microbes and popularization of germ theory, medical professionalization, the mass development of vaccines, and the rise of specialty medicine, to name just a few developments. When looking back on Civil War medicine from the vantage of the twentieth century, the army disease model reminded American physicians that the war's medical outcomes—when hundreds of thousands died from diseases that had become largely preventable or curable a few decades removed—could be chalked up to a mere lack of knowledge rather than more nefarious disregard of patient well-being. According to this line of thought, surgeons were simply unaware that hypodermic morphine carried the risk of addiction. Of course, this narrative implicitly required forgetting that antebellum doctors had developed a keen awareness of addiction.

The army disease narrative achieved remarkable staying power in the century elapsed since Marks, Terry, and Pellens articulated it. Addicted Civil War veterans have consistently appeared in the historiography of the Civil War and narratives of historical drug addiction for decades. In fact, the central premise of the army disease model—that morphine addiction was widespread among Civil War veterans and was largely the fault of military surgeons—is one of the longest-running, relatively unchallenged interpretations of any aspect of the Civil War history. Seemingly all angles of the war have been interpreted and reinterpreted by each generation of historians since Appomattox. But for more than a hundred years, offhanded references to the army disease have been standard fare in histories of the Civil War and scholarship on the history of drug addiction in America. As James M. McPherson observed in his Pulitzer Prize–winning 1988 synthesis of the Civil War, *Battle Cry of Freedom*, "Soldiers who suffered from anything from dysentery to constipation to malaria to a cold were dosed with calomel or tartar emetic or quinine or morphine or laudanum," as surgeons could do so little else beyond treating soldiers' symptoms. "Little wonder," McPherson reasoned, "that some became narcotics addicts."[18] The notion that Civil War surgeons caused soldiers to become addicted to opiates has played a prominent role in harsh portrayals of Civil War medicine by historians. Bertram Wyatt-Brown explained in 1997 that "as for medical services" during the Civil War, military "doctors might as well have been executioners, funeral directors, and dispensers to drug addicts, opium being the contemporary cure-all." Many scholars writing since the Progressive Era have echoed some version of these statements, which ultimately framed Civil War surgeons as butchers, an inaccurate characterization that has been rightfully critiqued in more recent scholarship on wartime medicine.[19]

That is not to say that the army disease model has been totally uncontested. During the 1970s, historian Mark A. Quinones mounted a short-lived challenge to the basic premise of the army disease, flatly rejecting the notion that Civil War veterans became widely addicted to opiates at all. Quinones reasoned that the hypodermic syringe, which became mainstream medical technology in the Gilded Age, was not in widespread use among Civil War surgeons, so it could not have been responsible for veterans' addiction. Furthermore, Quinones alleged that few cases of addicted veterans were recorded in the medical literature of the postwar decades, although he cited only a handful of postbellum sources to support these assertions. Consequently, Quinones argued, military medicine simply could not have caused widespread addiction among Civil War veterans. Instead, the army disease model was simply a "convenient scapegoat for the growth of addiction in America," concocted by Progressive Era intellectuals to justify the criminalization of opioids by the 1914 Harrison Narcotics Act.[20] Quinones's work sparked a debate about the extent of opiate addiction among Civil War veterans, but his position quickly became untenable. In a series of articles and books appearing in the late 1970s and 1980s, drug historian David T. Courtwright demonstrated that opiate addiction unquestionably occurred among Civil War veterans, citing several verifiable cases in a handful of postbellum medical journals and publications. Courtwright also pointed out that opiate addiction did not require the hypodermic syringe. Orally ingested opium, laudanum, and morphine, the most common opiate forms in the Civil War, were addictive in their own right. For his part, Courtwright also challenged the notion—first advocated by Marks, Terry, and Pellens—that the Civil War was the paramount cause of addiction in the nineteenth century. Most nineteenth-century opiate users were not veterans, Courtwright observed, thus the war could not have exclusively (or even mostly) caused the demographically broad Gilded Age addiction epidemic. In more recent years, most Civil War historians have embraced Courtwright's conclusions.[21] Major studies of veterans in postwar America by Eric T. Dean Jr., James Marten, Brian Matthew Jordan, and Diane Miller Sommerville note the occasional appearance of opiate-addicted veterans in the records of postbellum mental asylums and soldiers' homes, while accepting Courtwright's view that the Civil War was a relatively limited factor in late nineteenth-century opioid crisis.[22]

Yet the army disease narrative persists today because it retains its utility. The army disease reminds Americans in the twenty-first century of our own opioid addiction crisis and helps us come to grips with it.[23] With record levels of opioid overdose deaths, public interest in the deep historical origins of opioid addiction is at an all-time high. In this context, the memory of Civil War America's opioid crisis has again resurfaced and been used to advocate for various measures to tackle the ongoing opioid crisis. In a 2019 congressional hearing, Representative Alexandria Ocasio-Cortez, then a member of the US House of Representatives Committee on Oversight and Reform, reminded Americans that "the United States has a unique history with opioids. . . . And it starts with the US Civil War."[24] This well-meant historical reference called attention to the nation's long history of addiction and underscores the urgent need for a thorough investigation of this history.

Reckoning with opium slavery as experienced by Civil War veterans reveals disturbing parallels between past and present. Prescription opioids helped spark the US Civil War–era addiction crisis and that of today. During the 1860s–90s and again in the 1990s, pharmaceutical fraud enabled some Americans to profit from addiction while others suffered and perished. The more sympathetic depiction of white opioid users at the expense of Americans of color likewise reflects patterns established in the Civil War era, as does the continued underprescribing of opioid painkillers to Black Americans.[25] Ongoing efforts to curtail overprescribing, to expand rehab availability and harm-reduction measures, and to destigmatize addiction are not new developments either. Instead, these modern responses echo the solutions for addiction pioneered by nineteenth-century physicians after the Civil War. Ultimately, by recounting the history of opiate addiction in the Civil War era, we can not only gain a better sense of the war's terrible human costs in postwar America but also situate today's opioid epidemic within the long, tragic history of opioid crises in the United States.

Notes

Introduction

1. *Manual of Military Surgery*, 97.
2. Herzberg, *White Market Drugs*, 2, 48; Courtwright, "Preventing and Treating Narcotic Addiction," 2096.
3. Courtwright, "Opiate Addiction," 101–11; Marten, "Civil War Veterans," 620.
4. Courtwright, *Dark Paradise*, esp. 46, 54–55.
5. Examples of scholarship that directly or indirectly cites Courtwright's studies include McPherson, *Battle Cry of Freedom*, 486–87; Paludan, *People's Contest*, 337–38; Dean, *Shook over Hell*, 169–70; Marten, *Sing Not War*, 84, 111, 114; Jordan, *Marching Home*, 4, 180; Sommerville, *Aberration of Mind*, 161–62.
6. Faust aptly observes that the Civil War has "intoxicated" historians. Faust, "'We Should Grow Too Fond,'" 372–73. Faust and other scholars estimate that the number of books published about the Civil War stands at 60,000 to 70,000, not to mention the many thousands of articles and digital history projects. Reid, "Civil War, 1861–1865," 99; Wagner, Gallagher, and Finkelman, *Library of Congress Civil War Desk Reference*, 860.
7. See the discussion of "army disease" and "soldiers' disease" in the epilogue.
8. For example, writing in the 1990s, Eric T. Dean Jr. cross-referenced the admissions records of the Indiana Hospital for the Insane against the muster rolls of Indiana Civil War regiments to identify a sample of veterans who were patients at the asylum. This methodology was possible because both sets of records were housed at the Indiana State Archives. Dean then cross-referenced the resulting list with US Civil War pension records housed at the National Archives and Records Administration to obtain the veterans' military histories. This pre-digital research methodology, which took months of herculean research and was widely praised in reviews of Dean's book, generated a mere eight cases of opiate-addicted veterans out of Dean's 291-man "Indiana sample." Dean, *Shook over Hell*, app. A.
9. Eric T. Dean Jr., James Marten, and Diane Miller Sommerville provide the best snapshots of opiate addiction among Civil War veterans, situating veterans' addictions within the broader context of war trauma and readjustment into civilian life. The studies describe a limited number of cases, however. Dean, *Shook over Hell*, 169–79; Marten *Sing Not War*, 84, 111, 114; Sommerville, *Aberration of Mind*, 161–62.
10. Clarke, *War Stories*, 5–7.
11. Sternhell, "Revisionism Reinvented?"; Prokopowicz, "Common Soldier," 549–51.
12. Dean, *Shook over Hell*; Marten, *Sing Not War* and *America's Corporal*; Jordan, *Marching Home*; Sommerville, *Aberration of Mind*; Handley-Cousins, *Bodies in Blue*; McClurken, *Take Care of the Living*; Silkenat, *Moments of Despair*; M. Adams, *Living Hell*; Gordon, *Broken Regiment* and *Dread Danger*; Linderman, *Embattled Courage*; and Carroll, *Invisible Wounds*. These studies highlight emotional and psychological suffering among soldiers and civilians during and after the war. The landmark 2011 collection *Weirding the War*, edited by Stephen

Berry, enumerated many of these issues. Some older histories hinted at psychological trauma among combatants; see, for example, G. Adams, *Doctors in Blue*, 228. In 1981, Phillip Paludan broke ground by using psychological studies of Vietnam veterans to probe the psychological toll of Civil War atrocities, setting the tone for the emergence of war trauma as a key theme in the later historiography on veterans. See his *Victims*, xiv.

13. Bever, *At War with King Alcohol*; Foote, *Gentlemen and the Roughs*; Fialka, *Hope to Never See It*.

14. An illustrative example is Hsieh, "'Go to Your Gawd Like a Soldier,'" 555–59.

15. Sommerville recounts this debate at length in *Aberration of Mind*, 270–73nn11–13.

16. Dean, *Shook over Hell*; Sommerville, *Aberration of Mind*; Handley-Cousins, *Bodies in Blue*; and Carroll, *Invisible Wounds*, utilize asylum records to explore the postwar experiences of veterans and their families. Institutionalized veterans are not illustrative of all Civil War combatants, many of whom did not suffer from war trauma that might subject them to institutionalization. Yet asylum records are nonetheless invaluable sources for the war's social and medical history, providing insight not only into the lived experiences of traumatized veterans but also into the inimitable evidence produced by contemporary medical and community observers about the relationship between the Civil War and trauma.

17. Handley-Cousins et al., "Disability in the Civil War Era." Examples include Handley-Cousins, *Bodies in Blue*; Sommerville, *Aberration of Mind*; Carroll, *Invisible Wounds*. Although broadly focused, Marten, *Sing Not War*, and Jordan, *Marching Home*, also provide compelling analysis of nonvisible disabilities. On amputations, see Miller, *Empty Sleeves*.

18. Humphreys, *Marrow of Tragedy*, 1.

19. Humphreys, *Marrow of Tragedy* and *Intensely Human*; J. Downs, *Sick from Freedom*; Devine, *Learning from the Wounded*; Kiechle, *Smell Detectives*; Schultz, *Women at the Front*; Giesberg, *Civil War Sisterhood*; A. Taylor, *Embattled Freedom*; Browning and Silver, *Environmental History of the Civil War*.

20. Whites, *Civil War as a Crisis in Gender*.

21. Particularly helpful studies of manhood in the Civil War era include Linderman, *Embattled Courage*; Rotundo, *American Manhood*; Greenberg, *Manifest Manhood*; Kasson, *Perfect Man*; Nelson, *Ruin Nation*; Halttunen, *Confidence Men and Painted Women*; and Bederman, *Manliness and Civilization*.

22. Bederman, *Manliness and Civilization*, and Hickman, *Secret Leprosy of Modern Days*, are useful for framing veterans' drug use in the racial context of the Gilded Age. Cooper Owens, *Medical Bondage*, and Pernick, *Calculus of Suffering*, explore ideas about race, gender, and pain. Courtwright, *Dark Paradise*, and Ahmad, *Opium Debate and Chinese Exclusion Laws*, provide context on opium smoking and Chinese immigration.

23. Courtwright, *Dark Paradise*; Jaffe, *Addiction Reform in the Progressive Age*; Spillane, *Cocaine*; Hickman, *Secret Leprosy of Modern Days*; Herzberg, *White Market Drugs*; Gray, *Habit Forming*. Tracy, *Alcoholism in America*, focus on alcohol but provides a thorough overview of the inebriety movement. Clark, *Recovery Revolution*, carries this thread over to narcotics and links it to twentieth-century addiction treatments.

24. Pearson, "New Birth of Regulation"; Gabriel, "Restricting the Sale of 'Deadly Poisons.'"

25. Courtwright, *Dark Paradise*, sketches the early history of opiates at the beginning of the nineteenth century, but his focus is largely on the Gilded Age and Progressive Era. Hickman's *Secret Leprosy of Modern Days* concentrates on the Gilded Age but calls attention to antebellum abolitionism and temperance as formative for postbellum cultural discourse about addiction.

Gray's *Habit Forming* offers a more sustained treatment of opiates and other substances before midcentury. Although fruitful, none of these books have taken the Civil War or veterans as their primary focus.

26. Cypel, DePhilippis, and Davey, "Substance Use in US Vietnam War Era"; Teeters et al., "Substance Use Disorders in Military Veterans."

27. Courtwright, *Forces of Habit*; Kamienski, *Shooting Up*; Andreas, *Killer High*.

28. For instance, J. B. Mattison, "The Prevention of Opium Addiction," *Louisville Medical News*, February 23, 1884, 113–15. Additional examples appear throughout the book.

29. In 2019, the American Society of Addiction Medicine adopted language defining addiction as "a treatable, chronic medical disease involving complex interactions among brain circuits, genetics, the environment, and an individual's life experiences. People with addiction use substances or engage in behaviors that become compulsive and often continue despite harmful consequences." "Definition of Addiction," *American Society of Addiction Medicine*, updated September 15, 2019, www.asam.org/quality-care/definition-of-addiction.

30. Campbell, *OD*, 3. See also Kushner, "Taking Biology Seriously"; Lemon, *Addiction and Devotion*; and Room, Hellman, Stenius, "Addiction." Gray also implicitly notes the pragmatic benefits that historians can derive from meshing biological understandings of addiction with social history. See Gray, *Habit Forming*, 6–7.

31. Courtwright, "Addiction and the Science of History," 489.

32. Sommerville, *Aberration of Mind*, 11–12, 271n12, 272n13; Handley-Cousins, *Bodies in Blue*, 116–17; K. Williams, *I Saw Death Coming*, 285n22.

33. "The Opium Habit," *New-York Times*, March 2, 1878, 2; Rosenberg, "What Is an Epidemic?," 1.

34. Courtwright, "Preventing and Treating Narcotic Addiction"; Hickman, *Secret Leprosy of Modern Days*; Herzberg, *White Market Drugs*; N. Campbell, *OD*; Gray, *Habit Forming*. In *Cocaine*, Spillane also characterizes the Gilded Age as a period when drug use escalated sharply, warranting sustained public attention.

Chapter 1

1. Jacomet, "Plant Economy and Village Life," 47–59. Global histories of opium include Chouvy, *Opium*; Dormandy, *Opium*; and Booth, *Opium*. Histories that address opium in the context of other intoxicants include Breen, *Age of Intoxication*; Courtwright, *Forces of Habit*, 31–39; and Schivelbusch, *Tastes of Paradise*.

2. "Symposium on Drugs," 25.

3. Breen, *Age of Intoxication*, 157–59; Astyrakaki, Papaioannou, Askitopoulou, "References to Anesthesia, Pain, and Analgesia," 188–94; Galen, "On Antidotes," 196–97; Porter, *Greatest Benefit to Mankind*, 203, 262; Davenport-Hines, *Pursuit of Oblivion*, 35–37; Carter, *Inaugural Essay*, vi; *Medical and Surgical History*, pt. 2, 1:735.

4. J. Jones, *Plain Concise Practical Remarks*, 72.

5. Courtwright, *Dark Paradise*, 40.

6. Warner, *Therapeutic Perspective*, 136.

7. Quoted in Musto, "Iatrogenic Addiction," 695.

8. Cullen, *First Lines of the Practice of Physic*, 23–24, 70–71, 128.

9. Abrams, *Revolutionary Medicine*, 226–27. An 1804 prescription was for diarrhea; see Loewer, *Jefferson's Garden*, 151.

10. Rush quoted in D. Wilson, *Inaugural Dissertation*, 30–32. Wilson explained that Rush conveyed the case narrative in a letter.

11. Benjamin Rush to Bushrod Washington, May 2, 1812, Fred W. Smith National Library for the Study of George Washington, Mount Vernon, VA.

12. H. Levine, "Discovery of Addiction," 143–74.

13. Norwood *Trading Freedom*, 64; Courtwright, *Dark Paradise*, 19.

14. Beekman Family Recipe Book, 1800–1871 (bulk 1800–1832), New-York Historical Society, New York. Fifty-seven medicinal recipes are arranged in chronological order. Forty-nine recipes date or apparently date ca.1800–ca.1820, and eight recipes apparently from 1826 to 1831. Five (10.2 percent) of the pre-1826 recipes contain opiates, compared with three (37.5 percent) recipes from 1826 to 1831.

15. H. J. McLaurin, "On Opium," 3–4, Waring Historical Library Inaugural Theses Collection, Medical University of South Carolina, Charleston; Wood and Bache, *Dispensatory of the United States* (1845), 506–18.

16. Courtwright, *Forces of Habit*, 35; Kim, *Empires of Vice*, 3–4, 65, 74, table A.1; Andreas, *Killer High*, 143–47; Wood and Bache, *Dispensatory of the United States* (1845), 508–11.

17. For example, "The Opium Trade—England and China," *Morning Herald* (New York), May 4, 1840, 2–3. See also Su, "'Cause of Human Freedom,'" 465–96.

18. Courtwright, *Forces of Habit*, 33–34; Andreas, *Killer High*, 147–48; "Perkins and Company, 1–5; E. Gray, "Trade Off," 220–42.

19. Gray, *Habit Forming*, 24.

20. Whiskey and coffee prices in Rorabaugh, *Alcoholic Republic*, 76, 100.

21. J. Walker account, reel 4, frame 260, John William Ogilvie Medical Account Books, 1845–1870, Barnwell District, South Carolina, in *Records of Ante-Bellum Southern Plantations from the Revolution through the Civil War*, ser. A, pt. 2, miscellaneous collections, reels 3–4 (Frederick, MD: University Publications of America, 1985) (hereafter cited as OMAB).

22. See directions for making opium pills in Ewell, *Medical Companion* (1859), 675.

23. Gray agrees that laudanum was the most common preparation but contends that raw opium was rarely used. Gray, *Habit Forming*, 11.

24. George B. Green New Receipt Book, 1823–1862, Historical Medical Library, College of Physicians of Philadelphia. Recipe for "liquid laudanum" "as prepared Nov[ember] 1824" on p. 5.

25. Wood and Bache, *Dispensatory of the United States* (1833), 470.

26. Morphia first appeared in 1833 in Wood and Bache, *Dispensatory of the United States of America*, 897–904; see also Courtwright, *Forces of Habit*, 36–39.

27. Wood and Bache, *Dispensatory of the United States* (1833), 468, 471, 902.

28. Burnham, *Health Care in America*, 40, 43–45, 69–74.

29. Valenčius, *Health of the Country*.

30. Tomes, *Gospel of Germs*.

31. Warner, *Therapeutic Perspective*, 133–34; quotes in Rosenberg, "Therapeutic Revolution," 498.

32. Courtwright, "Hidden Epidemic," 63; Musto, *American Disease*, 1; and Cassedy, *Medicine in America*, 47; quote from Jameson, *American Domestic Medicine*, 475.

33. John P. Mushat, "On Opium," 14, Waring Historical Library Inaugural Theses Collection, Medical University of South Carolina, Charleston.

34. Arnold, "On the Uses of Opium," 183. Physicians believed that an individual's unique

constitution, shaped by myriad factors, including race, place, sex, age, and environment, helped determine the action of opium in individual bodies. A grain of opium taken by one person might not produce the same effects in another person; see Valenčius, *Health of the Country*, 71–74.

35. Kalant, "Opium Revisited," 271.
36. McGown, *Most Common Diseases of the South*, 349.
37. Valenčius, *Health of the Country*, 79–84, 91–132; Humphreys, *Yellow Fever and the South*, 45–76.
38. Rosenberg, *Cholera Years*.
39. Slack, "Opium in Cholera, Dysentery and Diarrhea," 530.
40. "On the Use of Opium," 156.
41. Courtwright, *Dark Paradise*, 45–46, 57, 62–63.
42. Slack, "Opium in Cholera, Dysentery, and Diarrhea," 530.
43. "Anti-Spasmodic Tincture," *Richmond Indiana Palladium*, September 23, 1837, 4.
44. "Specific for the Cholera," *Albany Journal*, June 22, 1832, 1; "No. 3. Van Swicten's Opium Mixture for the Cholera," Timothy Hall Recipe Book, 1823–1834, Historical Medical Library, College of Physicians of Philadelphia. The Beekman family of New York City cut and pasted into their recipe book a newspaper article, originally from the *New York Evening Journal* on July 29, 1831, that included an opium-based remedy for cholera. Beekman Family Recipe Book, 1800–1871 (bulk 1800–1832), New-York Historical Society, New York. See page 29.
45. Yandell, "Treatment of Epidemic Cholera," 221.
46. Courtwright also suggests that cholera helped escalate opiate use. Courtwright, *Dark Paradise*, 45–46.
47. On fatalism and palliation, see Warner, *Therapeutic Perspective*, 135–36, and Rosenberg, "Therapeutic Revolution," 499.
48. Thacher, *American Modern Practice* (1826), 341.
49. For topical application and ingestion, see Thacher, *American New Dispensatory*, 315, and Murray, *System of Materia Medica*, 78; for earache, Thacher, *American Modern Practice* (1826), 293.
50. Thomas DuBose Wilson, "On the Effects of Opium upon the System," 1857, 2, Waring Historical Library Inaugural Theses Collection, Medical University of South Carolina, Charleston.
51. J. Harrison, "Psychology of Opium Eating," 579; This belief had deep roots in Western medicine. See Breen, *Age of Intoxication*, 153.
52. Abraham Lincoln, "Inaugural Address, March 4, 1865," *Teaching American History*, https://teachingamericanhistory.org/document/second-inaugural-address/, accessed November 29, 2021.
53. Madison W. Drummond, "On Opium," 1856, 10, Waring Historical Library Inaugural Theses Collection, Medical University of South Carolina, Charleston.
54. Courtwright (*Dark Paradise*, 42–53) and Gray (*Habit Forming*, 20–65) also found that widespread medicinal use translated to an increasing rate and heightened visibility of addiction as the nineteenth century progressed. To deeply probe the medicinal use of opiates, I developed an unpublished dataset, the "Antebellum Opiate Therapies Database," sourcing data from a sample of thirty antebellum American medical textbooks, materia medica commentaries and formularies, medical handbooks and dictionaries, and home health guides published between 1813 and 1858. Six titles had multiple editions, indicating wide readership, while twenty-four titles were limited to a single run, as far as I could tell. Fifteen titles were intended primarily

for physicians and apothecaries, plus fifteen titles for laypeople. The dataset is drawn primarily from allopathic medical literature and does not necessarily reflect the diverse views of sectarian practitioners. All titles are digitized and available in full text via the Internet Archive, and most titles are cited in this chapter. I identified ailments for which opium, laudanum, morphine, Dover's powder, and black drop were indicated as suitable medical interventions, often in concert with other drugs or therapies. Opiates were most often indicated for managing symptoms like pain and diarrhea. But for many ailments, opiates were intended to correct constitutional imbalances that ostensibly caused the underlying malady. I excluded ambiguous, nonspecific illnesses like "general disease" from the count and consolidated instances where opiates were indicated for both causes and symptoms, for example, "bloody urine" and "bladder stones causing bloody urine." I obtained definitions and descriptions of various antebellum maladies from Dunglison, *Medical Lexicon*.

55. The preparation, along with morphine powders and paregoric, was billed to William Manner Bostich for his wife, "Mrs. B.," who was apparently nursing an infant in 1858–59. William Manner Bostich account, reel 4, frames 305, 329, OMAC.

56. "Snake bite," McFaddin Medical Diary, Medical University of South Carolina, Charleston.

57. Mushat, "On Opium," 20–21.

58. The exact figure is 45.7 percent. Allyn Merriam Hungerford Prescription Book, 1842–1845, Medical Historical Library, Yale University Medical School, New Haven, CT.

59. Out of 958 prescriptions sampled, opium appeared in 346 prescriptions. For comparison, ipecac appeared in 75 prescriptions and mercury (in various forms) appeared in 420 prescriptions. Of prescriptions that could be identified by sex, 48 percent were dispensed for women and 41 percent for men. Eighty-nine percent of prescriptions that could be identified by age were written for adults. Cowen, King, and Lordi, "Nineteenth Century Drug Therapy," 760; Cowen and Kent, "Medical and Pharmaceutical Practice," 94, 96.

60. Exact figures were 45.1 percent (1820s), 45.2 percent (1830s), and 62.6 percent (1850s). Warner, *Therapeutic Perspective*, 117, 135–41.

61. Warner, *Therapeutic Perspective*, 122–24.

62. Warner, *Therapeutic Perspective*, 308n22. The exact figure is 42.9 percent. Mercurials like calomel were the most prescribed drugs in the 1830s (50.8 percent) but were eclipsed by opiates in the 1840s.

63. Warner, *Therapeutic Perspective*, 307n12.

64. Warner, *Therapeutic Perspective*, 108–11, 119. The exact figures were 78.5 percent (1830s), 59.1 percent (1840s), and 53.2 percent (1850s).

65. Henry Hartshorne Account Books, vol. 1, 1848–1851, entries for October 21–26 and November 2, 1848, Historical Medical Library, College of Physicians of Philadelphia; J. Morris, "Obituary Notices," iii, v, vii.

66. Warner, *Therapeutic Perspective*, 140. The dose needed to poison a person varied widely according to individual tolerance and the strength of the opiate in question. Alkaloidal content varied in poppies grown in different regions, and adulteration was common, reducing the strength of some opium preparations. A modern medical study reported a near-fatal poisoning from a "pebble sized" amount of orally ingested crude opium. Garg, Hitawala, and Agarwal, "Cardiotoxic Effects of Raw Opium," 46–48. See also Martínez and Ballesteros, "Opium Poisoning in Modern Times," 1–10. For an example of adulteration, see "Spurious Opium," 483–84.

67. William S. Theodore, "An Essay on the Effects of Opium as a Drug upon the Human

System [. . .]" (1850), Drexel University College of Medicine Legacy Center, Archives and Special Collections, Philadelphia, 7–8.

68. Rothstein, *American Physicians*, 125–51 (quotation on 130); Rothstein, "Botanical Movements and Orthodox Medicine," 36–37, 41–46.

69. Warner, *Therapeutic Perspective*, 127–28, 135–41.

70. Malleck, *When Good Drugs Go Bad*, 24–25.

71. Sullivan, "Plantation Medicine and Health Care," 19–21.

72. Breslaw, *Lotions, Potions, Pills, and Magic*, 153–54. A testament to its wide readership, *Gunn's* had gone through twelve editions by 1838. Opiates are the most frequently referenced drugs in the second edition (1833). Excluding the index and table of contents, it contains at least 234 direct references to opiates in 552 pages, including 135 references for opium, 97 for laudanum, and 2 for morphia. By contrast, other frequently referenced medicines were camphor (19 references), ipecac (48 references), and calomel (140 references). Most references to opiates were positive endorsements, although *Gunn's* also frequently warned readers to avoid administering opiates for certain ailments. Quote from Gunn in *Gunn's Domestic Medicine, or Poor Man's Friend* (1847), 301.

73. Child, *Family Nurse*, 45–46, 95–46.

74. Clinton, *Plantation Mistress*, 144–45, 147.

75. Tully, "Experiments with Narcotine," 5–12.

76. Pickett, "Tartar-Emetic and Opium to Infants," 117.

77. Cutter, *Physiological Family Physician*, 98.

78. *Journal of Health* 1, no. 5 (November 11, 1829): 66.

79. *Alexandria Gazette*, April 13, 1849, 2.

80. Courtwright, *Dark Paradise*, 77–78; Herzberg, *White Market Drugs*, 26–27; Gabriel, "Restricting the Sale of 'Deadly Poisons,'" 330.

81. For example, New York's Rushton & Aspinwall hawked "8 cases Turkey opium" in the *Morning Herald*, September 14, 1837, 3. W. W. Swain, on Canal Street in New Orleans, advertised opium as "constantly on hand," in *True American*, March 22, 1839, 4.

82. Duffy, "Medical Practice," 65. One ounce equates to approximately 438 grains.

83. "Brinckerhoff & Penton, Druggists," *Chicago Daily Tribune*, December 16, 1853, 3.

84. Entry dated March 30, 1825, Daybook, Mansfield, Ohio, Daniel J. Swinney Papers, 1808–1827, Historical Medical Library, College of Physicians of Philadelphia.

85. Medical account book, 256, HM 75114, Huntington Library, San Marino, CA. One fluid ounce equates to over 591 drops.

86. Entries for Isaac R. Pratt, dated April 21, 1858, and June 20, 1858, 51, W. M. Parsons Ledger Book, 1858–1860, Huntington Library, San Marino, CA.

87. John B. Golding account, reel 4, frame 195, OMAB. The charge was dated November 18, 1852.

88. Moses Clarke White, "On the Abuses of Opium," 432, 451–53, in *Dissertations Read by the Candidates for the Degree of Doctor in Medicine in the Medical Institution of Yale College at the Annual Examination, January 25–26, 1854*, Medical Historical Library, Yale University Medical School, New Haven, CT. Warnings appeared in numerous antebellum medical texts. Wright, *Wright's Family Medicine* (1833), 155 (apoplexy); Ewell, *Medical Companion* (1847), 284 (dyspepsia); and 300 (loss of appetite, wasting of the body, and cravings); Murray, *System of Materia Medica and Pharmacy*, 83; Copland, *Dictionary of Practical Medicine*, 468 (yellow complexion); Murray, *System of Materia Medica and Pharmacy*, 83 (wasting of the body).

89. Thacher, *American Modern Practice* (1826), 216, 613. This warning had also appeared in the 1817 edition (p. 534).

90. Carpenter, *Carpenter's Family Medicine Chest Dispensatory*, 119. Similar warnings appear in Child, *Family Nurse*, 46, 80, 94–95, 132.

91. Kiechle, *Smell Detectives*, 34.

92. Courtwright, *Dark Paradise*, 26. See his discussion of methods on 15–28. Courtwright cautions that estimates should be read as a suggestive, not definitive. On opium smuggling, see Courtwright, *Dark Paradise*, 17–18; Norwood, *Trading Freedom*, 187–88; and Cohan, *Contraband*, 287–90.

93. Rorabaugh, *Alcoholic Republic*, 176.

94. Kraut, *Silent Travelers*, 31–49.

95. The exact figure is 4.26 percent. Figures calculated using transcriptions of New York City coroners' inquests, compiled in K. Scott, *Coroners' Reports, New York City, 1823–1842* and *Coroners' Reports, New York City, 1843–1849*. The age of one of the deceased was unknown.

96. Dozens of examples of rural opiate overdose deaths can be found through a keyword search of *CSI: Dixie*, https://csidixie.org, accessed June 25, 2021.

97. Barratt, "Successful Treatment by Flagellation," 197.

98. For example, "Suicidal Death from Opium," 284, and "News of the Day," *Alexandria Gazette*, June 3, 1856, 2.

99. K. Scott, *Coroners' Reports, New York City, 1843–1849*, 8.

100. Bailey, "Cases in Toxicology," *Medical and Surgical Reporter* 26 (January 27, 1872): 77. See also "Suicide of a Fireman," *New-York Times*, July 3, 1887, 2.

101. "Effects of Opium Eating," 128.

102. Thacher, *American Modern Practice* (1817), 487.

103. H. Campbell, *Caffeine as an Antidote*.

104. *Physician's Visiting List*, 8.

105. *Charleston Mercury*, August 14, 1830, 3; *Charleston Daily Courier*, August 31, 1830, 2.

106. "Suicide," *Charleston Mercury*, August 14, 1830, 3.

107. Copland, *Dictionary of Practical Medicine*, 470, 472.

108. N. Campbell, *OD*, 25–31.

109. Isaac H. Blair, "Opium," 12, Waring Historical Library Inaugural Theses Collection, Medical University of South Carolina, Charleston, https://waringlibrary.contentdm.oclc.org/digital/collection/wit/id/2636/rec/12; White, "On the Abuses of Opium," 448–49.

110. Rothstein, *American Medical Schools*, 32–33.

111. Josiah Phillips, "Modus Operandi of Opium," 13, Waring Historical Library Inaugural Theses Collection, Medical University of South Carolina, Charleston.

112. Drummond, "On Opium," 10, 23.

113. Drummond, "On Opium," 20–21.

114. Mushat, "On Opium," 21–22.

115. Howison, "Precautions in Prescribing Medicine," 263; Beach, *American Practice Condensed*, 23.

116. Copland, *Dictionary of Practical Medicine*, 468.

117. Beach, *American Practice Condensed*, 23. A case of extreme tolerance appears in Murray and Chapman, *System of Materia Medica*. Another example is "Deaths," *Charleston Daily Courier*, March 29, 1830, 2.

118. J. Harrison, "Psychology of Opium Eating," 579.

119. Perry, "Autopsy of an Opium Eater," 319–20. Dry drugs were typically measured in grains. One grain equals 64.7989 milligrams. For common dosages of opium at mid-century, see Flannery, *Civil War Pharmacy*, 290–91.

120. Nancy Campbell (*OD*, 7–10) and Elizabeth Kelly Gray (*Habit Forming*, 6) provide accessible introductions to opiate pharmacology. Extended overviews may be found in Kalant, "Opium Revisited"; Rosenblum et al., "Opioids and the Treatment of Chronic Pain," 405–16; and Boyer, "Management of Opioid Analgesic Overdose," 147.

Chapter 2

1. "Opium Eating" (September 4, 1833), 66. The article was unsigned and the patient anonymous. It is likely that the authors were the journal's editors: John Collins Warren, Walter Channing, and John Ware. See Streeter, "*Boston Medical and Surgical Journal*," 24. The article generated considerable attention, evidenced by the multiple replies from doctors published in subsequent issues of the journal and newspaper coverage. For example, see Seeger, "Opium Eating," 117–20.

2. To explain why white middle-class Americans addicted to "medicinal" drugs have historically been treated with sympathy while marginalized populations of drug users have been treated unsympathetically, historians have often focused on the early twentieth century. Several pioneering studies provide insight into the emergence of sympathetic and unsympathetic groups, informed by class, race, and gender. See Acker, *Creating the American Junkie*; Musto, *American Disease*; H. Morgan, *Drugs in America*, 7–8, 27; and Hickman, "'Mania Americana,'" 1269. Courtwright's *Dark Paradise* and Spillane's *Cocaine*, 90–122, classic studies that also call attention to the nineteenth century as a formative period in the history of drugs, have more recently been joined by Gray, *Habit Forming*, and Herzberg, *White Market Drugs*, 15–45.

3. "Opium Eating" (September 4, 1833), 66.

4. Quotation from "Effects of Opium Eating." See also "On the Influence of Opium-Eating," 252.

5. Courtwright also concludes that women comprised a majority among nineteenth-century American opiate addicts. Courtwright, "Opiate Addiction," 110–11, and *Dark Paradise*, chap. 2.

6. The exact figure was 54.7 percent. Calculated from inquests transcribed in K. Scott, *Coroners' Reports, New York City, 1823–1842*, and *Coroners' Reports, New York City, 1843–1849*.

7. *Annual Report of the Managers of the State Lunatic Asylum, Utica*, 16–23.

8. For example, between its founding in 1844 and 1865, the Pennsylvania Hospital for the Insane—one of the nation's flagship asylums, overseen by psychiatrist Thomas Kirkbride—treated 4,323 patients, yet only fifteen people were institutionalized for insanity attributed to opiate addiction. "Pennsylvania Hospital for the Insane," *Valley Spirit* (Franklin County, PA), March 1, 1865, 3.

9. Jarvis, *Comparative Liability of Males and Females to Insanity*.

10. I calculated this figure by searching for the keywords "opium," "morph" (to find instances of morphine and morphia) and "laudanum" in the *New England Journal of Medicine*'s full-text searchable archive, accessible at https://www.nejm.org. I read each article that contained the search terms, counting those that described opiate addiction or overdose.

11. "Effects of Opium Eating," 128. On De Quincey's influence, see Berridge, *Opium and the People*, 49–56; Padwa, *Social Poison*, 22–26; Courtwright, *Dark Paradise*, 58; Hickman, *Secret Leprosy of Modern Days*, 16–20; Gray, *Habit Forming*, 1–8, 126; Lowell, "An Opium Fantasy"; and "Opium-Eaters and Snuff-Chewers," 297.

12. Jarvis, *Comparative Liability of Males and Females to Insanity*, 11.

13. "Opium Eating" (September 4, 1833), 66. Courtwright, *Dark Paradise*, 36–37, and Gray, *Habit Forming*, 32, also find that gendered notions of pain helped foster higher levels of opiate use among women than men.

14. "Poisoning by Opium and Belladonna," 682.

15. K. Scott, *Coroners' Reports, New York City, 1823–1842*, 147.

16. On "fallen women," see L. Ginzberg, *Women and the Work of Benevolence*, 19–22.

17. "[Edward Aldrich to Mannevillette Brown] San Francisco [to Utica, New York] 15 Feb. 1854," in Aldrich, *Echoes from a Distant Frontier*, 282–84, 285.

18. For example, Charles W. Chesbrough died of a laudanum overdose in New York City in August 1842. The coroner noted that Chesbrough had "joined the Temperance Society last March," implying that he had perhaps switched from spirits to laudanum. K. Scott, *Coroners' Reports, New York City, 1823–1842*, 34.

19. Clinton, *Plantation Mistress*, 171–72; Courtwright, *Dark Paradise*, 59, Gray, *Habit Forming*.

20. Hening, *Statutes at Large*, 105; numerous examples of poisoning are explored in N. Taylor, *Brooding over Bloody Revenge*. See also Shearer, "Women of Violence," 181–97.

21. Chesnut, *Diary from Dixie*, 365–66. On refugees to freedom, see Taylor, *Embattled Freedom*; on arson, see Immerwahr, "Burning Down the House."

22. Cooper Owens, *Medical Bondage*, 44, 112.

23. Cartwright, "Diseases and Peculiarities of the Negro Race," 331–32. Edwards-Grossi provides a thorough analysis of Cartwright's work and influence in *Mad with Freedom*, 24–44. See also Willoughby, "Running Away from Drapetomania."

24. Ramsey, *Necrological Appearance of Southern Typhoid Fever*, 16–17.

25. Douglass, *Life of Frederick Douglas*, 59–60. See also E. Clark, "'Sacred Rights of the Weak,'" 463–93.

26. Savitt, *Medicine and Slavery*, chap. 5.

27. For example, on January 20, 1854, Ogilvie charged William M. Lipsey $4.50 to administer bleeding and laudanum to a "negro woman," returning the following two days to continue treatment. William M. Lipsey account, reel 4, frame 111, John William Ogilvie Medical Account Books, 1845–1870, Barnwell District, South Carolina, in *Records of Ante-Bellum Southern Plantations from the Revolution through the Civil War*, ser. A, pt. 2, miscellaneous collections, reels 3–4 (Frederick, MD: University Publications of America, 1985) (hereafter cited as OMAB). In some of these cases, the individuals' freedom status is not clear. In a few additional cases, the race of Ogilvie's patients is not clear. For example, he sold eight ounces of laudanum to J. N. Martin intended for "Old Grace" on May 22, 1852, perhaps an elderly enslaved woman. J. N. Martin account, reel 4, frame 183, OMAB.

28. Savitt, *Medicine and Slavery*, 83–110, 150–71.

29. Barclay, *Mark of Slavery*.

30. Savitt, *Medicine and Slavery*, 163.

31. Kolchin, *American Slavery*, 105; Fett, *Working Cures*, chaps. 3, 4.

32. L. Levine, *Black Culture and Black Consciousness*, 64–66; Savitt, *Medicine and Slavery*, 149–50, 171–84.

33. Coroners' Inquisitions, Virginia Open Data Portal, Library of Virginia, https://data.virginia.gov/Education/Coroners-Inquisitions/wx5a-uuyp, accessed July 5, 2022. This dataset includes of 1,325 inquests in which African Americans were named as the deceased or as persons of interest. I omitted 259 inquests for white deceased, "free" deceased whose race was not recorded, and inquests involving Black people as persons of interest only.

34. Figures calculated from inquests transcribed in K. Scott, *Coroners' Reports, New York City, 1823–1842*, and *Coroners' Reports, New York City, 1843–1849*.

35. Owens, *Medical Bondage*, 36–38; Fett, *Working Cures*, 152; Axelson, "Women as Victims of Medical Experimentation," 11. In contrast, Sims was extremely sensitive to white women's pain. In an 1872 surgery, Sims deemed one white woman too "feeble" to bear the same degree of pain that Anarcha and other enslaved subjects previously endured. He gave the white woman nitrous oxide and fifty drops of the opiate McMunn's elixir for pain relief. Sims also gave postoperative hypodermic morphine shots "for pain" to a white woman patient at St. Elizabeths Hospital in Washington, DC, on whom he had performed an ovariotomy under anesthesia in 1880. Two years later, Sims prescribed a wealthy white woman "morphine to quiet the pain" after surgery. Sims, *On Ovariotomy*, 48–49; Sims, *Treatment of Epithelioma of the Cervix Uteri*, 24, 27–28; Sims, *Bromide of Ethyl as an Anaesthetic*, 6. By comparison, Sims explicitly described administering opium to "lock up" his Black patients' bowels for up to four weeks after surgery, not to treat pain. Sims, *Treatment of Vesico-Vaginal Fistula*, 26–27. There has been some suggestion that Sims may have intentionally addicted his subjects to opiates. Wall, "Did J. Marion Sims Deliberately Addict?"

36. "Opium Eating" (September 4, 1833), 66; Seeger, "Opium Eating," 1.

37. "Victims of Opium," *New-York Times*, August 16, 1859, 3.

38. "Opium Eating" (September 4, 1833): 66; *New-York Daily Tribune*, August 8, 1843, 2.

39. Courtwright, *Dark Paradise*, 35–42; Spillane, *Cocaine*, 40–41; Hickman, *Secret Leprosy of Modern Days*, esp. 59–125; Herzberg, *White Market Drugs*, 19–24; Gray, *Habit Forming*, 194–240.

40. Herbert, *Gold Rush Manliness*, 17–45; Cashin, *Family Venture*, 32.

41. Greenberg, *Manifest Manhood*, 11–14.

42. On independence and masculinity, see Rotundo, *American Manhood*, 235–39. On chemical dependence and manhood, see Parsons, *Manhood Lost*, 43–44, 55.

43. Quoted in Morgan, *Yesterday's Addicts*, 5 (italics mine).

44. "Effects of Opium," 371.

45. "Opium Eating" (September 4, 1833), 66.

46. On ideals of the male physique, see Kasson, *Houdini, Tarzan, and the Perfect Man*, 49–68. On "incomplete" bodies, see Nelson, *Ruin Nation*, 188–200; Miller, *Empty Sleeves*, chaps. 2–3; and McLaren, *Impotence*, chap. 6, esp. 132–33.

47. White, "On the Abuses of Opium," 452.

48. "Opium Eater," 217.

49. "An Opium Eater," *Flag of Our Union*, January 19, 1856, 23. Similar accounts include "A Recent Confession of an Opium-Eater," *Harper's Weekly*, January 3, 1857, 4–5, and "Memoir of the Milford Bard," in *The Poetical and Prose Writings of Dr. John Lofland, the Milford Bard* [. . .] (Baltimore: John Murphy, 1853), 16–17.

50. "Opium-Eater in America," 47–57. See also, "Editor's Table," *Knickerbocker* 20 (1842): 93–94.

51. Cobb recorded his story in an 1867 letter to a friend. It is the only letter written by an antebellum male opium eater that I have located to date. Sylvanus Cobb to Robert, October

30, 1867, Letters of Sylvanus Cobb, 1827–1867, Albert and Shirley Small Special Collections, University of Virginia Library, Charlottesville.

52. "Use of Opium," *New-York Times*, November 6, 1852, 3.

53. "Effects of Opium," *Scientific American*, August 11, 1849, 371.

54. Quoted in McPherson, *Battle Cry of Freedom*, 92.

55. Sell, *Opium Habit*, 29.

56. W. J. Pohlman to John March, November 12, 1841, quoted in Marsh, *Temperance Recollections*, 110; see also Lazich, "American Missionaries and the Opium Trade." After the War of 1898, anti-opium missionaries played a key role in formulating American drug policy. Foster, "Opium, the United States, and the Civilizing Mission," and "Origins of Global Narcotics Prohibition."

57. "From the Canton Register," *Charleston Mercury*, May 12, 1830, 2.

58. For example, "Slavery and the Opium Trade," *Anti-Slavery Reporter* (London), December 1, 1859, 275–76; "Opium Eating in Siam," 193.

59. Ngai, *Chinese Question*, 137–43; B. Williams, *Chinese Must Go*.

60. "The Pacific Railroad—Steamships between San Francisco and China," *Congressional Globe*, January 9, 1855, 224–25.

61. White, "On the Abuses of Opium," 462–63.

62. Herbert, *Gold Rush Manliness*, 152–53.

63. White, "On the Abuses of Opium," 452. Additional examples include "An Opium Eater," 23, and Copland, *Dictionary of Practical Medicine*, 7:468–69.

64. Before the 1850s, media coverage of opium smoking usually described the phenomenon as occurring outside the United States. For example, see "Opium Eating," *Alexandria Gazette*, May 22, 1840, 3; *Charleston Mercury*, May 12, 1830; and "The Opium Trade—England and China," *Morning Herald* (New York), May 4, 1840, 2. During and after the Gold Rush–era influx of Chinese migrants, the American media, when discussing opium smoking, shifted focus to US cities. See Ahmad, *Opium Debate and Chinese Exclusion Laws*, 1–35.

65. For example, "An Opium-Smoking Saloon," *Harper's Weekly*, December 11, 1858, 798; "Opium Eating in Siam," 193; and "Opium Smoking in Borneo," *Chicago Daily Tribune*, October 28, 1853, 1.

66. See Ngai, *Chinese Question*, 137–43; B. Williams, *Chinese Must Go*, 17–88; and Herbert, *Gold Rush Manliness*, 58–59. On "miscegenation," see Ayers, *Thin Light of Freedom*, 193–94.

67. Stout, *Chinese Immigration*, 18, 24.

68. *New-York Times*, October 7, 1881, 4.

69. As the *New-York Times* explained, "Statements of the vicious influence of the Chinese . . . have had the effect of revising newspaper discussions of the opium habit." *New-York Times*, May 18, 1883, 4.

70. Chen, "'Seeds for a New Life,'" 452–53.

71. White, "On the Abuses of Opium," 463.

72. Walters, *American Reformers*, 123.

73. Opium eating also drew direct comparisons to tobacco use and gambling. "Opium Eating and Drinking," 373; "The Man about Town," *Harper's Weekly*, February 14, 1857, 9.

74. Beecher, *Six Sermons*, 41.

75. *American Temperance Magazine, and Sons of Temperance Offering*, 189, 261.

76. J. Harrison, "Psychology of Opium Eating," 579.

77. For example, Shaw, *Utility of Temperance Societies*, 31.

78. *Gunn's Domestic Medicine* (1833), 405.

79. Ewell, *Medical Companion* (1822), 21.

80. Temperance literature also deployed the rhetoric of slavery to describe the effects of alcohol abuse. Mattingly, *Well-Tempered Women*, 192.

81. "Our Fashionable Narcotics," *New-York Times*, January 10, 1854, 4.

82. Beecher, *Six Sermons*, 41; "An Opium Eater," *Boston Cultivator*, May 23, 1840, 4.

83. Hitchcock, *Essay on Temperance*, 3, 6.

84. "Opium Eating and Drinking," 373.

85. J. Harrison, "Psychology of Opium Eating," 579.

86. "An Opium Eater," *Boston Cultivator*, May 23, 1840, 4.

87. Galatians 5:19–23.

88. Henry Ward Beecher quoted in "Antidotes," *Christian Union*, May 2, 1877, 394.

89. "Opium Eating" (September 4, 1833), 66.

90. Schofield's accounts are in J. S. S., "Opium Eating," *New-York Times*, August 5, 1852, 1 and J. S. Schofield, "Opium Eating," *New-York Times*, November 4, 1852, 3. Follow up commentary, ostensibly by other doctors, included "Opium Eating in New York," *Scientific American*, November 13, 1852; "The Use of Opium," *New-York Times*, November 6, 1852, 3; and Candor, "Opium Eating," *New-York Times*, November 6, 1852, 1.

91. White, "On the Abuses of Opium," 470.

Chapter 3

1. Chappell's case reconstructed from A. M. Chappell to William R. Terry, May 24, 1886, Lee Camp Soldier's Home Correspondence, 1885–1894, Huntington Library, San Marino, CA; and Alpheus M. Chappell application, Confederate Disability Applications and Receipts, Library of Virginia, Richmond; Ayers, *Thin Light of Freedom*, 72.

2. A. M. Chappell to William R. Terry, May 24, 1886.

3. J. Edward Turner, *History of the First Inebriate Asylum*, 215; Saunt, *Unworthy Republic*, 296.

4. Bates, "Successful Treatment of Opium Eaters," 77.

5. Humphreys, *Marrow of Tragedy*, 208–42; Browning and Silver, *Environmental History of the Civil War*, 9–38. The Vicksburg campaigns also illustrate how disease left unchecked by medicine could cripple armies and undermine military operations. From November 1862 to June 1863, 20–30 percent of Grant's Army of the Tennessee and 30–50 percent of Confederate soldiers in the Department of Mississippi and East Louisiana were too sick to fight. Privette, *Surgeon's Battle*; Freemon, *Gangrene and Glory*, 118–19; McPherson, *Battle Cry of Freedom*, 487–88.

6. *Manual of Military Surgery*, 97; 7, 28–29 (pain); 12 (vomiting and diarrhea); 58 (internal bleeding); 34–35 (muscle spasms); 18, 98 (sedation).

7. J. Woodward, *Outlines of the Chief Camp Diseases*, 229 ("Control the frequency of the stools"); 217 ("simple diarrhea"); 222–23, 228, 230 (dysentery); 257–59, 261, 265 (chronic diarrhea); 221–22 (enteritis); 139–40, 146 (typhoid); 168, 178–79 (malaria); 280 (measles); 296–97 (catarrh); 311 (pneumonia); 329 (rheumatism); 148 ("in large doses").

8. *Manual of Military Surgery*. 7, 28–29 (pain); 12 (vomiting and diarrhea); 58 (internal bleeding); 34–35 (muscle spasms); 18, 98 (sedation). Opiates were also used in tetanus; see Adams, *Doctors in Blue*, 141–42.

9. Goldsmith, "Of the Duties of Surgeons," 3.

10. Long, *Doctoring Freedom*, 70–71.

11. Figures derived from "Abstract A," in "Report of the Surgeon General," 384–85.

12. G. Smith, *Medicines for the Union Army*, 3; *Medical and Surgical History*, pt. 1, 2:xxv.

13. Hacker, "Count of the Civil War Dead."

14. Flannery, "Medicine and Health Care," 597; G. Adams, *Doctors in Blue*, 226–28.

15. Flannery, *Civil War Pharmacy*, 116. Between 1863 and 1865, 1,287 cases of malaria occurred per 1,000 Union soldiers in Arkansas.

16. *Medical and Surgical History*. An illustrative case is that of twenty-year-old Robert Frazer of the 4th Illinois Cavalry, who was stabbed in the stomach with a bayonet in April 1865. There was little the surgeons could do except give hypodermic morphine shots to numb Frazer's "excruciating pain." When Frazier died thirty-six hours later, his case became a textbook study in the fearsome mortality of bayonet wounds, the hypodermic use of morphine, and the bitter irony of dying in the final days of the Civil War. *Medical and Surgical History*, pt. 2, 2:42.

17. *Richmond Dispatch*, August 3, 1861, 2.

18. Letterman, *Medical Recollections of the Army of the Potomac*, 89–90; Rutkow, *Bleeding Blue and Gray*, 151. Standard opium pills contained roughly 1.2 grains of opium. See *Pharmacopoeia of the United States* (1864), 258.

19. Act to Increase Duties on Imports, and for Other Purposes, Pub. L. No. 171, Stat. 13 (1864).

20. Hammond, *Military Medical and Surgical Essays*, 293, 362, 365–71, 373–74, 379–80 (diarrhea, dysentery, and vomiting); 222, 228 (fevers); 250 (perforations); 309, 325 (pneumonia); 390 ("freely"); 30 ("carry in his pocket").

21. "No. 80: Appendix," *Documents of the US Sanitary Commission*, [70].

22. Woodward, *Hospital Steward's Manual*, 285–91. On the role of stewards, see Flannery, *Civil War Pharmacy*, 80–86, and "Life of a Hospital Steward," 87–98. Hospital stewards often had unfettered access to opium, and unsurprisingly some became addicted.

23. Flannery, *Civil War Pharmacy*, 98–114.

24. See Schultz, *Women at the Front*; Giesberg, *Army at Home*; Glymph, *Women's Fight*; and Zipiro, *This Grand Experiment*.

25. Flannery, *Civil War Pharmacy*, 114.

26. Exactly how much is unknowable because many Confederate medical records were lost in an April 1865 fire accidentally begun by rebel soldiers. Enough records survived in other locations to support the production of the *Medical and Surgical History*, which features numerous Confederate surgical cases, but not enough material is extant to gauge Confederate opiate supplies as accurately as for the Union. See esp. *Medical and Surgical History*, pt. 1, 2:xxi. On the Richmond fire, see Sternhell, *War on Record*, 30.

27. Cunningham, *Doctors in Gray*, 146–60; Humphreys, *Marrow of Tragedy*, 208–42. Humphreys observes that hospitals in Virginia experienced the most severe supply shortages. Cunningham notes that many Confederate surgeons claimed to have had access to ample medical supplies.

28. Arthur Hopkins Rice to Maria Walker, May 29, 1863, Mississippi State University Libraries, https://scholarsjunction.msstate.edu/mss-rice-papers/14/. Nineteenth-century Americans regarded lettuce as a potential substitute for opium. In her antebellum health guide for women, Lydia Marie Child described lettuce leaf tea as a "gentle opiate," good for "check[ing] chronic diarrhea, allay[ing] coughs, and sooth[ing] nervous irritation." Childs, *Family Nurse*, 117.

29. Ayers, *In the Presence of Mine Enemies*, 268.

30. "The Confederate Evacuation of Chambersburg," *Richmond Daily Dispatch*, July 6, 1863.

31. Humphreys, *Marrow of Tragedy*, 204–5. This effort was part of the broader Confederate attempt to cultivate native plants as medical substitutes for drugs needed for the war, especially quinine.

32. Porcher, *Resources of the Southern Fields and Forests*, 23–28; for context, see Flannery, *Civil War Pharmacy*, 202–4, 224–29.

33. "Save All Poppy Seeds," *Richmond Christian Advocate*, November 13, 1862; "Resources of Our Southern Fields and Forests," *Richmond Semi-Weekly Examiner*, April 28, 1863, 1; "Poppies," *Tri-Weekly Telegraph* (Houston), January 14, 1864, 2.

34. Franke, "Official and Industrial Aspects of Pharmacy," 185–87; Legan, "Drugs for Louisiana," 193–202. The Confederate military established small laboratories in several cities across the South, where druggists examined medicines smuggled through the blockade and concocted remedies from indigenous, locally harvested plants, in keeping with Surgeon General Moore and Porcher's efforts. Flannery, *Civil War Pharmacy*, 202–8.

35. Sam'l Preston Moore, "Circular, Confederate States of America, Surgeon General's Office, Richmond Va., July 6, 1863," in *War of the Rebellion*, ser. 1, vol. 2, p. 442; Cunningham, *Doctors in Gray*, 150.

36. McCurry, *Confederate Reckoning*, 180.

37. "The 'Bermuda' at Savannah," *Harper's Weekly*, October 26, 1861, 675.

38. Warner, *Therapeutic Perspective*, 308n22.

39. There are numerous examples of opiates for sale in Confederate newspapers throughout the South. For Atlanta, see advertisements for Hamilton, Markley, & Joyner in *Daily Intelligencer*, July 30, 1861; *Daily Intelligencer*, August 12, 1862; *Daily Intelligencer*, June 25, 1863; and "Valuable Drugs Just Received from John Bull," *Southern Confederacy* (Atlanta), June 25, 1863, 2. For Richmond, see *Sentinel* (Richmond), May 30, 1864, 2; August 6, 1864, 2; and September 3, 1864, 7. For Charlotte, see *Sentinel* (Richmond), March 13, 1865, 2.

40. Flannery, *Civil War Pharmacy*, 195.

41. "A Secesh Female in the Drug Trade," *Valley Spirit* (Franklin County, PA), November 26, 1862, 5. Another example is in *Alexandria Gazette*, October 31, 1862, 1.

42. "Stealing Physic," *Richmond Daily Whig*, June 22, 1864, 2; "A Leak in the Drug Shop at Chimborazo," *Richmond Sentinel*, June 22, 1864, 1. Union hospital and pharmacy staff also stole opiates and resold them illicitly. In 1864, a Union surgeon sold a dram of morphine and some powdered opium to a Winchester, Missouri, shopkeeper. The wares were later found to have been stolen from a Union hospital. "Statement of Mr. Bowley in Regard to Purchasing Hospital Stores," Bowley, [Blank]—State: Missouri—Year: 1864, Papers Relating to Citizens, 1861–1867, RG 109, National Archives and Records Administration (hereafter cited as NARA), https://catalog.archives.gov/id/27574361, accessed July 15, 2022. Hospital steward Theodore E. Goetz was accused of stealing opium from the Union army's pharmaceutical lab in Astoria, New York, where he was tasked with making laudanum. He was dishonorably discharged in July 1863 after being found guilty of conduct prejudicial. NN5, box 1504, Court Martial Case Files, RG 153, Records of the Office of the Judge Advocate General (Army), NARA.

43. Humphreys, *Marrow of Tragedy*, 208–42. A doctor advocating for laws restricting the sale of opiates alleged in 1877 that opium had been so scarce in his part of the Confederacy that opium eaters switched to alcohol. "Rum and Opium," *Athens Georgian*, October 2, 1877, 2.

44. Register and Prescription Book of 210th Regiment, Pennsylvania Volunteers, Huntington Library, San Marino, CA. Twenty-two prescriptions contained opiates out of eighty-three total prescriptions dated between October 4 and 14, 1864.

45. Humphreys, *Marrow of Tragedy*, 36–42.

46. 2nd N.C. Hospital Prescription book, cited in Warner, *Therapeutic Perspective*, 99, 309n24, 309nn27–28.

47. Prescription and Diet Book, circa 1800s, Southern Historical Collection, Louis Round Wilson Special Collections Library, University of North Carolina, Chapel Hill. Records begin on August 1, 1864, but there is no end date listed.

48. See Black account, p. 722, and Elliott account, p. 761, Account Book, 1863–1873, William W. Rutherford Account Books, Historical Medical Library, College of Physicians of Philadelphia. Rutherford kept meticulous accounts, annotating wartime patient accounts with "soldier" or military ranks and usually recording prescriptions and procedures.

49. Milton Sawyer Diary, Western Michigan University Libraries, Kalamazoo. Entry for June 10, 1863, 106.

50. Quoted in Humphreys, *Marrow of Tragedy*, 219.

51. "Terpin" refers to turpentine, and "lodnum" to laudanum. Like many Confederate soldiers, Caldwell was semi-literate. I include the original spelling to illustrate the myriad spellings for opiates and other drugs that soldiers used in their letters and diaries. Robert C. Caldwell to Margaret Caldwell, October 29, 1863, *Private Voices*, https://altchive.org/node/9626, accessed July 22, 2022.

52. Humphreys, *Marrow of Tragedy*, 227; Browning and Silver, *Environmental History of the Civil War*, 62, 99.

53. "Treatment of Diarrhea and Dysentery," 239.

54. "Medical and Surgical Cases at Port Royal, S.C.," 271–72, 276.

55. John Thomas Parker Commonplace Book, 1859–1865, Virginia Historical Society, Richmond. Remedy on p. 88.

56. Ferdinand Sophus Winslow letters, September 1861–February 1862, Iowa Digital Library, University of Iowa Library, Iowa City, https://digital.lib.uiowa.edu/islandora/object/ui%3Atestcwd_17265. Entry dated January 15, 1862.

57. Devine, "Civil War Health and Medicine," 278–84.

58. *National Tribune*, December 1, 1877, 21.

59. Thaddeus Hildreth Daybook, 1865–1874, Historical Medical Library, College of Physicians of Philadelphia, entries for June 20, 1870, and August 15, 1870.

60. Johnson, *Muskets and Medicine*, 164–65.

61. Kiechle, *Smell Detectives*, 128.

62. Holt, *Surgeon's Civil War*, 71.

63. Browning and Silver, *Environmental History of the Civil War*, 18–19.

64. Mattison, "Opium Addiction among Medical Men," 622; "Experience with Morphine," 10–11; Collett, "Opioid Tolerance," 58–68.

65. Oliver, "Use and Abuse of Opium," 167.

66. J. Adams, "Substitutes for Opium in Chronic Diseases," 355.

67. Entry No. 12709, Case Books, vol. 44, Utica State Hospital Patient Case Files, 1843–1898, New York State Archives, Albany.

68. *Proceedings of the Board of Managers of the National Home for Disabled Volunteers*, 364.

69. Calkins, *Opium and the Opium Appetite*, 238–39.

70. Crothers, "New Sources of Danger," 339.
71. Hartsock, *Soldier of the Cross*, 219n7.
72. J. Mitchell, *Remote Consequences of Injuries*, 34.
73. "Medical and Surgical Cases at Port Royal," 273.
74. Quoted in Ash, *Rebel Richmond*, 213.
75. J. Mitchell, *Remote Consequences of Injuries*, 70–71.
76. J. Mitchell, *Remote Consequences of Injuries*, 73–74.
77. Holston, "Surgical Reminiscences of an Old Practitioner," 161.
78. Edinburgh physician Alexander Wood is credited with developing the subcutaneous method of injection around 1855, although other contemporary physicians also claimed credit. Early adopters of the hypodermic syringe sought a more efficient method of administering morphine, among other drugs, to treat painful nerve afflictions. London doctor Charles Hunter first used the label "hypodermic" to describe this new therapeutic method. Haller, "Hypodermic Medicine," 1671–79.
79. Billings, "Medical Reminisces of the Civil War," 115.
80. Arnold, *Managing the Shock and Reaction of Severe Surgical Injuries*, 5.
81. Billings, "Medical Reminisces of the Civil War," 116.
82. For example, at an October 5, 1864, meeting of the New York Academy of medicine, several doctors reported experimenting with hypodermic morphine with great success. "The Effects of the Hypodermic Application of Morphine," 318–21. In 1881, a Richmond doctor cited wartime experiments by Mitchell, Morehouse, and Keen as a catalyst for spreading the practice of hypodermic medicine to civilian doctors. Coggeshall, "Hypodermic Use of Sulphate of Morphia," 155.
83. "Report of the Surgeon General," 386. Surgeon figures in Flannery, "Medicine and Health Care," 590–91. Hypodermic morphine seems to have been far less common in the Confederacy, whose military did not systematically purchase or distribute hypodermic syringes. Warner, *Therapeutic Perspective*, 138, 140, 157; Courtwright, *Dark Paradise*, 46.
84. *Medical and Surgical History*, pt. 1, 1:312, and 2:646, 619.
85. Devine, *Learning from the Wounded*; Handley-Cousins, *Bodies in Blue*, 51–70.
86. S. Mitchell, *Injuries of Nerves*, 10–11. On Turner's Lane Hospital, see Devine, *Learning from the Wounded*, chap. 4; Freemon, "First Neurological Research Center," 135–42; and Middleton, "Turner's Lane Hospital," 14–42.
87. Mitchell, Keen, and Morehouse, "Antagonism of Atropia and Morphia," 721, 723–24.
88. Mitchell, Keen, and Morehouse, "Antagonism of Atropia and Morphia," 721; Mitchell, "Medical Department in the Civil War," 1149.
89. S. Mitchell, *Injuries of Nerves*, 285–86.
90. S. Mitchell, *Injuries of Nerves*, 298–302. On the context and significance of Mitchell's study, see Devine, *Learning from the Wounded*, 154–58.
91. Mattison, "Curious Case of Opium Addiction," 849.
92. Bartholow, *Treatment of Diseases by the Hypodermic Method*, 90. This passage does not appear in the first two editions of the book, initially published in 1869. On the influence of Bartholow's work, see Courtwright, *Dark Paradise*, 46, 207n89.
93. Hartwell, "Report on the Sale and Use of Opium," 143.
94. Hull, "Opium Habit," 539.
95. Pernick, *Calculus of Suffering*, pt. 3; Owens, *Medical Bondage*; M'Dowell, "Hospital Observations upon Negro Soldiers," 155–68.

96. "Kentucky—Second District. Extracts from Report of Dr. J. W. Compton," 368.

97. Versalle, *Eagles on Their Buttons*, 22–23.

98. Humphreys, *Intensely Human*, 11.

99. Register of Prescriptions, July–August 1865, Freedman's Hospital New Orleans, RG105, NARA. A digitized version is accessible at familysearch.org.

100. Downs, *Sick from Freedom*; Humphreys, *Intensely Human*, 57–79, 125–41.

101. See Downs, *Sick from Freedom*, 169; A. Taylor, *Embattled Freedom*, 7–8.

102. Stoler, *Along the Archival Grain*. See also Fuentes, *Dispossessed Lives*, and Cooper Owens, *Medical Bondage*, for archival silences surrounding slavery and medicine.

103. J. Roberts, "Opium Habit in the Negro" (italics mine). Edwards-Grossi explores white psychiatry's ideas about Blackness and insanity at length, although she does not address addiction, in *Mad with Freedom*, chap. 1.

104. Courtwright, "Hidden Epidemic," 57–72.

105. Tipton, "Negro Problem from a Medical Standpoint," 570.

106. Roberts, "Opium Habit in the Negro," 206–7.

107. Sommerville, *Aberration of Mind*, 85–88.

108. Farber, *Crack*, 17–18.

109. Swank, *Confederate Letters and Diaries*, 56–58. On the "good death," see Faust, *This Republic of Suffering*, 3–31.

110. Rotundo, *American Manhood*, 35, 42; Stott, *Jolly Fellows*, 5. Although Rotundo and Gail Bederman observe a late nineteenth-century celebration of physical vigor and toughness, Stott argues that inflicting pain became associated with the loss of respectability late in the nineteenth century. Bederman, *Manliness and Civilization*, chap. 5.

111. Ross, "Boxing Boys in Blue," 438–55.

112. Linderman, *Embattled Courage*, 27–30; Nelson, *Ruin Nation*, 185.

113. C. Stevens, *Berdan's United States Sharpshooters*, 521 (italics mine).

114. McGuire, "Last Wound of the Late Gen. Jackson (Stonewall)," 403–12; "How Gen. Jackson Was Wounded," *Staunton Spectator*, May 19, 1863, 2. On Jackson's death and the birth of the Lost Cause, see Purcell, *Spectacle of Grief*, chap. 1. Some scholars have uncritically repeated Lost Cause claims that Jackson refused opiates, for example, Richenbacher, "Demise of Stonewall Jackson," 649. Confederates wanted (and neo-Confederates continue to want) to see Jackson as transcending physical pain. In reality, in his 1866 account, McGuire recalled administering opium and morphine painkillers to Jackson at least twice.

115. Entry 63: Albert T. Shurtleff, Soldier and Sailor Contributions, Left-Handed Penmanship Contest, William Oland Bourne Papers, Library of Congress. Quote on 12.

116. On patterns of self-care, see Meier, *Nature's Civil War*.

117. J. W. Henderson to Sarah A. M. Henderson, August 7, 1862, J. Watson Henderson Collection, Special Collections, University of Mississippi Libraries, Oxford.

118. Brobst, *Well Mary*, 28.

119. Brewster, *When This Cruel War Is Over*, 327.

120. Lt. Shelton Diary, July 11 and July 20, 1864, Shelton Family Papers, 1864–1936, Iowa Digital Library, University of Iowa Library, Iowa City, https://digital.lib.uiowa.edu/islandora/object/ui%3Atestcwd_4275_3_4.

121. Quoted in Egerton, *Heirs of an Honorable Name*, 222.

122. Humphreys, *Marrow of Tragedy*, 44–45.

123. Polley, *Soldier's Letters to Charming Nellie*, 268.

124. Cummings, "Letters of Charles Cummings, 51.

125. George W. Nailer to Parents, Sisters, Brother & Friends, April 29, 1864, box 1, folder 1, George W. Nailer Papers, 1824–1864, Stuart A. Rose Manuscript, Archives, and Rare Book Library, Emory University, Atlanta.

126. "Wall Street," *Harper's Weekly*, February 7, 1863, 82.

127. Lord, *Civil War Sutlers and Their Wares*, 53.

128. Holt, *Surgeon's Civil War*, 127.

129. Wood, *Doctor to the Front*, 94–95.

130. McPherson, *Battle Cry of Freedom*, 486.

131. Soldiers in the 59th Georgia Infantry even composed a poem lauding their skillful, sympathetic surgeons. Miller, *Empty Sleeves*, 47–48.

132. George P. McClelland to "My Dear Sister Lizzie," December 20, 1862, quoted in Plumb, *Your Brother in Arms*, 62.

133. Lewis Branscomb to Dear Father, June 7, 1862, *Private Voices*, https://altchive.org/node/11369, accessed July 22, 1862.

134. Bierce, "What I Saw at Shiloh," 255.

135. Faust, *This Republic of Suffering*, chap. 7.

136. Dean, *Shook over Hell*; Anderson, "Dying of Nostalgia"; Sommerville, *Aberration of Mind*; Silkenat, *Moments of Despair*; Handley-Cousins, *Bodies in Blue*.

137. George Phillips Diary, September 6 and September 7, 1863, 87–88, Connecticut Historical Society, Hartford.

138. LL2571, box 748, Court Martial Case Files, RG 153, Records of the Office of the Judge Advocate General (Army), NARA.

139. Chassaignac, "Case of Opium Habit Cures," 258; Admissions Book and Index, vol. 38, 1879–1881, 336–37, Charity Hospital Records, MF GS36-58, City Archives, New Orleans.

140. On the "work of killing," see Faust, *This Republic of Suffering*, 32–60.

141. George H. Howes, Civil War Service Records, *Fold3*, www.fold3.com/image/8467267, accessed July 21, 2022. House's name is misspelled as "Howes." Misspellings are common in service records; see "9th Regiment, Alabama Infantry," *Civil War Soldiers and Database*, www.nps.gov/civilwar/search-battle-units-detail.htm?battleUnitCode=CAL0009RI, accessed July 21, 2022.

142. Chassaignac, "Case of Opium Habit Cures," 256–59; Admissions Book and Index, vol. 38, 336–37, Charity Hospital Records.

143. Benjamin Edward Stiles Jr. to Mary Ann Mackay Stiles, June 18, 1862, Mackay and Stiles Family Papers, 1743–1975, Southern Historical Collection, Louis Round Wilson Special Collections Library, University of North Carolina at Chapel Hill.

144. *War of the Rebellion*, ser. 1, vol. 36, pt. 1, p. 96.

145. "Rosecrans at Home," *Harper's Weekly*, November 7, 1863, 707; "The Removal of Rosecrans," *Richmond Daily Dispatch*, October 26, 1863; "Gen. Rosecrans," *Richmond Daily Dispatch*, October 31, 1863; *Alexandria Gazette*, October 27, 1863, 1; "A Letter from General Rosecrans," *United States Army and Navy Journal and Gazette of the Regular and Volunteer Forces*, December 24, 1864, 277.

146. On Bragg and Hood, see Lewy, "Army Disease," 113, and Seward, "Slander," *Harper's Weekly*, June 13, 1863, 371.

147. Shelden, *Washington Brotherhood*, 124–30.

148. Foote, *Gentlemen and the Roughs*, 17–40. Southerners, too, engaged in vice, alarming their officers and families. Rable, *Fredericksburg, Fredericksburg!*, 94.

149. Lt. Shelton Diary, Shelton Family Papers, 1864–1936, Iowa Digital Library, University of Iowa Library, Iowa City, https://digital.lib.uiowa.edu/islandora/object/ui%3Atestcwd_4275. On self-medication, see July 11 and July 28, 1864, entries. On the reading of *Confessions*, see November 7, 1864, entry.

150. On military justice and alcohol intoxication, see Bever, *At War with King Alcohol*. 81–84. Many of the patterns outlined by Bever carried over to opiate intoxication, although it was much less pervasive than drunkenness and was less cited in court-martial proceedings.

151. *United States Army and Navy Journal and Gazette of the Regular and Volunteer Forces*, February 11, 1865, 396; NN2844, box 1822, Court Martial Case Files, RG 153, Records of the Office of the Judge Advocate General (Army), NARA.

152. NN856, box 1604, Court Martial Case Files, RG 153, Records of the Office of the Judge Advocate General (Army), NARA.

153. LL151, box 427, Court Martial Case Files, RG 153, Records of the Office of the Judge Advocate General (Army), NARA.

154. LL3187, box 878, Court Martial Case Files, RG 153, Records of the Office of the Judge Advocate General (Army), NARA. Similarly, Private Joel Moffat of the 11th US Infantry was charged with sleeping while on guard duty at Richmond's Libby Prison in September 1866. He argued that a surgeon gave him opium and camphor for diarrhea, making him drowsy. Moffat was found guilty, but a sympathetic court nonetheless released the soldier from confinement and returned him to duty. MM3988, Box 1503, Court Martial Case Files, RG 153, Records of the Office of the Judge Advocate General (Army), NARA. Private George W. Bundy of the 153rd New York Infantry was likewise convicted but released from confinement and restored to duty after a general found that the soldier had "slept because [he was] stupified [sic] with opium, prescribed by the Assistant Surgeon of the Regiment." NN217, box 1526, Court Martial Case Files, RG 153, Records of the Office of the Judge Advocate General (Army), NARA.

155. Hayden was demoted after being found guilty of conduct prejudicial for sleeping on post. II974, box 326, Court Martial Case Files, RG 153, Records of the Office of the Judge Advocate General (Army), NARA. For Smith's case, see LL3190, box 878, Court Martial Case Files, RG 153, Records of the Office of the Judge Advocate General (Army), NARA.

156. NN2491, box 1780, Court Martial Case Files, RG 153, Records of the Office of the Judge Advocate General (Army), NARA; Samuel Horner to the Officer in Command Buccaneer Regiment of West Department Cumberland, February 2, 1863, Arthur Horner, Civil War Service Records, *Fold3*, www.fold3.com/image/229258608/horner-arthur-page-28-us-civil-war-service-records-cmsr-union-missouri-1861-1865.

157. LL2714, folder 2, box 780, Court Martial Case Files, RG 153, Records of the Office of the Judge Advocate General (Army), NARA.

158. *United States Army and Navy Journal and Gazette of the Regular and Volunteer Forces*, October 15, 1864, 122.

159. An example is the case of H. W. Willoughby, a surgeon assigned to the 1st USCT, who was dismissed from his post in August 1864 for the "intemperate use of whiskey and opium." *United States Army and Navy Journal and Gazette of the Regular and Volunteer Forces*, August 27, 1864, 10. Willoughby's case was also covered in Confederate newspapers. See "Miscellaneous," *Richmond Daily Dispatch*, August 22, 1864, 1.

160. Downs, "Properties of Opium and Belladonna," 159.
161. "Supposed Suicide," *Richmond Daily Dispatch*, March 19, 1861, 3.
162. Sommerville, *Aberration of Mind*, 30–36.
163. *Manual of Military Surgery*, 98.
164. *Buffalo Medical and Surgical Journal* 2 (1862–63): 273.
165. *Medical and Surgical History*, pt. 1, 2:194.
166. H. Downs, "Properties of Opium and Belladonna," 159.
167. H. Eaton, *This Birth Place of Souls*, 105.
168. Schultz, *Women at the Front*, 3.
169. Arnold, *Managing the Shock and Reaction of Severe Surgical Injuries*, iii–iv.
170. For example, Delavan, *To the Army of the United States*. See also Foote, *Gentlemen and the Roughs*, 17–40; S. Martin, "'Soldier Intoxicated,'" 66–87; and Giesberg, *Sex and the Civil War*.
171. "Opium Eating," *Worcester Evening Gazette*, September 21, 1876, 1. The article was reprinted from the *Providence (RI) Journal*.
172. "Opium Eating," *Voice of the West* (Buchanan, MI), March 16, 1869, 126.
173. "The Facts of an Alleged Suicide," *St. Louis Daily Dispatch*, June 8, 1867, 1; J. Jones, "Life and Death of Frank Clewell." There does not appear to have been large-scale domestic opium production in the South. "King Alcohol's Great Rival," *Greenville (OH) Democrat*, June 16, 1875, 1.
174. Frost, "Opium." For hypodermic morphine, 134; for "abuses," 143–44; for "surgical cases," 144–45; for "opium debases," 147. For Frost's enrollment board service, 55. See also Carleton P. Frost, Civil War Service Record, Fold3, https://www.fold3.com/file/312181585.
175. Lesley E. Keeley, for example, claimed that "some localities have a greater proportion" of opium users "than others, the South having more victims than the North. . . . The effects of the war upon the South were very marked in this matter, as since that time the habit has largely increased in the Southern States." Quoted in Cole, *Confessions of American Opium Eater*, 193.
176. "The Opium Habit: Some Extraordinary Series of the Extravagant Use of the Drug in Virginia—Correspondence of the Cincinnati Enquirer," *New-York Times*, March 2, 1878, 2.
177. The best analyses of the Shenandoah Valley during the war is Ayers, *In the Prescence of Mine Enemies* and *Thin Light of Freedom*. On the destructive 1864 campaigns, see 139–87, 227–43. Quote in *Thin Light of Freedom*, 126.
178. *The Ellijay (GA) Courier*, March 1, 1878, 1. This story was widely reprinted. For example, see the *Savannah Morning News*, February 18, 1878, 1.
179. "Opium Eaters," *Shenandoah Herald* (Woodstock, VA), January 30, 1878, 3.
180. "Refuting a Slander on Staunton," *Staunton Vindicator*, March 8, 1878, 2; "The Opium Eaters," *Staunton Vindicator*, February 1, 1878, 3.
181. "The Opium Flurry," *Staunton Spectator*, March 19,1878, 3.
182. For example, "Chinese Opium Smokers—A San Francisco Den," *Winchester Times*, August 23, 1871, 1.
183. *Staunton Vindicator*, January 25, 1878, 1, column 3; February 1, 1878, 4, column 4; and May 10, 1878, 4, column 4; "Opium and Morphine Habit Cured," *Staunton Vindicator*, March 8, 1878, 1, column 2.
184. An 1853 law required commissioners of revenue to record births and deaths. These registers did not entail investigations of the deaths recorded, unlike the coroners' inquests cited in chapters 1 and 2. The microfilmed registers are accessible at the Library of Virginia.

They have recently been digitized and are accessible at Family Search. See Death registers, 1853–1906 (Virginia), *Family Search*, www.familysearch.org/search/catalog/780106.

185. "Not Heart Disease," *National Tribune*, February 11, 1882, 6.

186. For example, Harnan, "Case of Morphine Narcosis."

187. Exceptions include Virginia, where birth, death, and marriage registers were kept between 1853 and 1896, and Massachusetts, which kept vital records from the colonial era onward.

188. Courtwright argues that the Civil War was only one of several factors contributing to the rising addiction rate in the Gilded Age. Further parsing this data, Courtwright estimates that the maximum rate of addiction to medicinal opiates stood at 3.25 per thousand. Courtwright, *Dark Paradise*, 9, 26–28, 36, 46–47, 54–55, 195n51.

189. Rothstein, *American Physicians*, 193.

190. For example, Calkins, "Opium and Its Victims," 25; and "The Opium Eaters," *Staunton Vindicator*, February 1, 1878.

191. "Use of Opium in the United States: American Druggists' Circular," *New York Observer and Chronicle*, December 20, 1866, 405.

192. H. Day, *Opium Habit*, 7. An additional example is "Opium and the Opium Trade," *National Review*, March 1870, 288.

193. H. James Brown, *Opium Cure*, 17. This claim seems self-serving, but the notion was widely echoed in medical circles.

194. "Opium-Eating," *Daily Evening Bulletin* (San Francisco), April 3, 1872, 1.

195. Courtwright, "Opiate Addiction," 110–11; Courtwright, *Dark Paradise*, 36–42.

196. Turner, *History of the First Inebriate Asylum*, 495.

197. Hull, "Opium Habit," 539.

198. Sommerville, *Aberration of Mind*, 221–25.

199. S. D. Armstrong to My Dear Friends, April 2, 1865, Captured Mail Collection, 1862–1865, Confederate Memorial Literary Society, Virginia Historical Society, Richmond. A similar case is found in Webster, "Opium Eating Cured by Belladonna Poisoning," 23–24.

200. *Papers of Jefferson Davis*, 611. A January 11, 1870, letter in the DeRosset Family Papers describes Marie DeRosset's prior opium use. DeRosset Family Papers, 1671–1940, Southern Historical Collection, Louis Round Wilson Special Collections Library, University of North Carolina at Chapel Hill.

201. Hubbard, *Opium Habit and Alcoholism*, 21–22.

202. See Hickman, *Secret Leprosy of Modern Days*, 80–91.

203. Oliver, "Use and Abuse of Opium," 173–74.

204. Crothers, "Inebriety Caused by Psychical Traumatism," 228. Crothers and other inebriety experts classified opiate addiction as a kind of inebriety, like alcohol addiction. See Mattison, "Remedy for the Diminution of Opium Inebriety," 207.

205. Fitz Hugh Ludlow, "What Shall They Do to Be Saved?," *Harper's New Monthly Magazine*, August 1867, 377–87.

206. D. A. Wedon, "Opium-Eating," *Zion's Herald*, November 19, 1868, 554.

207. "The Opium Poppy," *Scientific American*, March 18, 1876, 183.

208. A. Day, *Inebriety and Its Cure*, 8.

209. Weldon, "Opium Eating," 554.

210. Oliver, "Use and Abuse of Opium," 174–75.

211. "Champion Opium-Eater, *St. Louis Daily Globe-Democrat*, July 25, 1878, 2.

212. *Report of the Committee on Intemperance as a Disease*, 11.

213. "Effects of the Use of Intoxicating Liquor," 253.

214. Oliver, "Use and Abuse of Opium," 168.

215. The Iowa Board of Health's report is Hull, "Opium Habit." The Massachusetts Board of Health's 1888 report is Hartwell, "Report on the Sale and Use of Opium." The latter was expressly requested by the Massachusetts legislature in 1886. The fate of the Maryland Board of Health's report is unclear. The board sent questionnaires to physicians to ascertain the extent of opiate addiction in the state, but it is unknown whether the report was ever published. "Important Vital Investigations," *Baltimore Sun*, August 23, 1875, 4. For the methodology and findings of Marshall and Earle, see Courtwright, *Dark Paradise*, 10. For a distillation of Eaton's findings, see Virgil Eaton, "How the Opium Habit Is Acquired," *Popular Science Monthly*, September 1, 1888, 663.

216. De Forest, *Miss Ravenel's Conversion*, 297, 475; Casey, *New Men*, 17–47.

217. Roe, *Without a Home*, 479. Susan Zieger notes that Roe's novel, originally published in 1881, was the earliest book about hypodermic drugs published in the United States. She argues that Roe drew heavily on widely recognized themes common in Civil War–era drunkard narratives, like the loss of manhood through "slavery" to an external master—in this case, morphine. Zieger, *Inventing the Addict*, 98–123.

218. Cobbe, *Doctor Judas*.

219. Roe, *Without a Home*, vii.

220. Particularly useful studies of late nineteenth-century stereotypes include Hickman, *Secret Leprosy of Modern Days*, and Spillane, *Cocaine*.

221. *Opium Problem*, 47–48.

Chapter 4

1. Henley quoted in Woolley, *Opium Habit and Its Cure*, 16–18, 30; Albert W. Henley, Civil War Service Records, Fold3, www.fold3.com/image/20/84651882.

2. Andrews, "Cure of a Confirmed Opium-Eater," 68.

3. Pergolizzi, Raffa, and Rosenblatt, "Opioid Withdrawal Symptoms"; Kesten et al., "Changes in the Development of Opioid Tolerance."

4. Hubbard, *Opium Habit and Alcoholism*, 9.

5. *Opium Eating* (1876), 111–12.

6. "Morphiomania," 271–72.

7. Hull, "Opium Habit," 543–44.

8. Handley-Cousins, *Bodies in Blue*, 2.

9. Miller, *Empty Sleeves*, introduction; Nelson, *Ruin Nation*, chap. 4; Clarke, *War Stories*, chap. 6.

10. Bartholow, *Treatment of Diseases by the Hypodermic Method*, 90, 6.

11. "Opium slavery" was also widely used by and about non-veteran opium eaters. For example, see "Opium-Eating," *Lippincott's Magazine of Literature, Science and Education*, April 1868, 403–9, and Sewall, "Opium-Eating and Hypodermic Injection," 422.

12. *Theriaki*, July 1872, 53.

13. Collins, *Theriaki and Their Last Dose*, 15.

14. "Champion Opium-Eater," *St. Louis Daily Globe-Democrat*, July 25, 1878, 2.

15. Bartholow, *Treatment of Diseases by the Hypodermic Method*, 90.

16. Quoted in Dean, *Shook over Hell*, 170.

17. Hubbard, *Opium Habit and Alcoholism*, 6, 3–4.

18. Foote, *Inebriety and Opium Eating*, 9–10.

19. Mattison, "Opium Addiction among Medical Men," 622.

20. Mattison, "Ethics of Opium Habitués," 126.

21. Kalant, "Opium Revisited," 271–73; Dark, Larney, and Farrell, "Yes, People Can Die from Opiate Withdrawal," 199–200. Accessible overviews of opioid pharmacology and withdrawal are Pathan and Williams, "Basic Opioid Pharmacology"; Rosenblum et al., "Opioids and the Treatment of Chronic Pain"; and Pergolizzi, Raffa, and Rosenblatt, "Opioid Withdrawal Symptoms." Data about the number of Civil War veterans who relapsed were not collected, but many of the men in this study's sample relapsed, often repeatedly. I did not quantify a relapse rate for the sample because I did not have enough data to support an accurate count via a longitudinal study, one that tracks users over a life cycle in meticulous detail. However, based on the qualitative evidence presented throughout the book, it is also safe to assume that many users in the sample relapsed, and that many relapses occurred without appearing in the sources that are available to historians. Additionally, to gauge the frequency of relapse, we can weigh Civil War veterans against studies of male drug users from subsequent generations. In 1935, 823 male "narcotic drug addicts" were admitted for treatment at the Public Service Hospital, Lexington, Kentucky, a penitentiary-style "narcotics farm" operated by the federal government for the treatment (and confinement) of drug users. Of those 823 men, 346 were readmitted to the hospital by 1966, a readmission rate of 42 percent. Overall, between 1935 and 1966, "of the 33,479 males discharged, 22,430 were voluntary patients, and 11,049 were federal prisoners during their first admission. The rate of readmission for the male voluntary patients was 40.0 and the rate for the male prisoners was 36.1." This data does not represent a perfect substitute for statistics on relapses among Civil War veterans, for several reasons. Men admitted to the Lexington facility were not classified by drug of use but instead were labeled as "narcotics drug addicts." Heroin had been introduced around the turn of the century, and it is possible that heroin users relapsed at different rates than users of morphine, opium, and laudanum. But this Lexington data, particularly for the 1935 cohort of men, nevertheless allows for an approximation of potential relapse rates for opiate-addicted Civil War veterans, some of whom lived as late as the 1920s. Most of the Lexington data was generated prior to the 1960s–80s introduction of modern Medication-Assistance Treatment (MAT), which utilizes drugs such as buprenorphine, methadone, and naltrexone. Thus addiction treatment at the Lexington facility would have likely mirrored the withdrawal methods available to Gilded Age drug users at private inebriety clinics and mental asylums, as discussed in chapters 5 and 8. Men who were admitted/readmitted to the Lexington facility, especially the 1935 cohort, can stand in as a proxy for Civil War veterans who sought addiction care at asylums and inebriety clinics because both groups probably had similar treatment experiences and success rates. Ball, Thompson, and Allen, "Readmission Rates at Lexington Hospital for 43,215 Narcotic Drug Addicts," 610–13. On MAT, see Campbell, *OD*. On the Lexington facility, see Clarke, *Recovery Revolution*, 7–9.

22. Collins, *Theriaki and Their Last Dose*, 13.

23. Entry no. 11804, Case Books, vol. 36, Utica State Hospital Patient Case Files, 1843–1898, New York State Archives, Albany.

24. Chassaignac, "Case of Opium Habit Cures," 258.

25. Gould, "Opium Habit," 497.

26. Calkins, *Opium and the Opium Appetite*, 238–39.

27. "Chicago Opium-Eaters," *Christian Advocate*, November 11, 1880, 734.

28. Virgil Eaton, "How the Opium Habit Is Acquired," *Popular Science Monthly*, September 1, 1888, 663.

29. Roe, *Without a Home*, 479.

30. "Antidotes," *Christian Union*, May 2, 1877, 394.

31. "Unique Organization: How the Work of the Keeley League Is Retarded," *Boston Daily Globe*, January 8, 1896, 12.

32. "A Victim of Opium," *New-York Times*, October 24, 1885.

33. Gould, "Opium Habit," 496–97.

34. "Opium Eating," *Sanitarian*, February 1, 1876, 93; *Opium Eating*, 97.

35. On the cultural effects of panics, see Levy, *Freaks of Fortune*.

36. Parsons, *Manhood Lost*, 4, 13.

37. Rotundo, *American Manhood*, 178–85.

38. Keeley, *Morphine Eater*, 163.

39. Eventually, Richards obtained medical care for addiction through Leslie E. Keeley's Gold Cure, a patent medicine for drug and alcohol addiction, discussed at length in chapter 7.

40. Gould, "Opium Habit," 497.

41. Entry no. 12670, Case Books, vol. 42, Utica State Hospital Patient Case Files.

42. Entry no. 14073, Case Books, vol. 52, Utica State Hospital Patient Case Files.

43. Entry no. 12670, Case Books, vol. 42, Utica State Hospital Patient Case Files; Entry no. 14073, Case Books, vol. 52, Utica State Hospital Patient Case Files; *Opium Eating*, 111.

44. For boys and painful childhood games, see Rotundo, *American Manhood*, 34–42; for the work of killing and dying, see Faust, *This Republic of Suffering*.

45. Linderman, *Embattled Courage*, 27–30; Nelson, *Ruin Nation*, 185; and Handley-Cousins, *Bodies in Blue*, 88–92 (quotation from former New York governor Alonzo Cornell about Union veteran Henry Barnum on 92).

46. "Chicago Opium-Eaters," 734.

47. *Public Papers of Grover Cleveland*, 375.

48. *The Ohio Soldier*, September 29, 1888, 107; Marten, *Sing Not War*, 84.

49. Mitchell, *Injuries of Nerves*, 298–302.

50. J. L. Stewart to S. Weir Mitchell, January 28, 1891, Silas Weir Mitchell Papers, Historical Medical Library, College of Physicians of Philadelphia. The letter has been digitized and is available at https://mitchell.cppdigitallibrary.org/s/mitchell/item-set/16498.

51. *Report of Inspection of State Soldiers and Sailors' Homes for Year Ending June 30, 1894*, 250.

52. Abscesses were also reported among women who used hypodermic morphine. *Journal of Insanity* 28 (1871–72): 50. Similar commentary appears in the modern medical literature documenting the twenty-first-century opioid crisis. Fink et al., "Abscess and Self-Treatment," 523–31.

53. Sewall, "Opium-Eating and Hypodermic Morphine," 422.

54. Kane, *Drugs that Enslave*, 71.

55. Kane, *Hypodermic Injection of Morphia*, 35.

56. Haller, "Hypodermic Medicine," 1677; see also Coggeshall, "Hypodermic Use of Sulphate of Morphia," 152–53. When describing how to prepare morphine solution, Coggeshall emphasized the importance of cleaning hypodermic syringes between uses by flushing them with warm water to prevent tetanus. Unknown to Coggeshall, using unsterilized warm water might have introduced microbes.

57. Fleming, "Treatment of the Habit of Opium-Eating," 370.

58. Entry no. 12670, Case Books, vol. 42, Utica State Hospital Patient Case Files.

59. S. Mitchell, *Injuries of Nerves*, 300.

60. *Report of Inspection of State Soldiers and Sailors' Homes for Year Ending June 30, 1894*, 250. Gardner's weight loss was extreme but not unheard of. Another male morphine user of similar age dwindled to eighty pounds after years of addiction. Entry no. 15277, Case Books, vol 62, Utica State Hospital Patient Case Files. Weight loss was commonly reported by long-term opiate users in the same and attributed to opiates by veterans and their doctors. However, it is worth pointing out that other factors unrelated to opiate use could have contributed to emaciation, such as illness or malnutrition.

61. *Opium Eating*, 59, 64, 110.

62. Kalant, "Opium Revisited," 272. Another accessible overview is Baldini, Von Korff, and Lin, "Review of Potential Adverse Effects of Long-Term Opioid Therapy."

63. Kasson, *Perfect Man*, 49–68.

64. Stillman, *Life Insurance Examiner*, 37.

65. *Opium Eating*, 98.

66. Mann, "Cases Illustrative of the Treatment," 398.

67. *Theriaki*, July 1872, 26–27, 29–30.

68. Collins, *Theriaki: A Treatise*, 25–26.

69. Entry no. 14873, Case Books, vol. 58, Utica State Hospital Case Files.

70. *Opium Eating*, 57.

71. Mann, "Cases Illustrative of the Treatment," 399.

72. Rotundo, *American Manhood*, 167–74.

73. Entry no. 14873, Case Books, vol. 58, Utica State Hospital Patient Case Files.

74. Collins, *Theriaki and Their Last Dose*, 69–92.

75. Entry no. 12274, Case Books, vol. 40, Utica State Hospital Patient Case Files.

76. Collins, *Theriaki*, 49–50.

77. Dean, *Shook over Hell*, 170.

78. Rotundo, *American Manhood*, 178–85.

79. Parsons, "Risky Business," 285, and *Manhood Lost*, 61–62. Parsons applies this reasoning to alcohol abuse in Gilded Age Midwestern saloons, but the concept is transferrable to opiate addiction, which, like alcohol abuse, left men in a state of habitual intoxication.

80. Stanley, *From Bondage to Contract*, 98–137.

81. "Chicago Opium-Eaters," 734.

82. Cobbe, *Doctor Judas*, [3] (italics mine).

83. McClurken, *Take Care of the Living*, 68; Boydston, *Home and Work*, 55.

84. *Decisions of the Department of the Interior in Appealed Pension and Bounty-Land Claims*, 7:49–50.

85. Whites, *Gender Matters*, 11–24, and *Civil War as a Crisis in Gender*.

86. John Goolrick, Civil War Service Records, Fold3, www.fold3.com/image/9037851.

87. Quotes in Frances Goolrick to W. S. White, February 5, 1896, Goolrick Family Papers, 1859–1927, Virginia Historical Society, Richmond (hereafter cited as Goolrick Family Papers). Additional letters describe John's physical and mental state. Nora Goolrick to Frances Goolrick, March 8, 1986, Goolrick Family Papers.

88. Richard Lee Stout, ed. *Maud* (New York: Macmillan, 1939), 121–22. This is the edited diary of Isabella Maud Rittenhouse.

89. Dawson v. Dawson, 23 Mo. App. 169 (1886), Caselaw Access Project, https://cite.case.law/mo-app/23/169/, accessed August 6, 2022. An 1835 Missouri law allowed for divorce "when either party was addicted to habitual drunkenness for the space of two years." James Dawson successfully claimed that Eva Dawson's opiate "drunkenness" fell under the purview of this law.

90. W. S. White to Frances Goolrick, February 8, 1896, Goolrick Family Papers.

91. Nora Goolrick to Frances Goolrick, March 3, 1896, March 9, 1896, and March 10, 1896, Goolrick Family Papers.

92. Charles O'Conor Goolrick to Frances Goolrick, February 28, 1896, Goolrick Family Papers.

93. Isabella L. Hart to Frances Goolrick, January 5, 1915, Goolrick Family Papers.

94. "Judge John T. Goolrick," *Richmond Times-Dispatch*, September 18, 1925, 6.

95. John Tackett Goolrick, Certificate of Death, *Virginia, US, Death Records, 1912–2014*, Ancestry.com, www.ancestry.com/imageviewer/collections/9278/images/43004_162028006073_0104-00333, accessed August 5, 2022; Roy et al., "Opioid Drug Abuse and Modulation of Immune Function," 14–15; Pappritz and Van Linthout, "Opioid-Induced Immunomodulation," 335.

96. "Judge John T. Goolrick," 6.

97. W. S. White to Frances Goolrick, March 4, 1896, Goolrick Family Papers.

98. William Goolrick to Frances Goolrick, March 7, 1896, Goolrick Family Papers.

99. *Capitolian Advocate* (Baton Rouge), December 25, 1883, 1; *Galveston News*, December 23, 1863, 1.

100. Testimony of disability by R. W. Brisbeam, March 25, 1886, Alpheus M. Chappell application file, Confederate Disability Applications and Receipts, Library of Virginia, Richmond.

101. A. M. Chappell to William R. Terry, May 24, 1886, Lee Camp Soldier's Home Correspondence, 1885–1894, Huntington Library, San Marino, CA.

102. 1860 Federal Census, Delaware Township, Delaware County, Indiana, Fold3, www.fold3.com/image/51632949, accessed September 7, 2022; Joseph Depoy, Civil War Service Index, Fold3, www.fold3.com/image/294809007, accessed September 7, 2022; Claim by Lockhart & Stright [April 12, 1880], Delaware County Poor Relief Records, Archives and Special Collections, Ball State University Libraries, Muncie, IN, https://dmr.bsu.edu/digital/collection/PoRelRec/id/2954/rec/16, accessed September 7, 2022; Claim by Joseph LeFavour [May 29, 1884], Delaware County Poor Relief Records, https://dmr.bsu.edu/digital/collection/PoRelRec/id/4865/rec/10.

103. Claim by Tabitha Depoy, Delaware County Poor Relief Records, Archives and Special Collections, Ball State University Libraries, Muncie, IN, https://dmr.bsu.edu/digital/collection/PoRelRec/id/6998/rec/13, accessed September 7, 2022; Claim by Joseph LeFavour [May 29, 1884], Delaware County Poor Relief Records, https://dmr.bsu.edu/digital/collection/PoRelRec/id/4865/rec/1; Claim by Joseph LeFavour [November 25, 1886], Delaware County Poor Relief Records, https://dmr.bsu.edu/digital/collection/PoRelRec/id/6756/rec/9, accessed September 7, 2022; Claim by Lockhart & Stright [March 3, 1879], Delaware County Poor Relief Records, https://dmr.bsu.edu/digital/collection/PoRelRec/id/2030/rec/15, accessed September 7, 2022.

104. *Report of Inspection of State Soldiers and Sailors' Homes for the Year Ending June 30, 1894*, 231–32.

105. See, for example, Mattison, "Ethics of Opium Habitués," 125. Mattison believed there was a "better class of habitués," mostly medicinal opiate users who became addicted through doctors' prescriptions, who were distinct from "those who, viciously indulgent and lacking

alike in principle, take opium from mere sensual desire." The delineation tended to fall along class lines.

106. "Chicago Opium-Eaters," 734.

107. Morris, "Panorama of a Life," 61–62.

108. Mann, "Cases Illustrative of the Treatment," 398.

109. Fleming, "Treatment of the Habit of Opium-Eating," 368.

110. Allen, *Medical Examinations for Life Insurance*, 9, 11–12.

111. For example, Mulliner v. Guardian Mutual Life Insurance, 1 Thomp. & Cook 448 (1873), https://cite.case.law/thomp-cook/1/448/, accessed August 6, 2022.

112. Oliver, "Use and Abuse of Opium," 162.

113. Mann, "Cases Illustrative of the Treatment," 399.

114. Mattison, "Ethics of Opium Habitués," 125. Mattison rejected this view.

115. "Effects of Opium," 371.

116. *Theriaki*, July 1872, 23.

117. Oliver, "Use and Abuse of Opium," 176.

118. Entry no. 11804, Case Books, vol. 36, Utica State Hospital Patient Case Files, 1843–1898, New York State Archives, Albany.

119. For example, see "An Opium Eater," *Alexandria Gazette*, October 7, 1868, 1, and "The Opium Habit," *Sunny South* (Atlanta), April 26, 1879, 8.

120. "Hero's Sad End," *Boston Morning Journal*, December 6, 1897, 1.

121. "Death of Veteran Cyrus P. Harmon," *Akron Times-Democrat*, February 14, 1901, 8; "Died in the Pen," *Akron Beacon-Journal*, February 8, 1901; "In Columbus," *Akron Beacon-Journal*, February 11, 1901; "Inhuman," *Akron Beacon-Journal*, February 14, 1901.

122. Halttunen, *Confidence Men and Painted Women*, 34.

123. "Treatment of Opiamania and Morphiamania," 114.

124. *Report of Inspection of State Soldiers and Sailors' Homes for Year Ending June 30, 1896*, 321.

125. *Report of Inspection of State Soldiers and Sailors' Homes for Year Ending June 30, 1894*, 232.

126. Hubbard, *Opium Habit and Alcoholism*, 5.

127. Handley-Cousins, "'Wrestling at the Gates of Death,'" 224–25, 227–28.

128. McLaren, *Impotence*, chaps. 5–6.

129. John Burroughs, "Carlyle," *Century Illustrated Monthly Magazine*, May–October 1883, 543.

130. Diversion within the household is a well-documented twenty-first-century phenomenon. It stands to reason that nineteenth-century Americans may also have practiced household diversion.

131. The Jones's cases are entries 3127 and 3128, Dorothea Dix Hospital General Case Books, 18:1–3, North Carolina State Archives, Raleigh. The spine reads "Case Book Vol. 6," but the archival finding aid lists it as vol. 18. Andrew J. Jones, a native of Virginia according to his asylum record, matches several Virginia Confederate service records, thus it is difficult to determine which unit he served in. According to Andrew's asylum record, he was 49 in 1898, although such records sometimes approximated patients' ages. Accordingly, he would have been a teenager during the Civil War, old enough to serve in the Confederate military, but barely.

132. Thomas B. Chaplin to G. W. Aimar, February 3, 1877, Letters to G. W. Aimar, 1877–1880, South Carolina Historical Society, Charleston (hereafter cited as Letters to G. W. Aimar).

133. Thomas B. Chaplin to G. W. Aimar, March 31, 1877, Letters to G. W. Aimar.

134. Thomas B. Chaplin to G. W. Aimar, June 16, 1877, Letters to G. W. Aimar (underlining in the original).
135. Thomas B. Chaplin to G. W. Aimar, August 9, 1878, Letters to G. W. Aimar.
136. Thomas B. Chaplin to G. W. Aimar, September 27, 1878, Letters to G. W. Aimar.
137. Thomas B. Chaplin to G. W. Aimar, December 4, 1880, Letters to G. W. Aimar.
138. Beard, *Stimulants and Narcotics*, 47–48; see also Rotundo, *American Manhood*, 185–93. For a comparative perspective, see Hickman's analysis of H. H. Kane in *Secret Leprosy of Modern Days*, 66–72.
139. Coggeshall, "Hypodermic Use of Sulphate of Morphia," 158.
140. A. Day, *Inebriety and Its Cure*, 16–17.
141. On "race suicide," see Bederman, *Manliness and Civilization*, 199–203. On historical theories of hereditary, see Porter, *Genetics in the Madhouse*.
142. "Remarks on the Opium Habit," 436.
143. Happel, "Morphinism," 407.
144. On Gilded Age fears about white race decline, see Jacobson, *Barbarian Virtues*, 160–62, and *Whiteness of a Different Color*, 39–91.
145. "Inebriety as a Disease," *Scientific American*, January 27, 1877, 48.
146. Illustrative examples are "A Victim to Opium," *New-York Times*, December 12, 1881, and "Pretty but Depraved," *New-York Times*, November 12, 1884. On "white slavery," see Pliley, *Policing Sexuality*, 9–31.
147. *New-York Times*, May 18, 1883, 4.
148. "A Coroner's Jury and an 'Overdose' of Opium," *Brooklyn Daily Eagle*, March 7, 1874, 4.
149. "The Opium Habit," *Frank Leslie's Popular Monthly*, July 1877, 189, 191.
150. For estimates of the addicted population, see Courtwright, *Dark Paradise*, 26–28; on opium smoking among whites, see 61–84. On the crucial role white doctors played in Chinese exclusion, see Ahmad, "Opium Smoking, Anti-Chinese Attitudes," and Hickman, *Secret Leprosy of Modern Days*, 66–72.
151. For San Francisco, see Courtwright, *Dark Paradise*, 77. For Texas, see "Disorderly House."
152. For example, see "The 'Big Flat' Raided," *New-York Times*, December 8, 1884.
153. Cohen, "Jim Crow's Drug War"; Spillane, *Cocaine*, 120–22; Hickman, *Secret Leprosy of Modern Days*, 72–80.
154. Courtwright, "Opiate Addiction in the American West, 1850–1920," 28–29; Foster, "Opium, the United States, and the Civilizing Mission" and "Origins of Global Narcotics Prohibition."
155. "Union Army."
156. Costa, Yetter, and DeSomer, "Wartime Health Shocks"; Costa, Yetter, and DeSomer, "Intergenerational Transmission of Paternal Trauma," 11215–220. See also Pizarro, Silver, and Prause, "Physical and Mental Health Costs," 193–200. There is a growing social science literature documenting various facets of the Civil War's intergenerational health crisis. But the findings of these studies—which have been conducted mostly by social scientists, not historians—have not yet been well integrated into the medical historiography of the Civil War, in part because these studies were published in economics venues, not history journals.
157. Entry no. 14073, Case Books, vol. 52, Utica State Hospital Patient Case Files.
158. Kesten et al., "Changes in the Development of Opioid Tolerance."
159. *Press and Messenger* (Baltimore), November 30, 1874, 1.

160. An illustrative suicide is that of Edward Winfield Weeks, a veteran of the 41st Virginia Infantry. In August 1866, on the night of his death, Weeks entered his son's bedroom, kissed him, and said goodbye before turning to his wife, declaring his intention to die, and swallowing morphine pills. She "begged him not to do so." Petersburg (city), Misc. records, Coroner's inquests, 1826–1932, broken series, box 32, BC 1047087, 1-05-15-01-2, unbundled, Library of Virginia State Records Center, Charles City Road, Richmond.

161. Waldorf, Orlick, and Reinarman, *Morphine Maintenance*, 35.

162. Case Book no. 6, 1905–1910, vol. 285, p. 67, Records of Western State Hospital, 1825–2000, Library of Virginia, Richmond.

163. Dean, *Shook over Hell*, 169–70; Perry Bowser Pension Application, certificate no. 108546, quote from affidavit of October 25, 1869; Perry B. Bourer alias Bowser, United States National Homes for Disabled Volunteer Soldiers, 1866–1938, Family Search, www.familysearch.org/ark: /61903/1:1:VH4X-1NR?lang=en, accessed May 29, 2020.

164. McClurken, *Take Care of the Living*, 172.

165. Downs, *Sick from Freedom*; Humphreys, *Yellow Fever and the South*.

Chapter 5

1. Case Book no. 6, 1905–1910, vol. 285, p. 67, Records of Western State Hospital, Library of Virginia, Richmond; Certificate of Discharge, William Blankenbaker Confederate service record, Civil War Service Records, Fold3, www.fold3.com/image/20/7277127. According to his asylum medical record, Blankenbaker died of a mitral prolapse, a heart condition that can cause pain while breathing. Western Lunatic Asylum was renamed Western State Hospital in 1894.

2. On the historicity of mental illness and trauma, see F. Clarke, "So Lonesome I Could Die," 254. Clarke argues that the Civil War–era diagnosis of "nostalgia" was caused by homesickness, which was seen as traumatic for contemporary soldiers but less traumatic as understood by twenty-first-century scholars. However, addiction was both a recognizable condition in the Civil War era and seen as a manifestation of trauma. Although the use of psychiatric patient records provides great insight into the lives of addicted people, historians rightfully caution against the uncritical use of these records, which were recorded by doctors and thus reflect the bias of psychiatrists who often view their patients with disdain. Risse and Warner, "Reconstructing Patient Records."

3. Gerald N. Grob, *Mental Institutions in America*, describes nineteenth-century asylum doctors as the earliest American psychiatrists. I adopt this perspective here.

4. Studies that employ asylum records to assess the psychological legacy of the Civil War for veterans include Dean, *Shook over Hell*; McClurken, *Take Care of the Living*, 118–42; Sommerville, *Aberration of Mind*; Handley-Cousins, *Bodies in Blue*, 115–32; and Carroll, *Invisible Wounds*. Several recent works also utilize asylum records fruitfully to reconstruct the world of nineteenth-century asylums, including Summers, *Madness in the City*; Edwards-Grossi, *Mad with Freedom*; and Gonaver, *Making of Modern Psychiatry*. Dean controversially used retrospective diagnosis to describe Civil War veterans as suffering from PTSD. In contrast, McClurken, Sommerville, Handley-Cousins, and Carroll shy away from using the modern diagnostic category of PTSD, instead utilizing more flexible labels such as "war trauma." They do, however, present compelling evidence that many Americans of the Civil War generation believed the stressors of war could, and often did, manifest in serious psychological and emotional suffering. In many cases, although certainly not all, contemporary observers directly linked

Civil War veterans' emotional and mental breakdowns to wartime experiences. Drew Gilpin Faust also links the Civil War generation's traumatic experiences in the war, especially mass death, to profound changes in how Americans perceived and reacted to death in the postwar era. Faust, *This Republic of Suffering*. Studies on veterans' mental health can thus be understood as a manifestation of broader medical and cultural changes spawned by the Civil War.

5. Hsieh, "'Go to Your Gawd Like a Soldier'"; Clarke, "So Lonesome I Could Die," 254; Schantz, *Awaiting the Heavenly Country*. Clarke rightly cautions historians against the assumption that modern conceptions of trauma and corresponding psychiatric diagnoses like PTSD neatly correspond to nineteenth-century notions of trauma and associated diagnoses, such as nostalgia, without significant meaning being lost in translation. See also Marshall, "Great Exaggeration."

6. Some postwar physicians and patent medicine sellers rejected this belief, instead contending that addiction was a disease called "inebriety," the product of brain lesions, not a form of insanity. Yet this remained a minority viewpoint during the nineteenth century. This development is explored at length in chapter 8.

7. Sommerville, McClurkin, Handley-Cousins, and Carroll have successfully mined the records of certain mental institutions. Yet previous books have largely utilized a regional approach or focused on specific asylums. This chapter builds on such scholarship by drawing on a much larger and more expansive sample of asylum records, thus illuminating the transregional nature of war trauma.

8. Examples may be found in Woolley, *Opium Habit and Its Cure*, 28, and Hughes, "Opium Psycho-Neurosis."

9. These labels were manifestations of the movement to medicalize opium eating and deconstruct decades of cultural stigma around the condition, a trend explored in depth in chapter 8. Examples of these labels are "'Opiokapnism,' or Opium Smoking," 719; Hughes, "Opium Psycho-Neurosis"; Entry for Eugene L. Clemens, Register of Cases, 1855–1941, box 2, 126, Records of St. Elizabeths Hospital, RG 418, National Archives and Records Administration (hereafter cited as NARA).

10. *System of Medicine*, 316.

11. Conklin, "Climacteric Insanity," 365. Although the article appeared in 1871, Conklin was describing his wartime observations.

12. *Annual Report of the Board of Directors and Superintendent of the Longview Asylum to the Governor for the Year 1862*, 21.

13. Entry no. 16633, Case Books, vol. 72, Utica State Hospital Patient Case Files, 1843–1898, New York State Archives, Albany. Extant commitment papers are often bound between the pages of individual case histories in the casebooks. Although it is unclear when this screening question was first added to the questionnaire, I could not identify any antebellum examples.

14. *Report of the Trustees, Superintendent, Resident Physician and Treasurer of the Lunatic Asylum of the State of Georgia, for the Year 1867-8*, 10. Greene added more commentary on his views in *Report of the Trustees, Superintendent, Resident Physician and Treasurer of the Lunatic Asylum of the State of Georgia, for the Year 1868-9*, 10–11.

15. For Minnesota, *Journal of Insanity* 26 (1869–70): 363. For Massachusetts, *Journal of Insanity* 29 (1872–73): 116. In 1921, the journal was rebranded as the *American Journal of Psychiatry* and the organization renamed the American Psychiatric Association.

16. *Journal of Insanity* 25 (1868–69), 105.

17. *Journal of Insanity* 23 (1866–67): 572–73. Presumably, John Gray authored this commentary.

18. As Steven M. Stowe explains, "Because patients had many different kinds of healers to choose from, orthodox physicians thought twice about openly questioning their standard treatments. Disputes among physicians too easily spilled into public debate, raising the fears of already skeptical patients." Stowe, "Seeing Themselves at Work," 41. See also Grob, *Mental Institutions in America*, 146–47.

19. On Kirkbride's role in American medicine and the evolution of nineteenth-century asylum care, see Tomes, *Generous Confidence*.

20. Case Book no. 2, vol. 3: Female Patients, 1871–1874, Records of Western State Hospital. Alexander's case is on 559–73; her ultimate fate is not recorded.

21. On the Eastern Lunatic Asylum, see Gonaver, *Making of Modern Psychiatry*. On St. Elizabeths, see Summers, *Madness in the City*. Research by Catherine Clinton also investigates St. Elizabeths.

22. Figures calculated from thirty-six volumes of the Utica State Hospital Patient Case Files spanning the period 1843–98 and Utica State Hospital Admission, Discharge, and Parole Registers, 1843–1985, New York State Archives. The Utica asylum's patient registers do not reliably record opiate-addicted patients, thus determining the number of addiction cases at Utica required analyzing entries in both the admission registers and medical casebooks. I caution scholars to avoid over-relying on asylum admissions registers/books.

23. Figures calculated from vol. 247: Admissions Records, 1828–1868; vol. 248: Admission Register, 1868–1880; and vol. 249: Admissions Register, 1880–1889; vol. 277: Case Book, 1869–1874; vol. 278: Case Book, 1882–1889; vol. 287: Case Book, 1858–1869; vol. 288: Case Book, 1869–1888; vol. 289: Case Book, 1868–1871; and vol. 290: Case Book, 1871–1874, Records of Western State Hospital.

24. The only major exceptions to this rule in the sample were St. Elizabeths asylum in Washington, DC, and Willard Asylum for the Chronic Insane in New York. St. Elizabeths, also known as the Government Asylum for the Insane, was the federal government's primary repository for insane soldiers as well as insane veterans who were removed from the National Home for Disabled Volunteer Soldiers (NHDVS). The asylum also served the indigent insane of Washington, DC. Staff at St. Elizabeths typically recorded the regiments in which veterans had served during the Civil War in the asylum's admissions books. At Willard, asylum staff often, but not always, identified Civil War veterans by writing "soldier" at the top of patients' medical records in bold black ink, underlined in red ink, and listed the patients' former units. However, this practice was not universal at Willard, and it is unclear why only some patients were flagged in this way. See, for example, Case Book no. 1, p. 6, Willard State Hospital Patient Case Files, 1869–1938, New York State Archives, Albany.

25. Sheehan-Dean, *Why Confederates Fought*, 3. This figure references military-aged white males in Confederate Virginia.

26. Examples of the printed commitment questionnaires from 1886 are pasted between the pages of Case Books, for example, vol. 68, Utica State Hospital Patient Case Files. This question is on the first page.

27. Entry no. 16196, Case Books, vol. 68, Utica State Hospital Patient Case Files. The letter, dated March 22, 1886, is inserted between the pages of the man's medical records.

28. The Indiana and South Carolina cases were identified in Dean, *Shook over Hell*, and Sommerville, *Aberration of Mind*, and supplemented with primary source material. All other cases were identified via the admissions registers/books and medical casebooks of the asylums, cited individually throughout the book.

29. For Pennsylvania, New York, South Carolina, and Virginia, respectively, see Tomes, *Generous Confidence*, 103–19; Dwyer, *Homes for the Mad*, 86–98, and Dwyer, "Civil Commitment Laws"; McCandless, *Moonlight, Magnolias, and Madness*, 69, 74, 266–67; and *Report of the Board of Directors and Physician and Superintendent of the Western Lunatic Asylum of Virginia, for the Fiscal Year 1874-'75*, 8–10.

30. A useful source for historians interested in nineteenth-century commitment laws is G. Harrison, *Collection of All the Lunacy Laws*.

31. W. S. White to Frances Goolrick, February 8, 1896; W. S. White to Frances Goolrick, February 25, 1896, Goolrick Family Papers, Virginia Historical Society, Richmond (hereafter cited as Goolrick Family Papers).

32. Nora Goolrick to Frances Goolrick, March 3, 1896, Goolrick Family Papers.

33. Nora Goolrick to Frances Goolrick, March 9, 1896, Goolrick Family Papers.

34. Nora Goolrick to Frances Goolrick, March 10, 1896, Goolrick Family Papers.

35. W. S. White to Frances Goolrick, March 4, 1896, Goolrick Family Papers.

36. Nora Goolrick to Frances Goolrick, March 8, 1896, Goolrick Family Papers.

37. William Goolrick to Frances Goolrick, March 7, 1896, Goolrick Family Papers.

38. H. W. W. Martin to Frances Goolrick, March 18, 1896, Goolrick Family Papers.

39. John Goolrick to Frances Goolrick, April 26, 1896, Goolrick Family Papers.

40. Robert. B. Andrews, Civil War Service Records, Fold3, www.fold3.com/image/73192936; R. B. Andrews, Lunacy Records, 1881–1916, Wake County Miscellaneous Records, 1772–1948, North Carolina State Archives, Raleigh; entry for R. B. Andrews, General Case Books, 13:174, Dorothea Dix Hospital Admissions Book, North Carolina State Archives; entry no. 2067, Dorothea Dix Hospital Admissions Book, North Carolina State Archives. The asylum doctors diagnosed Andrews with long-standing dementia, which they attributed to his opium addiction.

41. Entry no. 13126, Case Books, vol. 46, Utica State Hospital Patient Case Files. The young man's enlistment form records his age as 19. But the September 1860 census entry for his family records the boy's age as 12 on the eve of the Civil War. Assuming the correctness of the census, the boy would have been only 15 when he enlisted. 1st Veteran Cavalry, Company B, 146, New York Civil War Muster Roll Abstracts, Fold3, www.fold3.com/image/316340888; 1860 Census, Greene Village, Chenango, New York, Fold3, www.fold3.com/image/44964234?rec=44964533.

42. Entry no. 16196, Case Books, vol. 68, Utica State Hospital Patient Case Files.

43. Entry no. 63, vol. 1, Willard State Hospital Patient Case Files.

44. Affidavit of P. J. Watters, February 11, 1897, Samuel M. Martin Pension File, certificate 237259, Pension Application Files Based upon Service in the Civil War and Spanish American War, RG 15: Records of the Veterans Administration, 1783–1985, National Archives and Records Administration. Portions of Martin's asylum medical record were transcribed in the affidavit.

45. Vol. 285, p. 279, Case Book, 1905–1910, Records of Western State Hospital.

46. "Champion Opium-Eater," *St. Louis Daily Globe-Democrat*, July 25, 1878, 2.

47. "Dr. Wishard," *Star Tribune* (Minneapolis), February 19, 1877, 1; "The Opium Eater," *Sandersville (GA) Herald*, March 1, 1877, 1; *Indiana Herald* (Huntington), February 21, 1877, 2; "A Victim to the Opium Habit," *Weston (WV) Democrat*, March 10, 1877, 1; "The Opium Eater," *LaGrange (GA) Reporter*, March 1, 1877, 1; Milton M. Wishard, Civil War Service Index, Fold3, www.fold3.com/image/294922318; Milton M. Wishard to Mrs. Hiram Meck, July 10, 1863, Civil War "Widow's Pensions," Fold3, www.fold3.com/image/300801765. Wishard signs this letter in his capacity as a hospital steward, a role that carried largely unfettered access to opium. Wishard, at least in the newspapers that carried a transcript of his suicide note, did not

ascribe his addiction to the Civil War but stated that it "was contracted more than ten years ago," before 1867. This quote and "half crazed" are from "The Opium Eater," *Sandersville (GA) Herald*. "Opium is the cause" from "A Victim to the Opium Habit," *Weston (WV) Democrat*, March 10, 1877, 1. Newspaper accounts slightly differed in the transcription of Wishard's letter.

48. A Massachusetts doctor reported in 1880 that two of his morphine-addicted patients "committ[ed] suicide because they were unable to break their terrible bonds" of morphine slavery. Quoted in Kane, *Hypodermic Injection of Morphia*, 278. A similar account is "A Cool Suicide," *Pantagraph* (Bloomington, IL), March 10, 1886, 1.

49. Entry no. 14710, Case Books, vol. 58, Utica State Hospital Patient Case Files.

50. Silkenat, *Moments of Despair*, chaps. 1–3; Sommerville, *Aberration of Mind*, chaps. 1–5.

51. Vol. 278, p. 709, Case Book, 1882–1889, Records of Western State Hospital.

52. "Suicide of an Army Surgeon," *New-York Times*, October 12, 1865, 5.

53. J. Mitchell, *Remote Consequences of Injuries*, 187–88. For his part, Mitchell, the son of S. Weir Mitchell, did not attribute the veteran's insanity, suicidal ideation, or death to his war wound. In contrast, J. G. P.'s comments, as recorded in Mitchell's case report, indicate that the veteran attributed much of his suffering to the painful war wound.

54. Quotes from Coddington, *Faces of the Civil War Navies*, 95–100. Matthews did not leave a suicide note explaining an intent to die or his potential motive. But considering his imminent arrival at the asylum the next day, a suicide to avoid being institutionalized is a reasonable explanation and fits the broader pattern of suicides among opium eaters.

55. Sommerville, *Aberration of Mind*, 8–9.

56. "The Facts of an Alleged Suicide," *St. Louis Daily Dispatch*; "Suicide," *Atlanta Daily Intelligencer*, May 2, 1867, 4; *Memphis Daily Avalanche*, April 30, 1867, 1; "Remorse and Suicide," *Chicago Tribune*, April 30 1867, 3; "Suicide from Remorse," undated clipping from unknown St. Louis newspaper, Francis C. Clewell Papers, North Carolina State Archives, Raleigh; "Capt. F. C. Clewell," undated clipping from unknown St. Louis newspaper, Francis Clewell Papers; "Another Suicide," *St. Louis Republican* [n.d.], Francis Clewell Papers.

57. "Remorse and Suicide."

58. "Facts of an Alleged Suicide."

59. Letter dated May 11, 1864, Francis Clewell Papers, North Carolina State Archives.

60. Entry no. 11156, Case Books, vol. 34, Utica State Hospital Patient Case Files. Letter dated April 1, 1874. The note never reached the man's wife, as it was intercepted by the Utica asylum staff and eventually placed between the pages of the man's medical casebook entry, where it can be found today.

61. Entry no. 12709, Case Books, vol. 44, Utica State Hospital Patient Case Files. The quotation is from a letter pasted between the pages of the man's case history.

62. Entry for R. B. Andrews, General Case Books, 13:174, Dorothea Dix Hospital, North Carolina State Archives; entry no. 2067, Dorothea Dix Hospital Admissions Book, North Carolina State Archives.

63. St. Elizabeths Hospital Registers of Cases, 1855–1941, box 4, 62, RG 418, NARA.

64. Entry no. 63, Case Books, vol. 1, Willard State Hospital Patient Case Files. The patient's medical history leaves off after an 1890 entry, so his fate is unknown.

65. Grob, *Mental Illness in American Society*, 8.

66. Entry nos. 9497 and 10051, St. Elizabeths Hospital Registers of Cases, 1855–1941, box 4, 60, 82, RG 418, NARA.

67. Grob, *Mental Illness in American Society*, 9–10.

68. Dwyer, *Homes for the Mad*, 86, 116.

69. This argument has been made most prominently by historian David J. Rothman in *Discovery of the Asylum*, although he does not address drug addiction in the context of asylums. Rothman's model is controversial. See Tomes, *Generous Confidence*, introduction. Here, I aim for a balanced treatment of asylums that examines both the institutions' pragmatic function within communities as well as asylums' prominent role in the state carceral apparatus.

70. William A. Hammond, T. D. Crothers, Elon N. Carpenter, Cyrus Edson, "Is Drunkenness Curable?" *North American Review* (September 1891): 346–74; quote on 350. Hammond was referring to alcohol in this passage, but the broader article dealt with substance use more broadly, including the "opium habit," cases of which Hammond claims to have personally treated on 352. Hammond became a critic of institutional psychiatry in the postwar era, a position discussed in chapter 8.

71. "An Act for the Better Regulation and Discipline of the New York State Inebriate Asylum," passed March 31, 1865, quoted in *Superintendent's Report to the Board of Trustees*, 32.

72. Quoted in American Association for the Cure of Inebriates, *Proceedings of the First Meeting*, 79.

73. "Opium Eating" (June 20, 1872), 412; "Opium Eating," *Druggists' Circular & Chemical Gazette*, March 1, 1873, 1. For context on the Kentucky law, see Jones, "'Died from Eating Too Much Morphine.'"

74. The Pinel Hospital was empowered "to receive and retain all inebriates, opium-eaters and insane," including public and private patients. Although the hospital operated as a for-profit corporation, it was expressly charged by the state legislature with accepting public patients on the state's dime. "Act to Incorporate the Pinel Hospital," 248–50.

75. Brock, *Virginia and Virginians*, 2:698–99.

76. "Pinel Hospital," 303.

77. "Document No, 8. Statement of the Name, Age, Sex, Color, Duration of the Attack, and Character of the Insanity of the Lunatics Confined in Jails and Other Places in the Commonwealth than Lunatic Asylums," in *Annual Reports of Officers, Boards and Institutions of the Commonwealth of Virginia, for the Year Ending September 30, 1880*. It is unclear when the hospital closed, but the *Richmond Dispatch* advertised its facility as available to rent in 1892. *Richmond Dispatch*, June 19, 1892, 9.

78. Jaffe, *Addiction Reform in the Progressive Age*, 68–69. Jaffe does not speculate on the decline of these institutions. But the effects of the Harrison Narcotics Act, the growth of morphine maintenance clinics, and the nationwide prohibition of alcohol in the early twentieth century made these institutions redundant. On the Foxborough hospital, see Tracy, *Alcoholism in America*, 147–95.

79. *Annual Reports of the Board of Visitors*, 24–25. The superintendent is referring to both opiate and alcohol inebriates in this passage. The Ohio legislature considered a similar bill in 1890. See *Journal of the Senate of the State of Ohio* 86 (1890): 664.

80. Entry no. 11804, Case Books, vol. 36, Utica State Hospital Patient Case Files.

81. Fisher, "Habitual Drunkenness," 11.

82. See McCandless, *Moonlight, Magnolias, and Madness*, 276–77; Grob, *Mental Institutions in America*, 340–42; and Tomes, *Generous Confidence*, 296–311.

83. Averages in Grob, *Mental Institutions in America*, app. 3.

84. Figures from Grob, *Mental Institutions in America*, 395. Grob's statistical analysis of asylum annual reports reveals a sweeping decline in "cure" rates between 1860 and 1875.

85. *Report of the Trustees, Superintendent, Resident Physician and Treasurer of the Lunatic Asylum of the State of Georgia, for the Year 1866-7*, 5-6.

86. *Report of the Board of Directors and Medical Superintendent of the Western Lunatic Asylum Staunton, VA. For the Fiscal Year 1869-1870*, 8-9.

87. McCandless, *Moonlight, Magnolias, and Madness*, 272.

88. Grob, *Mental Illness and American Society*, 53-55.

89. Dwyer, *Homes for the Mad*, 14-16, 22-23.

90. Case Book, vol. 1, pp. 411, 494, Willard State Hospital Patient Case Files.

91. McCandless, *Moonlight, Magnolias, and Madness*, 273.

92. Entry no. 63, Case Book, vol. 1, Willard State Hospital Patient Case Files.

93. Redmond Walsh or Welsh, no. 2354, Registers of Patients, box 1, 95, RG 418, Records of St. Elizabeths Hospital; Mary Walsh to C. H. Nichols, July 18, 1873, Case Files of Patients, no. 2354 [Redmond Walsh or Welsh], Records of St. Elizabeths Hospital. The success of Mary Walsh's efforts is unclear in the records.

94. Seguin, "Right of the Insane to Liberty," quoted in Grob, *Mental Institutions in America*, 166. Gilded Age neurologists were frequent critics of psychiatry and mental asylums. See Tomes, *Generous Confidence*, 290-91.

95. *Reports of the Board of Directors and of the Physician and Superintendent of the Virginia Western Lunatic Asylum, for the Fiscal Years 1875-76, 1876-77*, 9, 11. According to the asylum superintendent, the man was not suicidal before his furlough.

96. Entry for George W. Long, no. 8246, Registers of Cases, box 3, 10, RG 418, Records of St. Elizabeths Hospital.

Chapter 6

1. "Break off the morphine habit" quoted from Perry Bowser to Commissioner of Pensions, October 6, 1893, Perry B. Bowser Pension File, certificate 108546, Pension Application Files Based upon Service in the Civil War and Spanish American War, RG 15, Records of the Veterans Administration, 1783-1985, National Archives and Records Administration (hereafter cited as NARA); Milwaukee, Wisconsin, Register no. 11500-12999, United States National Homes for Disabled Volunteer Soldiers, 1866-1938, FamilySearch, image 672 of 777; Dayton, Ohio, Register no. 19500-20999, United States National Homes for Disabled Volunteer Soldiers, 1866-1938, FamilySearch, image 502 of 790; Marion, Indiana, Register no. 04500-05999, United States National Homes for Disabled Volunteer Soldiers, 1866-1938, FamilySearch, image 384 of 784.

2. The Harrison Narcotics Tax Act, enacted in 1914 after more than a decade of lobbying by anti-opium activists, is often credited as inaugurating America's war on drugs by criminalizing addiction on a national scale. It was presaged by state and local regulations, as well as international opium trafficking restrictions to which the United States became a party in the decades preceding 1914. While the Harrison Act was not intended to punish addicted Americans for their condition but to regulate the distribution of opiates at the national level, the act's interpretation and implementation by US Treasury Department officials and law enforcement effectively criminalized opiate use without a doctor's prescription. In effect, the Harrison Act formalized the long-standing cultural distinction between sympathetic and unsympathetic drug users that first emerged in the antebellum era, explored in chapter 2. As one element of a broader progressive agenda to address the perceived ills plaguing American

society in the late nineteenth and early twentieth centuries, the Harrison Act was shortly followed by the federal prohibition of alcohol through the Eighteenth Amendment to the US Constitution and the Volstead Act. A classic account of the origins of narcotics control in the United States is Musto, *American Disease*, esp. 91–150. See also Courtwright, *Dark Paradise*, 100–104. For the Harrison Act within the context of previous drug debates and the effects of the Harrison Act on narcotics markets and users, see Herzberg, *White Market Drugs*, 29–57; Acker, *Creating the American Junkie*, 14–15; Spillane, *Cocaine*, 5–6; and Hickman, *Secret Leprosy of Modern Days*, 93–125.

3. Rothman, *Discovery of the Asylum*; Kelly, *Creating a National Home*, esp. 94–96, 166–68; and Marten, *Sing Not War*, 159–98. Margot Canaday makes a similarly framed argument about state policing of sexuality through the WW1-era military bureaucracy in *Straight State*, 56–59.

4. Gerstle, "Civil War and State-Building."

5. Handley-Cousins, *Bodies in Blue*, 9.

6. Handley-Cousins, *Bodies in Blue*, 106.

7. Jordan, *Marching Home*, 156. In her landmark account of the US Pension Bureau, Theda Skocpol likewise notes that "Civil War pensions were idealized as that which was justly due to the righteous core of a generation of men (and survivors of dead men)." Skocpol, *Protecting Soldiers and Mothers*, 149. Only those veterans deemed "righteous" by Pension Bureau agents were deemed as deserving of pensions.

8. Marten, *Sing Not War*, 97–98.

9. Jordan, *Marching Home*, 106, 218–26; entry 63, Albert T. Shurtleff, Soldier and Sailor Contributions, Left-Handed Penmanship Contest, William Oland Bourne Papers, Library of Congress, Washington, DC (quotation on 12). Shurtleff's fate is unclear. He does not describe postwar morphine use but certainly fit the patterns laid out in previous chapters that facilitated addiction among many veterans in his circumstances. Clarke urges scholars to take the patriotism and sentimental suffering expressed by the left-handed penmanship contestants at face value, and there is merit to this interpretation. See Clarke, *War Stories*, 146. Still, it is hard to imagine that the trauma these veterans expressed was entirely mitigated by patriotism or sentimentalism. These sources are also multidimensional, capable of expressing sincere sentimentalism and sheer suffering simultaneously.

10. Crothers, "Some New Studies of the Opium Disease," 105; Hickman shows how the addiction-as-intemperance model was universally accepted by physicians, in *Secret Leprosy of Modern Days*.

11. Parsons, *Manhood Lost*, 61–62; Marten, *Sing Not War*, 100–120.

12. During heated Gilded Age debates about the pension program, in December 1882 the US Senate demanded that the secretary of the interior provide a list of all veterans receiving pensions from the federal government. The list was delivered in five volumes in March 1883, recording every pensioner on the rolls as of January 1, 1883. Most pensioners were Civil War veterans, but the roll included a handful of veterans of the Mexican-American War and the War of 1812. The roll recorded pensioners' names, post office addresses, pension certificate numbers, the amount of the award, initial date awarded, as well as the disability for which pensioners received their awards. The 1883 pension roll is an invaluable resource for historians of Civil War veterans seeking to understand why veterans received pensions before the 1890 Dependent Pension Act. A keyword search of Hathi Trust's full-text version for the keywords "opium" and "morphine" and common abbreviations "opi" and "morph" yields zero hits, which I verified manually. *List of Pensioners on the Roll January 1, 1883*.

13. Scholars have put forth several interpretations, not necessarily mutually exclusive, of the pension program's origins. Theda Skocpol, *Protecting Soldiers and Mothers*, 102–51, convincingly argues that the pension program presaged New Deal–era welfare programs. Skocpol attributes the liberalization of the pension program in 1890 to the Republican Party's decades-long effort to attract the Union veteran vote, to offset unpopular surpluses generated by tariffs, and, to a lesser degree, to effective lobbying by veterans' organizations. Brian Matthew Jordan gives more weight to the lobbying of the Grand Army of the Republic, culminating in the 1890 Dependent Pension Act. See Jordan, *Marching Home*, 151–70. Megan J. McClintock argued that dependents' pensions for Union veterans resulted from the government's efforts to encourage voluntary enlistment in the Union army by guaranteeing that the government would care for volunteers' families if soldiers died during the Civil War. McClintock, "Civil War Pensions," 459.

14. In 1893, the Commissioner of Pension's Order no. 241 enacted a policy that veterans of age 75 "shall receive the maximum ($12) for senility alone, if there are no special pensionable disabilities shown" beyond old age. Quoted in the *National Tribune Soldier's Handbook*, 100.

15. The first pensions for disabled Union soldiers were awarded in 1862. An accessible overview of the Civil War pension system is Prechtel-Kluskens, "'Reasonable Degree of Promptitude.'"

16. Quoted in Skocpol, *Protecting Soldiers and Mothers*, 128.

17. "An Act Granting Pensions to Soldiers and Sailors, 182–83. On the law's political context, see Skocpol, *Protecting Soldiers and Mothers*, 109, 128–29. GAR Pension Committee quoted in Skocpol, 128.

18. *Report of the Commissioner of Pensions to the Secretary of the Interior for the Year Ended June 30, 1894*, 3–5.

19. "An Act Granting Pensions to Soldiers and Sailors," 182.

20. Handley-Cousins, *Bodies in Blue*, 95–99 (quote is on 99).

21. For example, "Editorial Article 7—No Title," *New-York Times*, October 8, 1881.

22. This ruling affirmed the rejection of a pension claim originally denied because the "surgeons who examined this claimant state there has been an 'entire disregard of all hygienic rules,' and that this 'with the excessive use of tobacco, is responsible for claimant's condition.'" *Decisions of the Department of the Interior in Appealed Pension and Bounty-Land Claims*, 7:402–3.

23. "Vicious Habits—Evidence—Act June 27, 1890," in *Decisions of the Department of the Interior in Appealed Pension and Bounty-Land Claims*, 7:578, 581.

24. The context for this quote was the reversal of a denial of a veteran's pension on grounds of vicious habits. The full quote reads: "In the case of Morris Hess (9 P.D., 252), his claim under the act of June 27, 1890, was rejected on the ground that a ratable disability was not shown independent of rupture; that the claimant was unable to prove that the latter was not due to vicious habits. On appeal I held that there being nothing in the case to arouse a suspicion that the disability was in any way due to vicious habits, or that the claimant had ever been addicted to vicious habits, or that his statement as to the circumstances under which the disability was incurred was untrue, the rejection on the ground stated was error, and was set aside." *Appeals in Pension Cases*, 14.

25. Commissioner of Pensions, *Treatise on the Practice of the Pension Bureau*, 99.

26. On pension exams, see Handley-Cousins, *Bodies in Blue*, 107–12, and Prechtel-Kluskens, "'Reasonable Degree of Promptitude.'"

27. Joseph A. Lazelle Pension File, certificate 1047963, Pension Application Files Based upon Service in the Civil War and Spanish American War, Record Group 15: Records of the Veterans Administration, 1783–1985, NARA.

28. Perry B. Bowser Pension File, certificate 108546, NARA. Bowser received a pension award for chronic diarrhea at four dollars per month sometime in the early 1870s. His rate was increased in January 1879 to eight dollars per month. The Pension Bureau also suspected that Bowser suffered from syphilis. Bowser petitioned unsuccessfully during the late 1880s to have the Pension Bureau increase his pension rate. "We did not feel justified," "chronic diarrhea all the time," "cannot do any manual labor at all," "it is stated," "please strip him," "nervous system is impaired" and "he acquired habit" in Surgeon's Certificate, April 1, 1891; "Was carried home" in Perry B. Bowser to Pension Bureau, April 24, 1896.

29. Martin's Pea Ridge injury is recorded in "Army of the South-West," 152; Deposition of January 29, 1893, Samuel M. Martin Pension File, certificate 237259, Pension Application Files Based upon Service in the Civil War and Spanish American War, Record Group 15: Records of the Veterans Administration, 1783–1985, NARA.

30. Invalid Pension Application September 1892, Samuel M. Martin Pension File.

31. Medical Report March 21, 1894, Samuel M. Martin Pension File.

32. Noble B. Howard affidavit July 24, 1896, Samuel M. Martin Pension File; Samuel M. Martin deposition July 21, 1896, Samuel M. Martin Pension File.

33. Special Examiner's Report February 13, 1897, Samuel M. Martin Pension File. Martin's wife, Florence, filed an application for a widow's pension on November 17, 1897, so he must have been dead by November. Florence H. Martin Widow's Pension Affidavit, Samuel M. Martin Pension File, certificate 237259.

34. The wording of the "vicious habits" clause evolved slightly over the late nineteenth century, but the substance remained intact across the various versions of the pension application surgeon's affidavits. The National Archives has digitized sample Civil War pension files, which are accessible online: Case Files of Approved Pension Applications of Veterans Who Served in the Army and Navy Mainly in the Civil War and the War with Spain ("Civil War and Later Survivors' Certificates"), Nos. SC 9,487–999,999, 1861–1934, NARA, https://catalog.archives.gov/id/300019, accessed September 24, 2022. See, for example, Surgeon's Certificate November 30, 1898, Approved Pension File for Private Ephraim Reynolds, Company D, 151st Pennsylvania Infantry Regiment (SC-357317), image 37 of 117, Case Files of Approved Pension Applications.

35. Crothers, "Some New Studies of the Opium Disease," 108. This passage also appeared in American Association for the Study and Cure of Inebriety, *Disease of Inebriety*, 323.

36. Pray's surname is misspelled as "Bray" in the NHDVS report, but he is correctly identified as a member of the 24th Ohio Infantry. *Proceedings of the Board of Managers of the National Home*, 2:364. Pray's pension index card, which notes his service in the 24th Ohio, confirms his identity as the same veteran recorded in the NHDVS report. Frank E. Pray, Civil War Pension Index, *Fold3*, www.fold3.com/image/5844555. One of Pray's general index cards notes that he had spent time as a hospital steward while in the 88th Ohio. Frank E. Pray, Civil War Service Index, *Fold3*, www.fold3.com/image/292442732. Frank E. Pray Pension File, certificate 385070, Pension Application Files Based upon Service in the Civil War and Spanish American War, RG 15, NARA.

37. Wirt Morris Pension File, certificate 582310, Pension Application Files Based upon Service in the Civil War and Spanish American War, RG 15, NARA; "Hero's Sad End," *Boston Morning Journal*, December 6, 1897.

38. *National Tribune Soldier's Handbook*, 100–102. On the *National Tribune*'s relationship with the GAR, see Marten, *Sing Not War*, 147.

39. *The Congressional Globe: Containing the Debates and Proceedings of the Second Session Forty-Second Congress; An Appendix, Embracing the Laws Passed at that Session*, 468. The congressman was Leonard Myers of Pennsylvania.

40. United States Pension Bureau, *General Instructions to Special Examiners*, 19, 21–22. James Marten and Eric T. Dean Jr. make similar arguments about the pension bureau's stance on substance use. Dean, *Shook over Hell*, 149–50; Marten, *Sing Not War*, 16. In contrast, Jonathan Lewy asserts without substantiating evidence that "the Bureau of Pensions had no policy towards addiction, and veterans were not prone to lose their pensions if they were found addicted to drugs." Lewy, "Army Disease," 115.

41. On Confederate pensions, see Miller, *Empty Sleeves*, 141–72, and McClurken, *Take Care of the Living*, 143–72.

42. Pension Board Minutes, 1891–1939, A summary, 2651, Arkansas Ex-Confederate Pension Records, 1891–1939, FamilySearch, www.familysearch.org/search/collection/1921864, digitized from records housed at State Auditor's Office, Little Rock, Arkansas.

43. Sample Soldier's Pension Application, Tennessee Confederate Pension Applications: Soldiers and Widows, Tennessee State Library and Archives, https://sos.tn.gov/products/tsla/tennessee-confederate-pension-application-soldiers-application, accessed May 10, 2019 (no longer available); Kentucky Confederate Pension Applications, 1912–1950, FamilySearch, www.familysearch.org/search/collection/1916017, digitized from records housed at the Kentucky Historical Society, Frankfort. For a sample application, see William Thomson Brasher pension application, 0001-00086, image 2 of 349, Louisiana Confederate Pensions, 1898–1950, FamilySearch, www.familysearch.org/search/collection/1838535, digitized from records housed at Louisiana State Archives, Baton Rouge; for another sample application, see Joshua Aarons pension application, Aarons, Joshua–Aldrich, L. E., image 4 of 1358, Louisiana Confederate Pensions, 1898–1950, FamilySearch.

44. Alabama, Confederate Pension Applications, ca. 1880–1939, *FamilySearch*, www.familysearch.org/search/collection/3029256, digitized from records housed at the Alabama Department of Archives and History, Montgomery. For a sample application, see Isaac Fortenberry pension application, image number 00232, digital folder no. 008494163, Missouri, Confederate Pension Applications and Soldiers Home Applications, 1861–1938, *FamilySearch*, www.familysearch.org/search/collection/1865475, digitized from records housed at Missouri Department of Records and Archives, Jefferson City. For a sample application, see Isaac Fortenberry pension application, Pension Applications—Approved, Houchen, James J.–Hyde, J. B., image 12 of 270, Confederate Pension Records, Oklahoma Digital Prairie, www.digitalprairie.ok.gov/digital/collection/pensions. For other sample applications, see Andrew Abercrombie, Confederate Pension Records, Oklahoma Digital Prairie, www.digitalprairie.ok.gov/digital/collection/pensions/id/925/rec/5; North Carolina, Confederate Soldiers and Widows Pension Applications, 1885–1953, *FamilySearch*, www.familysearch.org/search/collection/1911763, digitized from records housed at the North Carolina State Archives, Raleigh, and W. A. Aaron pension application, Aarant, Sam A.–Alexander, Benjamin, image 9 of 1096.

45. As Kathleen Gorman has observed in the case of Georgia, Confederate veterans who failed to obtain positive character references from community members had little prospect of ultimately securing a pension. Gorman, "Confederate Pensions as Southern Social Welfare," 24–39.

46. "The Soldier's Budget," *Vermont Watchman & State Journal*, April 8, 1865, 6.

47. *Compilation of the Messages and Papers of the Presidents*, 6169; Parker, *Recollections of Grover Cleveland*, 118.

48. *Public Papers of Grover Cleveland*, 128 (italics mine).

49. *Decisions of the Department of the Interior in Appealed Pension and Retirement Claims*, 1:110–11; *Public Papers of Grover Cleveland*, 131.

50. *Public Papers of Grover Cleveland*, 131.

51. *Decisions of the Department of the Interior in Appealed Pension and Bounty-Land Claims*, 9:440–41.

52. *Decisions of the Department of the Interior in Appealed Pension and Bounty-Land Claims*,8:131–33.

53. *Decisions of the Department of the Interior in Appealed Pension and Bounty-Land Claims*, 7:49–50.

54. *Decisions of the Department of the Interior in Appealed Pension and Bounty-Land Claims*, 3:183–87.

55. *Decisions of the Department of the Interior in Appealed Pension and Bounty-Land Claims*, 1:108–11.

56. Skocpol, *Protecting Soldiers and Mothers*, 102.

57. About 100,000 Union veterans eventually took up residence in the federally funded NHDVS system or in smaller state-funded soldiers' homes scattered throughout the North and the West. In the former Confederate states and in some border states, about 20,000 Confederate veterans found refuge in soldiers' homes. Marten, *Sing Not War*, 15.

58. Rosenburg, *Living Monuments*, 78–92.

59. Tennessee Confederate Soldiers' Home: Applications and Ledgers, Tennessee State Library and Archives, Nashville. A sample application is viewable at http://sostngovbuckets.s3.amazonaws.com/tsla/history/military/civil_war/csh-application.pdf, accessed March 8, 2020.

60. Rosenburg, *Living Monuments*, 82–83.

61. North Carolina, Confederate Soldiers and Widows Pension Applications, 1885–1953, Hays, N.T.–Herron, Calvin, image 93 of 1884.

62. Missouri, Confederate Pension Applications and Soldiers Home Applications, 1911–1938, Soldiers Home Applications—Disapproved: Adams, James E.–Wright, Vergil S., image 3 of 1020.

63. Soldiers' Home Association: Hospital Patients, 1908–1916, North Carolina Digital Collections, https://digital.ncdcr.gov/Documents/Detail/soldiers-home-association-hospital-patients-1908-1916/585426: "cancer," 171; "softening of the brain," 171; insanity, 169; dysentery, 149; sore legs, 166; tuberculosis, 159; apoplexy, 180; asthma, 144.

64. The applications are viewable at FamilySearch. Soldiers Home Applications—Disapproved, Missouri, Confederate Pension Applications and Soldiers Home Applications, 1911–1938, FamilySearch, www.familysearch.org/en/search/image/index?owc=M8V3-TZ9%3A168965901%3Fcc%3D1865475&cc=1865475.

65. *Report of the Board of Managers of the National Home for Disabled Volunteer Soldiers for the Fiscal Year Ending June 30, 1896*, 74, 90, 108, 124, 141, 158, 172, 254, 264, 276, 289, 301, 315, 325, 335, 344, 354, 366, 376, 410, 419, 428, 438. Such reports of opiate-addicted veterans are found in many NHDVS annual reports dating from the 1870s onward. The figure is drawn from hospital data included in a report by William W. Averell, the NHDVS inspector general, who, along with subordinates, surveyed the facilities.

66. Kelly, *Creating a National Home*, 94–96, 166–68. Kelly contests the Foucauldian interpretation of asylums and similar state-funded institutions, which interprets the institutions primarily as state mechanisms for enforcing normative social behaviors and cultural mores. Instead, Kelly argues, institutions like the NHDVS, which kept ailing poor veterans fed, clothed, housed, and off the dangerous streets of America's growing cities, also served a pragmatic function by filling social needs.

67. On daily life and discipline in the NHDVS, see Marten, *Sing Not War*, 159–98; Jordan, *Marching Home*, 170–91; Trevor K. Plante, "The National Home for Disabled Volunteer Soldiers" *Prologue Magazine*, Spring 2004, www.archives.gov/publications/prologue/2004/spring/soldiers-home.html, accessed October 2, 2022; Kelly, *Creating a National Home*, 140–68.

68. *Report of Inspection of State Soldiers and Sailors' Homes for Year Ending June 30, 1894*, 231–32.

69. Marten observes a similar pattern of expulsions affecting habitually drunk NHDVS residents, in *Sing Not War*, 104.

70. St. Elizabeths Hospital Register of Cases, box 2, 32, NARA.

71. St. Elizabeths Hospital Register of Cases, box 3, 71, NARA.

72. Figure calculated from St. Elizabeths Hospital Register of Cases, boxes 1–4, NARA. Medical staff at St. Elizabeths usually, although not always, identified veterans as such in the asylum's admissions registers and often recorded the various NHDVS branches as places from which patients had been sent. Scores of opiate-addicted men and women were committed to St. Elizabeths during the postwar decades, so it is possible there were additional cases of NHDVS residents among this broader population of opiate-addicted patients that were not identified as such by asylum staff in the registers.

73. *Report of Inspection of State Soldiers and Sailors' Homes for Year Ending June 30, 1895*, 264–65; Charles L. Williams, Application for Admission to the Michigan Soldiers' Home, Michigan Soldiers Home Reel 25, M-2378, Grand Rapids Public Library.

74. *Report of Inspection of State Soldiers and Sailors' Homes for Year Ending June 30, 1894*, 123.

75. *Report of Inspection of State Soldiers and Sailors' Homes for Year Ending June 30, 1894*, 135.

76. *Report of the Board of Managers of the National Home for Disabled Volunteer Soldiers for the Fiscal Year Ending June 30, 1893*, 400, 404.

77. *Report of Inspection of State Soldiers and Sailors' Homes for Year Ending June 30, 1894*, 123.

78. *Report of Inspection of State Soldiers and Sailors' Homes for Year Ending June 30, 1894*, 37. An example of an inquiry about the Gold Cure is found in "Our Correspondents," *National Tribune*, February 15, 1894.

79. *Report of the Board of Managers of the National Home for Disabled Volunteer Soldiers*, 11.

80. Marten, *Sing Not War*, 111–13.

81. *Report of the Board of Managers of the National Home for Disabled Volunteer Soldiers for the Fiscal Year Ended June 30, 1895*, 265.

82. Charles L. Williams Application for Admission to the Michigan Soldiers' Home, Michigan Soldiers Home Reel 25, M-2378, Grand Rapids Public Library.

83. Veterans seeking liberalized medical care for addiction and sympathy from NHDVS doctors and administrators fit the broader pattern of veteran lobbying, such as for pension reform. See Jordan, *Marching Home*, chap. 6.

84. Cole, *Confessions of an American Opium Eater*, 6.

85. Undated letter from Perry Bowser, received July 23, 1900, Perry B. Bowser Pension File, certificate 108546.

Chapter 7

1. Hon, "Coca in the Opium Habit," 63–64; "Coca in the Opium-Habit," 246.
2. Hon, "Coca in the Opium Habit," 63–64. The article does not describe how J. T. B. first encountered patent medicine addiction remedies. To piece together this narrative, I relied on testimonies authored by addicted veterans, patent medicine advertising pamphlets, and historian James Harvey Young's descriptions of the marketing and distribution of patent medicines in nineteenth-century America. Young, *Toadstool Millionaires*.
3. *The Free Press* (Cartersville, GA), November 25, 1880, 1.
4. Keeley, *Morphine Eater*, 120, 166. Keeley's aim of selling his own "Gold Cure" means we should be careful about accepting this figure uncritically. The cost of $2,500 in 1881, when this account was published, is about $78,382 in 2025.
5. Marten, "Civil War Veterans," 619, Jordan, "Veterans in New Fields," 308.
6. On prosthetic limbs, see Nelson, *Ruin Nation*, 211–26, and Miller, *Empty Sleeves*, 146–58. On undertaking and embalming, see Faust, *This Republic of Suffering*, 91–99, and Browning and Silver, *Environmental History of the Civil War*, 144–47. On pension attorneys, see Skocpol, *Protecting Soldiers and Mothers*, 114, 116–17, 145–46.
7. Lears, *Fables of Abundance*, 143.
8. Monetizing negative views about illness and sick people in the interest of selling health and cleaning products was a frequently adopted strategy in the late nineteenth- and early twentieth-century United States. See Tomes, *Gospel of Germs*.
9. Burnham, *Health Care in America*, 81–83. An example of Dr. M'Munn's Elixir of Opium being linked to an overdose death is "Suicide of the Murderer Macdonald," *Harper's Weekly*, May 26, 1860, 326–37; on Mrs. Winslow's Soothing Syrup, see Sommerville, *Aberration of Mind*, 221–25.
10. Burnham, *Health Care in America*, 83, 114; Schuster, "Rise of a Modern Concept of 'Health,'" 261.
11. Burnham, *Health Care in America*, 80–83; Young, *Toadstool Millionaires*, chap. 7; Miller, *Empty Sleeves*, 141–58.
12. An example advertisement is in the *New York Herald*, October 30, 1859. Zell's occupation is listed as "butcher" in *Doggett's New York City Directory for 1845 & 1846*, 407.
13. Mattison, "'Opium Antidotes,'" 568.
14. Oliver, "Use and Abuse of Opium," 167.
15. "The Opium Habit," *Frank Leslie's Popular Monthly*, July 1877, 191. The same story appeared *Scientific American*, February 19, 1876.
16. *Theriaki*, July 1872, 54.
17. *Theriaki*, July 1872, 56.
18. On theriac, see Snowden, *Epidemics and Society*, 76. On exoticism in advertising, see Lears, *Fables of Abundance*, 144–49. "Theriaki" also bears a marked similarity to the Farsi word for opium, *taryak*.
19. Collins, *Theriaki: An Annual*, 78–85, 7–8.
20. "1860 United States Federal Census for Samul D Collins," 1860 United States Federal

Census, Ancestry.com, www.ancestry.com/imageviewer/collections/7667/images/4217606_00094. Collins's first name and middle initial are incorrectly listed in this census, but the place of birth, age, his spouse, and the census location confirm his identity.

21. "1870 United States Federal Census for Samuel B Collins," 1870 United States Federal Census, Ancestry.com, www.ancestry.com/imageviewer/collections/7163/images/4263406_00302.

22. Packard, *History of La Porte County, Indiana*, 442.

23. A photograph of the mansion appears in *Historic Architecture of La Porte, Indiana*, 167–68.

24. Packard, *History of La Porte County, Indiana*, 442. Collins purchased a full-page advertisement in this volume. The book's glowing coverage of his enterprise is not coincidental. Daniels, *Record of La Porte County, Indiana*, 242.

25. Claims by vendors that their products contained gold reflected a centuries-old tactic of conflating medicine with gold, a strategy intended to lend credence to the medicine's purported efficacy.

26. Analyses of Keeley's Gold Cure in the context of the nineteenth-century temperance movement and the medicalization of alcoholism include Hickman, "Leslie E. Keeley, the Gold Cure"; Warsh, "Adventures in Maritime Quackery"; and H. Morgan, "'No, Thank You. I've Been to Dwight.'"

27. According to Sarah W. Tracy, Keeley's Gold Cure and his insistence that addiction was a disease rooted in the body, not the soul, "arguably helped popularize the disease concept more than the efforts of the [American Association for the Study and Cure of Inebriety]," the primary medical organization behind the medicalization movement that is the subject of chapter 8. Tracy, *Alcoholism in America*, 21.

28. The official was O. R. Weaver, a GAR department inspector. *Proceedings of the Twenty-Seventh National Encampment of the Grand Army*, 121.

29. Marten, *Sing Not War*, 114–20; *Keeley Institutes*, 10; *Daily Morning Union* (Grass Valley, CA), June 30, 1897, 4.

30. *Chicago Daily Tribune*, February 8, 1880, 5; March 26, 1884, 8; February 29, 1880, 5; April 16, 1899, 6; September 14, 1893, 8.

31. *Confederate Veteran* 5, no. 1 (January 1897), 46. For other examples of advertisements for opium addiction cures, see *National Tribune*, May 24, 1883, 8; *National Tribune*, March 26, 1885, 7; *National Tribune*, February 18, 1887, 7; *National Tribune*, August 14, 1887, 7; *National Tribune*, November 30, 1893, 2; and *National Tribune*, August 22, 1907, 7. The Stephens figure was calculated through a keyword search for the term "J. Stephens" in the full-text issues of the *National Tribune* via the Library of Congress's Chronicling America database at https://chroniclingamerica.loc.gov, accessed January 17, 2019.

32. Woolley, *Opium Habit and Its Cure*, 36. On Atlanta as a New South city, see Link, *Atlanta, Cradle of the New South*.

33. James Hamblin, "Why We Took Cocaine out of Soda," *Atlantic*, January 31, 2013, www.theatlantic.com/health/archive/2013/01/why-we-took-cocaine-out-of-soda/272694/; King, "Dr. John S. Pemberton"; Pendergrast, *For God, Country, and Coca-Cola*, 25–27. Pendergrast cites the "drug fiend" testimony as solid evidence of Pemberton's morphine addiction without closely scrutinizing the timing or motivation behind the allegation.

34. Perry Bowser to His Excellency Ulysses Grant, October 5, 1875, Perry B. Bowser Pension File, certificate 108546, Pension Application Files Based Upon Service in the Civil War and

Spanish American War, RG 15, Records of the Veterans Administration, National Archives and Records Administration.

35. Collins, *Positive Cure for the Opium Habit*, 22–26.
36. Collins, *Positive Cure for the Opium Habit*, 23.
37. Collins, *Positive Cure for the Opium Habit*, 24–26.
38. Collins, *Theriaki and Their Last Dose*, 11; William H. Chappell, Civil War Service Records, Fold3, www.fold3.com/image/20/6869761.
39. Keeley, *Morphine Eater*, 121, 166; Collins, *Theriaki: A Treatise*, 25–26.
40. Collins, *Positive Cure for the Opium Habit*, 23.
41. Lears, *Fables of Abundance*, 44.
42. "Testimony from One of the 'Fourth Estate,'" *Sunday Gazette* (Atlanta), January 11, 1880, 4.
43. Lears, *Fables of Abundance*, 143.
44. Collins, *Positive Cure for the Opium Habit*, 25. For examples of such temperance narratives, see John W. Crowley, "Slaves to the Bottle." Keeley's 1881 pamphlet *The Morphine Eater, or, From Bondage to Freedom* recalls the title of Frederick Douglass's 1855 narrative *My Bondage and My Freedom*.
45. Hopkins, "Intoxicant Habit," 204.
46. Woolley, *Opium Habit and Its Cure*, 17; *Theriaki*, July 1872, 53, 54.
47. *Theriaki*, July 1872, 26–27.
48. Surgeon's Certificate March 30, 1892, and Certificate of Death, Michigan Soldiers' Home, May 24, 1895, Joseph C. Darrow Pension File, certificate 415496, Pension Application Files Based upon Service in the Civil War and Spanish American War, RG 15, Records of the Veterans Administration, 1783–1985, National Archives and Records Administration.
49. "An Opium-Eater's Cure," *Galaxy: A Magazine of Entertaining Reading*, January 1875, 127; *History of Wages in the United States*, 225. A twenty-eight-year-old Baltimore woman swallowed 5,840 ounces of laudanum in two years, for which she paid $1,160. "Excessive Opium Eating," 56.
50. *Annual Report of the Commissioner of Pensions to the Secretary of the Interior for the Year Ended June 30, 1890*, 4.
51. Collins, *Theriaki: A Treatise*, 12.
52. *History of Warren County, Ohio*, 781–82.
53. Thomas Sweeting to Joseph L. Stephens, March 21, 1887, Ohio Historical Society, Columbus, Ohio. A Thomas P. Sweeting served in the 37th Georgia Infantry. Thomas P. Sweeting, Civil War Service Records, Fold3, www.fold3.com/image/49924341. There are no other men named Thomas Sweeting that appear in a search of Fold3's Civil War records. A Thomas Sweeting also appears in the 1880 census for Key West, Florida, which notes that the man was born in the Bahamas. 1880 United States Federal Census for Thomas Sweeting, Ancestry.com, www.ancestry.com/search/collections/6742/records/39559177. Considering that the letter from Sweeting to Stephens was sent from the Bahamas to Ohio and no other individuals named Thomas Sweeting appears to have served in the Civil War, I suspect the Confederate veteran and the 1887 letter writer were the same individual.
54. Hon, "Coca in the Opium Habit," 63–64; undated letter from Perry Bowser, received July 23, 1900, Perry B. Bowser Pension File, certificate 108546.
55. Entry no. 47775, Case Books, vol. 14, Willard State Hospital Patient Case Files, 1869–1938, New York State Archives, Albany.

56. The clipping is located inside the back cover of Charles A. Hentz Diary, 1887, Hentz Family Papers, 1782–1932, Southern Historical Collection, Louis Round Wilson Special Collections Library, University of North Carolina at Chapel Hill. The name of the newspaper from which the clipping originated is unclear, but the same classified advertisement appeared in the *Newnan (GA) Herald*, February 15, 1887, 2. Hentz recorded attending to a friend who suffered from opium addiction in 1870–71. "My Autobiography, Vol. 2," unpublished manuscript, 81–85, Hentz Family Papers, 1782–1932, Southern Historical Collection.

57. Medical Society of South Carolina Meeting Minutes: 1881–1897, Waring Historical Library, Medical University of South Carolina, Charleston, 400.

58. Collins, *Positive Cure for the Opium Habit*, 12–14.

59. Mattison, "'Opium Antidotes,'" 569.

60. "Remarks on the Opium Habit," 436.

61. "'Opium Antidotes' Exposed," 500–501.

62. Mattison, "'Opium Antidotes,'" 568.

63. "Soldiers' Home Mismanaged," *Los Angeles Times*, April 16, 1896, 3; "Western Soldiers' Home: Serious Charges Made against President," *New-York Times*, March 8, 1896, 9; "Compelled to Take the Cure," *Washington Post*, December 10, 1896, 3; quotes from undated letter from Perry Bowser, received July 23, 1900. In a previous letter, Perry Bowser to Pension Bureau, April 6, 1896, Bowser described taking the Gold Cure, which is likely the cure being referenced in the 1900 letter, although it is possible Bowser was referring to another brand of cures, or even potentially his own failed brand from the 1870s. Perry B. Bowser Pension File, certificate 108546.

64. Adams, *Great American Fraud*, 111–12, 119.

65. Young, *Toadstool Millionaires*, chaps. 13–14.

Chapter 8

1. *Medical and Surgical History*, pt. 2, 1:728–52. Woodward's critique of physicians who overprescribed opiates was part of a broader analysis of the efficacy of opiates as used during the war and lesson learned therein. "With a freedom which borders on recklessness" on 744. "Chronic opium intoxication" on 747, 749. "The more I learn of the behavior" on 750.

2. Humphreys, *Marrow of Tragedy*, 273.

3. On the growth of drug use among "respectable" Americans during the Gilded Age, see Herzberg, *White Market Drugs*, 21–25.

4. Courtwright and Gabriel call attention to several additional factors in the 1890s and early 1900s that reduced opiate prescribing rates. The development of new painkillers, better diagnostic techniques for chronic and painful ailments that reduced the need for cure-alls, and a growing acceptance of germ theory that helped usher in the decline of chronic gastrointestinal illnesses relative to the Civil War era all meant that Americans became less reliant on opiates. Physicians and pharmacists also lobbied for state-level legislation regulations on the sale of opiate pharmaceuticals so as to reduce addiction, death by suicide, and accidental poisonings. And, critically, the younger generation of American physicians, who were increasingly better educated than their elders, paid more attention to the addictive potential of opiates and, consequently, moved away from prescribing the drugs. Courtwright, *Dark Paradise*, 51–52; Gabriel, "Restricting the Sale of 'Deadly Poisons,'" 330.

5. Fleming, "Treatment of the Habit of Opium-Eating," 368.
6. Calkins, *Opium and the Opium Appetite*, 55.
7. "Opium Eating in Maine," *Days' Doings*, January 9, 1869, 83.
8. Quoted in H. Day, *Opium Habit*, 251.
9. "The Curse of Opium Eating," *Banner of Light*, September 5, 1874, 2.
10. A. M. Chappell to William R. Terry, May 24, 1886, Lee Camp Soldier's Home Correspondence, 1885–1894, Huntington Library, San Marino, CA.
11. "Surgeon's Certificate," Charles L. Williams Application for Admission to the Michigan Soldiers' Home, Michigan Soldiers' Home Reel 25, file M-2378, Grand Rapids Public Library.
12. *Opium Eating*, 58–59.
13. Cobbe, *Doctor Judas*, 18–26. Cobbe claimed that he served in the Civil War and in the postwar US Navy, although I could not locate a military service record. A 1907 obituary corroborates Cobbe's navy service but does not specify when he enlisted. "Drink Cure Author Dies Liquor Derelict," *Inter Ocean* (Chicago), January 2, 1907, 3. Regardless of the details of his military service, Cobbe's claimed identity as a veteran amplified his public platform in a society populated by millions of veterans and obsessed with veterans' issues. Cobbe's book received widespread attention in the contemporary media. Dormandy, *Opium*, 188; Hickman, *Secret Leprosy of Modern Days*, 66–72.
14. Cobbe, *Doctor Judas*, 13.
15. William Rosser Cobbe, "Slave of the Drug: Horrors of the Use of Opium as Told by a Habitué," *Chicago Tribune*, April 22, 1894, 41–42.
16. Skocpol, *Protecting Soldiers and Mothers*, 111; Jordan, *Marching Home*, 151–69. Courtwright also observed an upward trend in warnings about physician-caused opiate addiction in medical literature from the 1870s to the 1890s but does not connect this trend to the Civil War or veterans. Courtwright, *Dark Paradise*, 49–50.
17. On the "cult of the fallen soldier," see Blight, *Race and Reunion*, chap. 1.
18. "Opium Eating," *Penn Monthly*, December 1, 1875, 944–45; "Opium Eating" (December 9, 1875), 679. The public health periodical *Sanitarium* likewise panned *Opium Eating*, condemning the veteran author for "choosing a quack instead of a physician." "Opium Eating," *Sanitarian*, February 1, 1876, 93.
19. "Books of the Day—Dr. Judas: A Portrayal of the Opium Habit," *Arena*, April 1895, 5; *Chicago Tribune*, October 5, 1895, 11.
20. *Theriaki*, July 1872, 45.
21. "Once Opium's Slaves, Nearly One Thousand Victims of the Drug Cured," *Chicago Tribune*, February 13, 1894, 10.
22. *Slave of the Drug: Horrors of the Use of Opium as Told by a Habitué* ([Dwight, IL?], [1894?]).
23. Hubbard, *Opium Habit and Alcoholism*, 4.
24. Hull, "Opium Habit," 537–38.
25. "Nerves and Narcotics," *Scientific American*, August 15, 1891, 100. Additional examples include "The Opium Habit's Power," *New-York Times*, December 30, 1877, 8, and "Dangerous Drugs: How to Control Effectually All Such Horrible Habits," *Puck*, November 10, 1886, 70.
26. V. Eaton, "How the Opium Habit Is Acquired," 663.
27. V. Eaton, "How the Opium Habit Is Acquired," 663.
28. "How the Opium Habit Is Acquired," 419–20.
29. Fleming, "Treatment of the Habit of Opium-Eating," 368.

30. Bartholow, *Manual of Hypodermic Medicine*, 71–72.

31. Sewall, "Opium-Eating and Hypodermic Injection," 422.

32. Bartholow, *Treatment of Diseases by the Hypodermic Method*, 90.

33. Beard, *Stimulants and Narcotics*, 153.

34. Oliver, "Use and Abuse of Opium," 168–74.

35. *Medical and Surgical History*, pt. 2, 1:746, 750.

36. Bartholow, *Treatment of Diseases by the Hypodermic Method*, 6.

37. Sell, *Opium Habit*, 8.

38. "Some Observations on the Deep Injection of Morphia," 212–14.

39. Quoted in Kane, *Hypodermic Injection of Morphia*, 277. Rejecting Noble's assertion, Kane used this case to illustrate the "danger of contracting the [morphine] habit" when doctors overprescribed morphine.

40. Woodbury, "Physic-Tippling and Medicine-Bibbling," 195.

41. J. C. Wilson, "Causes and Prevention of the Opium Habit," 506.

42. S. Mitchell, *Doctor and Patient*, 93.

43. J. Adams, "Substitutes for Opium in Chronic Diseases," 351–56.

44. "Morphiomania," 271. Similar remarks are in Hull, "Opium Habit," 537–45.

45. *Chicago Medical Examiner* 26 (1869): 29.

46. *BMSJ* 6 (1866–67): 421.

47. *Report of the Committee on Intemperance*, 14–15.

48. *Buffalo Medical and Surgical Journal* 7 (1867–68): 108. During the 1850s, Cornell reported that he relied on opium to treat epilepsy in his antebellum medical practice. See Cornell, *Observations on Epilepsy*, 29, and Cornell, "Muriate of Opium," 279–80. In the 1860s, he received much praise for his work on epilepsy. Cornell, *Sabbath, Or Lord's Day*, [67–72].

49. For context, see Devine, *Learning from the Wounded*, esp. chaps. 1, 4.

50. Henry, "Disease Known as 'Chorea,'" 66.

51. Mitchell to "the Governor Soldiers' Home Hampton—Va.," April 15, 1890, Silas Weir Mitchell Papers, Historical Medical Library, College of Physicians of Philadelphia, available at https://mitchell.cppdigitallibrary.org/s/mitchell/item/16414#?c=0&m=0&s=0&cv=0&xywh=-213%2C49%2C5688%2C3508.

52. Marten, *Sing Not War*, 80–81; Journet, "Phantom Limbs and 'Body-Ego,'" 87–99. The story appeared in the July 1866 issue of *Atlantic Monthly*.

53. Mitchell, Keen, and Moorhouse, "On the Antagonism of Atropia and Morphia," 118.

54. Mitchell, *Injuries of Nerves*, 298–302.

55. Swann, A. F., identifier Z10 40 series 2, folder 44, Turner's Lane Hospital; case and follow-up studies of peripheral nerve disorders, including correspondence addressed to S. W. Mitchell: Philadelphia, 1861–1892, Silas Weir Mitchell Papers, available at https://mitchell.cppdigitallibrary.org/s/mitchell/item-set/16498.

56. See Pappert, "Philadelphia Infirmity for Nervous Diseases," 1847–53.

57. Philadelphia Orthopaedic Hospital and Infirmary for Nervous Diseases Casebook, 1885–1917, David M. Rubenstein Rare Book and Manuscript Library, Duke University, Durham, NC. On Mitchell's Friday clinics, see Hinsdale, "S. Weir Mitchell," 3.

58. Da Costa attributed irritable heart to the physical manifestations of stress. The condition was sometimes called "Da Costa's syndrome." Dean, *Shook over Hell*, 130–31; Devine, *Learning from the Wounded*, 158–64; Bowen-Murphy, "'All Broke Down,'" 198–200.

59. Da Costa, "On Irritable Heart," 48.

60. J. M. Da Costa, Medical Clinic Records, Jefferson Medical College, 1870–1875, 3 vols., Medical Historical Library, Yale University Medical School, New Haven, CT; Warner, *Therapeutic Perspective*, Table 1 and 136–37. Warner notes how the opiate prescription rate varied by region and by professional training. I selected Boston's Massachusetts General Hospital as a comparison because of its similarities to Philadelphia's Jefferson College medical clinic. Both were Northeastern hospitals that treated public patients and were staffed by medical students overseen by elite physicians.

61. Da Costa, *Medical Diagnosis*, 903.

62. J. C. Wilson, "Causes and Prevention of the Opium Habit," 506. Three Union surgeons had the initials "J. C. Wilson." It is unclear which of the three men authored "Causes and Prevention of the Opium Habit," but considering the rhetoric espoused in the paper, I strongly suspect the author was the same J. C. Wilson as Da Costa's subordinate at the Jefferson College medical clinic. Straight, *Roster of All Regimental Surgeons and Assistant Surgeons*, 111, 172, 259.

63. J. Adams, "Substitutes for Opium in Chronic Diseases," 351–56. Adams was appointed an acting assistant surgeon aboard the USS *James L. Davis* in February 1864, serving until January 1865. *Register of Commissioned and Warrant Officers*, 164, 172. He had previously served as a army medical cadet in Washington, DC. "Death of Dr. J. F. A. Adams," *Springfield (MA) Weekly Republican*, July 30, 1914.

64. J. Adams, "Substitutes for Opium in Chronic Diseases," 351–56.

65. J. Adams, "Substitutes for Opium in Chronic Diseases," 351–56.

66. "Opium Habit," 94.

67. Hartwell, "Report on the Sale and Use of Opium," 142.

68. On the introduction of chloral and its use in nineteenth-century America, see Snelders, Kaplan, and Pieters, "On Cannabis, Chloral Hydrate, and Career Cycles," 95–114.

69. E. Clarke, "Hydrate of Chloral," 449–57. For opium eating, see 456. Clarke praised Mitchell and Hammond's wartime research on nerve wounds and neurology in his 1876 history of American medicine, coauthored with Henry J. Bigelow et al., *Century of American Medicine*, 54–57.

70. Hughes, "Hydrate of Chloral in Trismus and Tetanus," 190. Several journals ran this same article, including *Baltimore Physician and Surgeon* 2, no. 9 (September 1874): 71, and *Medical News* 31–32 (1873): 124.

71. Watson, "Use of Chloral Hydrate," 77. Similar comments appear in "Clinic of the Month" and "Notes and Queries."

72. *Journal of Insanity* 31 (1874–75): 231. See also 44–50.

73. "Proceedings of the Association of Medical Superintendents," 208–9, 236.

74. Hull, "Opium Habit," 545.

75. Watson, "Caution in the Use of Chloral Hydrate," 77.

76. *Decisions of the Department of the Interior*, 3:191–94.

77. *Decisions of the Department of the Interior*, 3:342–44.

78. Dorothea Dix Hospital General Case Books, 13:10–11, North Carolina State Archives, Raleigh.

79. Spillane, *Cocaine*, 1–24.

80. Da Costa, "Use of the Hydrochlorate of Cocaine," 48. Da Costa's article was widely read and reprinted. See, for example, *The Epitome: A Monthly Retrospect of American Practical Medicine*, March 1885, 14–15, and *Pharmacology of the Newer Materia Medica*, 435–38. Spillane, *Cocaine*, 13–14.

81. Noble B. Howard affidavit July 24, 1896, and Samuel B. Boots affidavit July 22, 1896, Samuel M. Martin Pension File, certificate 237259, Pension Application Files Based upon Service in the Civil War and Spanish American War, Record Group 15: Records of the Veterans Administration, 1783–1985, National Archives and Records Administration.

82. Spillane, *Cocaine*, 20–22.

83. "Cocaine in Inebriety," 127.

84. Crothers, "Cocaine Inebriety," 16–22; Mattison, Blanchard, Day, Parrish, and Mason quoted in "Annual Meeting of the American Association for the Cure of Inebriates," 12–15. Such warnings about the dangers of cocaine, especially when used as a substitute for opium, appeared with increasing frequency in the last two decades of the nineteenth century. See, for example, "Cocaine in Inebriety," 127, and "Cocaine Dosage and Cocaine Addiction," 123–24.

85. Spillane, *Cocaine*; Courtwright, "Hidden Epidemic"; and Hickman, *Secret Leprosy of Modern Days*, 72–80. An illustrative account is Hammond, "Remarks on Cocaine," 754–58.

86. Some prescription records, especially in the form of daybooks, are well-preserved and accessible. But such factors as inconsistent recordkeeping and poor handwriting complicate the use of these materials to quantify prescribing patterns.

87. Warner, *Therapeutic Perspective*, table 1 and figure 12. See also figure 10.

88. Courtwright, *Dark Paradise*, 201n27.

89. Warner, *Therapeutic Perspective*, 142–43. Warner notes that "unlike their counterparts in Cincinnati, practitioners at the [Massachusetts General Hospital] expressed considerable sensitivity in the case records to the problem of iatrogenic opiate addiction."

90. "Sixty-Fifth Annual Report of the Superintendent of the McLean Asylum," 49.

91. A major factor in the decline of opiates was the introduction of alternative drugs like choral hydrate and cocaine during the 1870s, which offered more options for physicians to choose from when selecting drugs to prescribe. Of course, prescribing newly available drugs was often part of doctors' efforts to mitigate iatrogenic opiate addiction.

92. The original *Harper's New Monthly Magazine* article, published in August 1867, was Ludlow, "What Shall They Do to Be Saved?" It was republished in H. Day, *Opium Habit*, 250–84; quote on 260. Day's volume also included an 1868 essay by Ludlow describing a medicalized plan for treating opiate addiction, which Ludlow argued could best be accomplished in an inebriate "home" as opposed to a mental asylum. *Opium Habit*, 286–335. Ludlow was widely known in Civil War–era American literary circles as the author of *The Hasheesh Eater*, an 1857 autobiography depicting Ludlow's cannabis use, written in the style of De Quincey's 1821 *Confessions of an English Opium-Eater*. See Gray, *Habit Forming*, 77–81.

93. "Domestic Intelligence-Medical Society," 104.

94. *Physicians and Surgeons of the United States*, 440–41.

95. An advertisement describing the sanitarium is found in Parrish, *Probe*.

96. *Physicians and Surgeons of the United States*, 548.

97. *Physicians and Surgeons of the United States*, 680–81.

98. *Report of the Committee on Intemperance*. The report was published in pamphlet form in 1869 and was also printed or abstracted in medical journals, including the *Chicago Medical Journal* in November 1869, *American Eclectic Medical Review* in December 1869, the Medical Society of the State of Pennsylvania's *Transactions* in 1870, and the *Journal of Insanity* in 1871.

99. *Report of the Committee on Intemperance*, 14.

100. *Report of the Committee on Intemperance*, 7.

101. *Report of the Committee on Intemperance*, 11.

102. *Report of the Committee on Intemperance*, 12.
103. *Report of the Committee on Intemperance*, 3.
104. *Report of the Committee on Intemperance*, 14.
105. *Report of the Committee on Intemperance*, 7–8.
106. See, for example, *Thirteenth Annual Report of the State Hospital Commission July 1, 1917, to June 30, 1918*, 370; Grob, *Inner World of American Psychiatry*, 14–15.
107. The group originally formed under the name American Association for the Cure of Inebriates. The name changed to the American Association for the Study and Cure of Inebriety in 1888 in an effort to foreground the society's interest in the scientific study of inebriety. Jaffe, *Addiction Reform in the Progressive Age*.
108. At this time, Parrish was director of the Pennsylvania Sanitarium in Media, Pennsylvania, a private facility that treated inebriates. Parker was a noted surgeon and president of the New York State Inebriate Asylum at Binghamton, the nation's first publicly funded institution for treating alcohol and drug addiction. On the founding of the AASCI, see Tracy, *Alcoholism in America*, 1–5, and Blumberg, "American Association for the Study and Cure of Inebriety," 235.
109. Willard Parker quoted in Tracy, *Alcoholism in America*, 3.
110. Blumberg, "American Association for the Study and Cure of Inebriety," 235–36.
111. The AASCI's principles quoted from Blumberg, "American Association for the Study and Cure of Inebriety," 235.
112. Mann, "Plea for Medical Jurisprudence to Keep Pace," 67–68.
113. Crothers, "Inebriety and Its Symptomology," 193.
114. *American Association for the Cure of Inebriates. Proceedings of the Second Meeting*, 114.
115. Claire D. Clark defines inebriety as "a medical explanation for the habitual and compulsive consumption of psychoactive substances" that "gained ground in the decades following the American Civil War." Clark, *Recovery Revolution*, 3. Although it has declined in use, the term "inebriety" remains familiar in the modern lexicon of addiction.
116. Joint Special Committee to Consider Inebriation as a Disease, 2.
117. Crothers, "Medical Treatment of Inebriety," 993.
118. Crothers, "New Sources of Danger," 338.
119. Crothers, "Inebriety and Its Symptomology," 195.
120. "Classification of Inebriety," 115.
121. An example of this view is James Parton, "Inebriate Asylums, and a Visit to One," 385.
122. Crothers, "Inebriety and Its Symptomology," 196.
123. Beard, *Stimulants and Narcotics*, 19, 38, 64, 129, 149; Blumberg, "American Association for the Study and Cure of Inebriety," 237; Jaffe, *Addiction Reform in the Progressive Age*, 17–20, 24, 30–34; Baumohl, "Inebriate Institutions in North America," 1185–1204.
124. Mattison, "Opium Addiction among Medical Men," 621–22.
125. Burnham, *Healthcare in America*, 131–33, 184–86; Grob, *Mental Institutions in America*, 135–50.
126. The journal's name changed in 1907 to the *Journal of Inebriety*. Thirty-five volumes and 141 issues were published, containing 801 major and 4,694 minor papers. Weiner and White, "*The Journal of Inebriety* (1876–1914)," 15–16; Dewey, "American Association for the Study and Cure of Inebriety," 123. See also Blumberg, "American Association for the Study and Cure of Inebriety," 235–36.
127. Jaffe, *Addiction Reform in the Progressive Age*, 34–35.
128. A. Day, *Journal of Inebriety—Extra*.

129. Tracy, *Alcoholism in America*, 3.

130. *Journal of Insanity* 18 (1861–62): 318.

131. Mann, "Cases Illustrative of the Treatment," 393.

132. Quoted in "Recognition of Inebriety," 37.

133. *Quarterly Journal of Inebriety* 11 (1889): 295.

134. See Tracy, *Alcoholism in America*, 16–18, and chaps. 3, 5–6, and E. Brown, "'What Shall We Do with the Inebriate?,'" 48–59. Clark also draws a direct lineage between Gilded Age inebriate institutions and the rehabilitation centers and twelve-step recovery programs of the twentieth century. Clark, *Recovery Revolution*, 3.

135. One notable example of an early call for the establishment of "asylums for inebriates" is M. B. Wright, *Drunkenness, Its Nature and Cure*.

136. For an overview of the Binghamton asylum's founding, see Crowley and White, *Drunkard's Refuge*.

137. *Superintendent's Report to the Board of Trustees*, 24.

138. James Parton, "Inebriate Asylums, and a Visit to One," *Atlantic Monthly*, October 1868, 385–404.

139. Crothers, "The Late Dr. Albert Day," 51–55; Crowley and White, *Drunkard's Refuge*, 57–59.

140. "Document No. 26," 7.

141. E. Brown, "'What Shall We Do with the Inebriate?,'" 50–53.

142. *Superintendent's Report to the Board of Trustees*, 24; Parton, "Inebriate Asylums, and a Visit to One." 385; Hedrick, *Harriet Beecher Stowe*, 336. Stowe's daughter, Georgiana, also suffered from morphine addiction. Courtwright, *Dark Paradise*, 40.

143. "Document No. 26," 7–8.

144. E. Brown, "'What Shall We Do with the Inebriate?,'" 54; Tracy, *Alcoholism in America*, 108–11.

145. Parton, "Inebriate Asylums, and a Visit to One," 385.

146. *Report of the Committee on Intemperance*, 12.

147. *Report of the Committee on Intemperance*, 15.

148. There is no comprehensive list of clinics. Brown estimates there were 100 clinics by 1900. E. Brown, "'What Shall We Do with the Inebriate?,'" 56. Morgan estimates about one hundred sanitariums in 1910, not including the scores of Keeley clinics also in operation. H. Morgan, *Drugs in America*, 74.

149. Quoted from Blumberg, "American Association for the Study and Cure of Inebriety," 235. Between 1876 and 1914, at least seventy-eight institutions for the treatment of inebriety were advertised in the *Quarterly Journal of Inebriety*. Weiner and White, "*Journal of Inebriety*," 20.

150. The best historical sketch of a public inebriate asylum is Sarah W. Tracy's account of the Massachusetts Hospital for Dipsomaniacs and Inebriates at Foxborough. Tracy, *Alcoholism in America*, chap. 5.

151. Jaffe, *Addiction Reform in the Progressive Age*, 26–27; Brown, "'What Shall We Do with the Inebriate?,'" 52.

152. "Annual Report of the Inebriates' Home," 1.

153. *Congressional Record*, January 19, 1875, 590.

154. *Quarterly Journal of Inebriety* 4, no. 1 (January 1880): [81].

155. Mattison, "Opium Addiction among Medical Men," 621. Mattison echoed the widely voiced contemporary observation that physicians were overly represented among

opiate-addicted Americans. "Inebriates Home for Kings Co.," 102–3; "The Inebriates Home Fort Hamilton," 13.

156. Mattison, "Curability of Opium Addiction," 252–53.
157. Mattison, "Opium Addiction among Medical Men," 622–23.
158. No comprehensive list of inebriety clinics exits. William L. White has self-published a list of American addiction treatment centers predating 1950, including several dozen inebriate clinics. William White, "American Institutions Specializing in the Treatment," WilliamWhitePapers.com, https://deriu82xba14l.cloudfront.net/file/1263/Early%20American%20Institutions%20Specializing%20in%20the%20Treatment%20of%20Alcohol%20and%20Drug%20Addiction%202023%20Update.pdf, accessed May 13, 2025.
159. Joint Special Committee to Consider Inebriation as a Disease, *Report*, 8–9.
160. "Opium Eating" (June 20, 1872), 412.
161. Rogers, "Medical History of Kentucky," 211–12.
162. On the depression stemming from the Panic of 1873, see Foner, *Reconstruction*, 512–24 (quotation on 524).
163. Baumohl, "Inebriate Institutions in North America, 1840–1920," 1187–1204.
164. An advertisement for Parrish Hall is in *Quarterly Journal of Inebriety* 2, no. 4 (1878). Kings County asylum remained open without Mattison until 1898. Baumohl, "Inebriate Institutions in North America," 1191.
165. "Some Private Asylums and Homes," 99; Jaffe, *Addiction Reform in the Progressive Age*, 41.
166. E. Brown, "'What Shall We Do with the Inebriate?,'" 56.
167. *Biographical Dictionary of Contemporary American Physicians and Surgeons*, 362.
168. Crothers, "Inebriety and Its Symptomology," 198.
169. The institution was originally called the Walnut Hill Asylum, renamed to Walnut Lodge Hospital in 1878. Crothers's system of care at Walnut Lodge is described in Crothers, "New Studies of the Opium Disease," 137–47, and Crothers, *Drug Habits and Their Treatments*.
170. Figure from Weiner and White, "History of Addiction/Recovery-Related Periodical," 18.
171. Crothers, "New Sources of Danger," 339.
172. Hickman, *Secret Leprosy of Modern Days*, 48–50.
173. "Remarks on the Opium Habit," 436.
174. Baumohl, "Inebriate Institutions in North America," 1195.
175. Jaffe, *Addiction Reform in the Progressive Age*, 34–35.
176. "Death of Dr. Albert Day," 815; "Recent Deaths," 456.
177. "Fighting the devil in the morphine bottle" in "A New Crusade," *State Journal* (Lincoln, NE), March 12, 1894, 4; Tyrell, *Woman's World/Woman's Empire*, 148–50, 169. Quoting "Mrs. James Haven of Indiana," 149.
178. "Anti Opium Department of the World's W.C.T.U. Dr. S. B. Collins's . . . Painless Opium Antidote . . . A Boon to Humanity," Ephemera Binder, box 2, folder 14, Helfand Collection, Library Company of Philadelphia.
179. "A Cure for Grip," *State Journal* (Lincoln, NE), March 12, 1894, 4.
180. "Church of Our Savior: The Question of Hell," *New York Herald*, November 9, 1874, 8.
181. "Cured by Faith Alone," *New-York Times*, March 28, 1884, 1.
182. "An Opium-Eater's Confession," *Times-Picayune* (New Orleans), September 11, 1880, 1.
183. Herzberg, *White Market Drugs*, chaps. 1–2.
184. Clark, *Recovery Revolution*, 5.

185. Tracy, *Alcoholism in America*, 3–4. On the Harrison Act and morphine maintenance clinics, see Musto, *American Disease*, chaps. 3 and 5, and Herzberg, *White Market Drugs*, 46–84.

186. Courtwright, "Preventing and Treating Narcotic Addiction," 2095–97.

187. On the transition from iatrogenic addiction to nonmedical addiction in the early twentieth-century United States, see Courtwright, *Dark Paradise*, 61–144. On the new addict stereotypes, see Keire, "Dope Fiends and Degenerates"; Hickman, *Secret Leprosy of Modern Days*, 59–92; Acker, *Creating the American Junkie*; and Herzberg, *White Market Drugs*, chaps. 1–2. Heroin addiction among World War I veterans is an understudied topic that warrants more attention.

188. Rosenberg, "What Is an Epidemic?," 8–9.

Epilogue

1. The Civil War generation did not use "army disease" and "soldier's disease" as shorthand for opiate addiction among Civil War soldiers or veterans. I was unable to find a single instance of "army disease" or "soldier's disease" being used as a descriptor for opiate addiction during the nineteenth century in an extensive review of Civil War–era primary sources, including medical journals, pamphlets, and books; hospital and asylum records; military records; pension applications; records of soldiers' homes; newspapers and popular periodicals; medical advertisements; and drug users' letters. The use of these labels for opiate addiction among Civil War veterans appears to have originated in the twentieth century.

2. Marks, *Leviathan*, 173; see also 179. Reviewers in contemporary medical journals lauded the book for its depiction of drug addiction. See *Medical Council* [Philadelphia] 19 (1914): 280, and *New Charlotte Medical Journal* 69–70 (1914): 246.

3. Herzberg, *White Market Drugs*, 32–45.

4. Marks, "Curse of Narcotism in America," 314–15.

5. Jeannette Marks, "Narcotism and the War," *North American Review*, December 1917, 879–84.

6. Kolb and Du Mez, "Prevalence and Trend of Drug Addiction," 1181. See also Courtwright, *Dark Paradise*, 15, 63.

7. "Mayor of Durham Explains Arrest," *Twin-City Daily Sentinel*, November 26, 1921, 7. See also E. Williams, *Opiate Addiction*, 33, 36, 61.

8. Committee on the Judiciary, House, *Establishment of Two Federal Narcotics Farms*, 49–50. The metaphor of drug users as an "army" was also prevalent. For example, see Lineberger, *Milestones in the War*, 8.

9. Terry and Pellens, *Opium Problem*, 69. Additional contemporary examples of the army disease model include Bishop, *Narcotic Drug Problem*, 117–18, 120–21, and Kolb and Du Mez, "Prevalence and Trend of Drug Addiction," 1198. On Terry and Pellens's work, see N. Campbell, *Discovering Addiction*.

10. United States Commission on Marihuana and Drug Abuse, *Drug Use in America*, 15. For context on the commission, also known as the Shafer Commission, see Musto, *American Disease*, 256–57.

11. Foster, *Long War on Drugs*, chap. 9; Lassiter, *Suburban Crisis*, 260–62.

12. Armed Forces Information Service, *Drug Abuse*, 4, 7.

13. *Little House on the Prairie*, season 2, episode 21, "Soldier's Return," written by Blanche Hanalis, Laura Ingalls Wilder, and B. W. Sandefur, directed by William F. Claxton, aired March

24, 1976, on NBC. The episode is available for viewing at www.imdb.com/title/tt0633070/?ref_=ttfc_fc_tt.

14. Jenny Stevens, "'I Was a Bad Influence on the Beatles': James Taylor on Lennon, Love and Recovery," *Guardian*, February 17, 2020, www.theguardian.com/music/2020/feb/17/james-taylor-i-was-a-bad-influence-on-the-beatles-lennon-love-and-a-life-in-song.

15. National Institute on Drug Abuse, *Research Issues 26*, 11.

16. Maurer and Vogel, *Narcotics and Narcotic Addiction*, 6.

17. Examples include Lindesmith, *Addiction and Opiates*, 225, and Dai, *Opium Addiction in Chicago*, 35, 153.

18. McPherson, *Battle Cry of Freedom*, 487. Although he framed morphine addiction as a by-product of Civil War medicine, McPherson mostly viewed military medicine in a positive light, concluding that Civil War medicine did more good than harm.

19. Wyatt-Brown, "War as Hell," 734–35. See also Adams, *Living Hell*, 200, and Schroeder-Lein, *Encyclopedia of Civil War Medicine*. For a critical analysis of the butcher trope, see Miller, *Empty Sleeves*, 18–49.

20. Quinones, "Drug Abuse during the Civil War." See also Swatos, "Opiate Addiction in the Late Nineteenth Century."

21. Exceptions include Bollet, *Civil War Medicine*, 241–42; "Opiate Use and Addiction," in Schroeder-Lein, *Encyclopedia of Civil War Medicine*, 240–41; and Lewy, "Army Disease."

22. Dean, *Shook over Hell*, 169–70; Marten, *Sing Not War*, 84, 111, 114; Jordan, *Marching Home*, 4, 180; Sommerville, *Aberration of Mind*, 161–62.

23. A memory history example is Macy, *Dopesick*. PBS's *Mercy Street* also prominently featured hypodermic morphine addiction among soldiers and surgeons.

24. Committee on Oversight and Reform, *Medical Experts*, n.p.

25. Netherland and Hansen, "White Opioids"; Hoffman et al., "Racial Bias in Pain Assessment."

Bibliography

Primary Sources

Manuscript Collections

Archives and Special Collections, Ball State University Libraries, Muncie, Indiana
    Delaware County Poor Relief Records
Bentley Historical Library, University of Michigan, Ann Arbor, Michigan
    Department of Medicine and Surgery (University of Michigan) theses, 1851–1878
        Eleazer Hall, "Opium[:] A Thesis by Eleazer Hall Respectfully Submitted to the Medical Faculty of the University of Michigan Feb[ruary] 12th 1866," Samuel DuBois Medical Thesis, 1855
City Archives, New Orleans, Louisiana
    Charity Hospital Records
        Admissions Book and Index, vol. 38: 1879–1881, MF GS36-58
Connecticut Historical Society, Hartford, Connecticut
    George Phillips Diary, 1863
Drexel University College of Medicine Legacy Center, Archives and Special Collections, Philadelphia, Pennsylvania
    William S. Theodore, "An Essay on the Effects of Opium as a Drug upon the Human System, Respectfully Submitted to the Faculty of the Homeopathic Medical College of Pennsylvania. February 22 A.D. 1850. For the Doctorate in Medicine"
Fred W. Smith National Library for the Study of George Washington, Mount Vernon, Virginia
    Benjamin Rush to Bushrod Washington, May 2, 1812
Georgia Department of Archives and History, Morrow, Georgia
    Record Group 26-12-29: Central State Hospital, Admissions Registers, 1842–1957, microfilm series, vol. 3, box 19 (October 19, 1860–July 31, 1873)
Grand Rapids Public Library, Grand Rapids, Michigan
    Michigan Soldiers' Home Reel 25, M-2378
Historical Medical Library, The College of Physicians of Philadelphia, Pennsylvania
    George B. Green New Receipt Book, 1823–1862
    Timothy Hall Recipe Book, 1823–1834
    Henry Hartshorne Account Books, vol. 1, 1848–1851
    Thaddeus Hildreth Daybook, 1865–1874
    The Silas Weir Mitchell Papers
    William W. Rutherford Account Books
        Account Book, 1863–1873
    Daniel J. Swinney Papers, 1808–1827

The Huntington Library, San Marino, California
   Lee Camp Soldier's Home Correspondence, 1885–1894
   Medical account book, HM 75114
   W. M. Parsons Ledger Book, 1858–1860
   Register and Prescription Book of 210th Regiment, Pennsylvania Volunteers
Iowa Digital Library, University of Iowa Library, Iowa City, Iowa
   Shelton Family Papers, 1864–1936, https://digital.lib.uiowa.edu/islandora/object/ui%3Atestcwd_4275
   Ferdinand Sophus Winslow letters, September 1861–February 1862, https://digital.lib.uiowa.edu/islandora/object/ui%3Atestcwd_17265
Library Company of Philadelphia, Philadelphia, Pennsylvania
   Helfand Collection
Library of Congress, Washington, DC
   William Oland Bourne Papers
     Soldier and Sailor Contributions, Left-Handed Penmanship Contest
       Albert T. Shurtleff
The Library of Virginia, Richmond, Virginia
   Confederate Disability Applications and Receipts
   Petersburg (city), Misc. records, Coroner's inquests
   Records of Eastern State Hospital, 1770–2009
   Records of Western State Hospital, 1825–2000
Louis Round Wilson Special Collections Library, University of North Carolina at Chapel Hill, Chapel Hill, North Carolina
   Southern Historical Collection
     DeRosset Family Papers, 1671–1940
     Hentz Family Papers, 1782–1932
       Charles A. Hentz Diary, 1887
       "My Autobiography, Vol. 2," unpublished manuscript
     Mackay and Stiles Family Papers, 1743–1975
     Prescription and Diet Book, circa 1800s
Medical Historical Library, Yale University Medical School, New Haven, Connecticut
   J. M. Da Costa, Medical Clinic Records, Jefferson Medical College, 1870–1875
   Allyn Merriam Hungerford Prescription Book, 1842–1845
   Moses Clarke White, "On the Abuses of Opium," in *Dissertations Read by the Candidates for the Degree of Doctor in Medicine in the Medical Institution of Yale College at the Annual Examination, January 25–26, 1854*
Mississippi State University Libraries, Starkville, Mississippi
   Rice (Nannie Herndon) Family Papers
   Arthur Hopkins Rice to Maria Walker, May 29, 1863, https://scholarsjunction.msstate.edu/mss-rice-papers/14/
National Archives and Records Administration, Washington, DC
   Record Group 15: Records of the Veterans Administration, 1783–1985
     Pension Application Files Based upon Service in the Civil War and Spanish American War
       Perry B. Bowser Pension File, certificate 108546

    Joseph C. Darrow Pension File, certificate 415496
    Joseph A. Lazelle Pension File, certificate 1047963
    Samuel M. Martin Pension File, certificate 237259
    Wirt Morris Pension File, certificate 582310
    Frank E. Pray Pension File, certificate 385070
  Record Group 109: War Department Collection of Confederate Records, 1825–1927
    Papers Relating to Citizens, 1861–1867
      Missouri, 1864: Bowley, [blank,] "Statement of Mr. Bowley in regard to purchasing hospital stores," https://catalog.archives.gov/id/27574361
  Record Group 153: Records of the Office of the Judge Advocate General (Army)
    Court Martial Case Files
  Record Group 418: Records of St. Elizabeths Hospital
    Registers of Cases, 1855–1941, boxes 1–4
    Case Records of Patients, 2354–2481, box 5
New-York Historical Society, New York, New York
  Beekman Family Recipe Book, 1800–1871
New York State Archives, Albany, New York
  Utica State Hospital Admission, Discharge, and Parole Registers, 1843–1985
  Utica State Hospital Patient Case Files, 1843–1898, 104 volumes
  Willard State Hospital Patient Case Files, 1869–1938, 17 volumes
North Carolina State Archives, Raleigh, North Carolina
  Francis C. Clewell Papers, 1860–1867
  Dorothea Dix Hospital Admissions Book
  Dorothea Dix Hospital General Case Books, vols. 13–19, 1887–1902
  Soldiers' Home Association: Hospital Patients, 1908–1916, North Carolina Digital Collections, https://digital.ncdcr.gov/Documents/Detail/soldiers-home-association-hospital-patients-1908-1916/585426
  Wake County Miscellaneous Records, 1772–1948
    Lunacy Records, 1881–1916 (broken series)
Ohio History Center, Columbus, Ohio
  Thomas Sweeting to Joseph L. Stephens, March 21, 1887
David M. Rubenstein Rare Book and Manuscript Library, Duke University, Durham, North Carolina
  Philadelphia Orthopaedic Hospital and Infirmary for Nervous Diseases Casebook, 1885–1917
South Carolina Historical Society, Charleston, South Carolina
  Letters to G. W. Aimar, 1877–1880
Special Collections, University of Mississippi Libraries, Oxford, Mississippi
  J. Watson Henderson Collection
Special Collections Libraries, University of Georgia, Athens, Georgia
  Isaiah Smith Papers
    Diary, 1860–1867, https://dlg.usg.edu/record/dlg_turningpoint_harg3302-001-001
Stuart A. Rose Manuscript, Archives, and Rare Book Library, Emory University, Atlanta, Georgia
  George W. Nailer Papers, 1824–1864

Tennessee State Library and Archives, Nashville, Tennessee
   Sample Tennessee Confederate Pension Applications: Soldiers and Widows, https://sos.tn.gov/products/tsla/tennessee-confederate-pension-application-soldiers-application (no longer available)
   Tennessee Confederate Soldiers' Home: Applications and Ledgers
University of Virginia Library, Charlottesville, Virginia
   The Albert and Shirley Small Special Collections Library
      Letters of Sylvanus Cobb, 1827–1867
Virginia Historical Society, Richmond, Virginia
   Captured Mail Collection, 1862–1865
   Goolrick Family Papers, 1859–1927
   John Thomas Parker Commonplace Book, 1859–1865
Waring Historical Library, Medical University of South Carolina, Charleston
   McFaddin Medical Diary, 1841–1854
   Medical Society of South Carolina Meeting Minutes: 1881–1897
   Waring Historical Library Inaugural Theses Collection
      Isaac H. Blair, "Opium," 1855, https://waringlibrary.contentdm.oclc.org/digital/collection/wit/id/2636/rec/12
      Madison W. Drummond, "On Opium," 1856, https://cdm16606.contentdm.oclc.org/digital/collection/wit/id/2824
      H. J. McLaurin, "On Opium," 1860, https://cdm16606.contentdm.oclc.org/digital/collection/wit/id/3012
      John P. Mushat, "On Opium," 1855, https://cdm16606.contentdm.oclc.org/digital/collection/wit/id/2716
      Josiah Phillips, "On the Modus Operandi of Opium," 1843, https://cdm16606.contentdm.oclc.org/digital/collection/wit/id/1045
      Thomas DuBose Wilson, "On the Effects of Opium upon the System," 1857, https://cdm16606.contentdm.oclc.org/digital/collection/wit/id/2754/rec/1
University of Michigan Library Digital Collections
   Civil War Collection
      Milton Sawyer Diary, 1863 https://quod.lib.umich.edu/c/civilwar1/USCW005.0001.001?view=toc

Databases Consulted

Alabama, Confederate Pension Applications, ca. 1880–1930s. Family Search. www.familysearch.org/search/collection/3029256.
Arkansas, Ex-Confederate Pension Records, 1891–1939. Family Search. www.familysearch.org/search/collection/1921864.
Case Law Access Project. https://case.law.
Chronicling America. Library of Congress. https://chroniclingamerica.loc.gov.
Civil War Richmond. https://civilwarrichmond.com.
Confederate Disability Applications. Library of Virginia Online. https://lva-virginia.libguides.com/confederate-disability.
Confederate Pension Records. Oklahoma Digital Prairie. www.digitalprairie.ok.gov/digital/collection/pensions.

Coroner's Inquisitions. Virginia Open Data Portal. https://data.virginia.gov/Education/Coroners-Inquisitions/wx5a-uuyp.
CSI: Dixie. https://csidixie.org.
Death Registers, 1853–1906 (Virginia). Family Search. www.familysearch.org/search/catalog/780106.
1860 United States Federal Census. Ancestry. www.ancestry.com/search/collections/7667.
1870 United States Federal Census. Ancestry. www.ancestry.com/search/collections/7163.
1880 United States Federal Census. Ancestry. www.ancestry.com/search/collections/6742.
1890 Veterans Schedules of the US Federal Census. Ancestry. www.ancestry.com/search/collections/8667.
Find A Grave. www.findagrave.com.
Georgia Historic Newspapers. Digital Library of Georgia. https://dlg.usg.edu/collection/dlg_ghn.
Historical American Medical Journals. Medical Heritage Library. www.medicalheritage.org/content/historical-american-medical-journals/. No longer available.
Kentucky, Confederate Pension Applications, 1912–1950. Family Search. www.familysearch.org/search/collection/1916017.
Louisiana, Confederate Pensions, 1898–1950. Family Search. www.familysearch.org/search/collection/1838535.
Missouri, Confederate Pension Applications and Soldiers Home Applications, 1861–1939. Family Search. www.familysearch.org/search/collection/1865475.
New York Civil War Muster Roll Abstracts. Fold3. www.fold3.com/publication/924/us-new-york-civil-war-muster-roll-abstracts-1861-1900.
North Carolina, Confederate Soldiers and Widows Pension Applications, 1885–1953. Family Search. www.familysearch.org/search/collection/1911763.
Private Voices. University of Georgia. https://altchive.org.
Union Army Data Set. National Bureau of Economic Research. *Early Indicators of Later Work Levels, Disease, and Death*. www.nber.org/research/data/union-army-data-set.
United States, National Homes for Disabled Volunteer Soldiers, 1866–1938. Family Search. www.familysearch.org/search/collection/1916230.
US Census—Federal, 1860. Fold3. www.fold3.com/publication/19/us-census-federal-1860.
US Civil War. Fold3. www.fold3.com/collection/us-civil-war.
US Civil War Pension Index, 1861–1900. Fold3. www.fold3.com/publication/57/us-civil-war-pensions-index-1861-1900.
US Civil War "Widow's Pensions." Fold3. www.fold3.com/publication/24/us-civil-war-widows-pensions-1861-1910.
The Valley of the Shadow: Two Communities in the American Civil War. Virginia Center for Digital History. https://valley.newamericanhistory.org.
Virginia Chronicle. Library of Virginia. https://virginiachronicle.com.

Published Government Reports

"An Act Granting Pensions to Soldiers and Sailors Who Are Incapacitated for the Performance of Manual Labor, and Providing for Pensions to Widows, Minor Children, and Dependent Parents." In *The Statutes at Large of the United States of America*. Vol. 26. Washington, DC: Government Printing Office, 1891.

"An Act to Incorporate the Pinel Hospital." In *Acts and Joint Resolutions Passed by the General Assembly of the State of Virginia at the Session of 1875–6*, 248–51. Richmond: R. F. Walker, Superintendent Public Printing, 1876.

Annual Report of the Board of Directors and Superintendent of the Longview Asylum to the Governor for the Year 1862. Columbus: Richard Nevins, State Printer, 1863.

Annual Report of the Commissioner of Pensions to the Secretary of the Interior for the Year Ended June 30, 1890. Washington, DC: Government Printing Office, 1890.

"Annual Report of the Inebriates' Home for Kings County, for 1870." *Documents of the Assembly of the State of New York: Ninety-Fourth Session—1871.* Vol. 3. Albany: Argus, 1871.

Annual Report of the Managers of the State Lunatic Asylum, Utica, N.Y., for the Year 1874. Albany, NY: Weed, Parsons, 1875.

Annual Reports of the Board of Visitors, Trustees, Superintendent, Treasurer, and Financial Agent of the New Hampshire Asylum for the Insane to the Governor and Council, June 1887. Manchester, NH: John B. Clarke, 1887.

Annual Reports of the Department of the Interior. Washington, DC: Government Printing Office, 1868.

Annual Reports of the Officers, Boards and Institutions of the Commonwealth of Virginia, for the Year Ending September 30, 1880. Richmond: R. F. Walker, Superintendent of Public Printing, 1881.

Appeals in Pension Cases. Report of Assistant Secretary Webster Davis to the Secretary of the Interior for the Fiscal Year ended June 30, 1898. Washington, DC: Government Printing Office, 1898.

Committee on Oversight and Reform, House of Representatives, 116th Congress. *Medical Experts: Inadequate Federal Approach to Opioid Treatment and the Need to Expand Care.* Serial No. 116-35. Washington, DC: Government Printing Office, 2019.

Committee on the Judiciary, House of Representatives, 70th Congress. *Establishment of Two Federal Narcotics Farms, April 26, 27, 28, 1928.* Serial 29. Washington, DC: Government Printing Office, 1928.

"Correspondence Concerning the Effects of the Use of Intoxicating Liquor." In *Second Annual Report of the State Board of Health of Massachusetts*, 245–348. Boston: Wright & Potter, 1871.

Decisions of the Department of the Interior in Appealed Pension and Bounty-Land Claims. Vol. 3. Washington, DC: Government Printing Office, 1890.

Decisions of the Department of the Interior in Appealed Pension and Bounty-Land Claims. Vol. 7. Washington, DC: Government Printing Office, 1895.

Decisions of the Department of the Interior in Appealed Pension and Bounty-Land Claims. Vol. 8. Washington, DC: Government Printing Office, 1897.

Decisions of the Department of the Interior in Appealed Pension and Bounty-Land Claims. Vol. 9. Washington, DC: Government Printing Office, 1898.

Decisions of the Department of the Interior in Appealed Pension and Retirement Claims. Vol. 1. Washington, DC: Government Printing Office, 1887.

"Document No. 26: Report of the Trustees of the State Inebriate Asylum." In *Documents of the Assembly of the State of New York. Ninetieth Session—1867.* Vol. 2. Albany: Printing House of C. Van Benthuysen & Sons, 1867.

Graham, B. *Report of Superintendent of the Texas State Lunatic Asylum, from October 1868 to October 1869*. Austin: Tracy, Seimering, 1870.

Hartwell, B. H. "Report on the Sale and Use of Opium in Massachusetts." In *Twentieth Annual Report of the State Board of Health of Massachusetts*, 135–58. Boston: Wright and Potter, 1889.

Henry, Joseph. "Circular in Regard to the Disease Known as 'Chorea.'" In *Annual Report of the Board of Regents of the Smithsonian Institution, Showing the Operations, Expenditures, and Condition of the Institution for the Year 1874*. Washington, DC: Government Printing Office, 1875.

History of Wages in the United States from Colonial Times to 1928. Revision of Bulletin No. 499 with Supplement, 1929–1933. Washington, DC: Government Printing Office, 1934.

Hull, J. M. "The Opium Habit." In *Third Biennial Report of the Board of Health of the State of Iowa for the Fiscal Period Ending June 30, 1885*, 537–45. Des Moines, IA: George F. Roberts, State Printer, 1885.

Joint Special Committee to Consider Inebriation as a Disease. *Report*. [Boston?], May 1868. https://catalog.hathitrust.org/Record/011534148.

"Kentucky—Second District. Extracts from Report of Dr. J. W. Compton." In *Statistics Medical and Anthropological of the Provost-Marshal-General's Bureau*. 1: 365–69, edited by J. W. Baxter. Washington DC: Government Printing Office, 1875.

The Medical and Surgical History of the War of the Rebellion. Vols. 1–6. Washington, DC: Government Printing Office, 1870–88.

Oliver, F. E. "The Use and Abuse of Opium." In *Massachusetts State Board of Health Third Annual Report*, 162–77. Boston: Wright and Potter State Printers, 1872.

Opium Problem: Message from the President of the United States Transmitting from the Secretary of State a Report on the International Opium Commission and On the Opium Problem as Seen within the United States and Its Possessions, Prepared by Hamilton Wright on Behalf of the American Delegates to the Said Commission, Held at Shanghai in February, 1909. Washington, DC: Government Printing Office, 1910.

Proceedings of the Board of Managers of the National Home for Disabled Volunteers. Vol. 2. Washington, DC.: Public Documents Library, 1902.

Report of Inspection of State Soldiers and Sailors' Homes for Year Ending June 30, 1894. Washington, DC: Government Printing Office, 1894.

Report of Inspection of State Soldiers and Sailors' Homes for Year Ending June 30, 1895. Washington, DC: Government Printing Office, 1895.

Report of Inspection of State Soldiers and Sailors' Homes for Year Ending June 30, 1896. Washington, DC: Government Printing Office, 1896.

Report of Inspection of State Soldiers and Sailors' Homes for Year Ending June 30, 1897. Washington, DC: Government Printing Office, 1897.

Report of the Board of Directors and Medical Superintendent of the Western Lunatic Asylum Staunton, VA. For the Fiscal Year 1869–1870. Richmond: C. A. Schaffter, Superintendent Public Printing, 1870.

Report of the Board of Directors and Physician and Superintendent of the Western Lunatic Asylum of Virginia, for the Fiscal Year 1874–'75. Richmond: R. F. Walker, Superintendent Public Printing, 1875.

Report of the Board of Managers of the National Home for Disabled Volunteer Soldiers. March 2, 1877. House of Representatives, 44th Congress, 2nd Session, Mis. Doc. no. 45.

Report of the Board of Managers of the National Home for Disabled Volunteer Soldiers for the Fiscal Year Ending June 30, 1893. Washington, DC: Government Printing Office, 1893.

Report of the Board of Managers of the National Home for Disabled Volunteer Soldiers for the Fiscal Year Ending June 30, 1895. Washington, DC: Government Printing Office, 1895.

Report of the Board of Managers of the National Home for Disabled Volunteer Soldiers for the Fiscal Year Ending June 30, 1896. Washington, DC: Government Printing Office, 1896.

Report of the Commissioner of Pensions to the Secretary of the Interior for the Year Ended June 30, 1894. Washington, DC: Government Printing Office, 1894.

"Report of the Surgeon General." *Annual Report of the Secretary of War.* Washington, DC: Government Printing Office, 1866.

Report of the Trustees, Superintendent and Resident Physician of the Lunatic Asylum of the State of Georgia, for the Year 1864-5. Milledgeville, GA: Boughton, Nisbet, Barnes & Moore, 1866.

Report of the Trustees, Superintendent and Resident Physician of the Lunatic Asylum of the State of Georgia, for the Year 1866-7. Milledgeville, GA: Federal Union Book and Job Office, 1868.

Report of the Trustees, Superintendent, Resident Physician and Treasurer of the Lunatic Asylum of the State of Georgia, for the Year 1867-8. Milledgeville, GA: Federal Union Book and Job Office, 1869.

Report of the Trustees, Superintendent, Resident Physician and Treasurer of the Lunatic Asylum of the State of Georgia, for the Year 1868-9. Milledgeville, GA: Federal Union Book and Job Office, 1870.

Report of the Trustees, Superintendent, Resident Physician and Treasurer of the Lunatic Asylum of the State of Georgia, for the Year 1866-7: With Supplemental Report to Gov. Ruger. Milledgeville, GA: Federal Union Book and Job Office, 1868.

Reports of the Board of Directors and of the Physician and Superintendent of the Virginia Western Lunatic Asylum, for the Fiscal Years 1875-76, 1876-77. Richmond: R. F. Walker, Superintendent Public Printing, 1877.

"Sixty-Fifth Annual Report of the Superintendent of the McLean Asylum for the Insane to the Trustees of the Mass. General Hospital, for the Year 1882." In *Sixty-Ninth Annual Report of the Trustees of the Massachusetts General Hospital and McLean Asylum, 1882.* Boston: Geo. H. Ellis, 1883.

Statistics, Medical and Anthropological, of the Provost-Marshal-General's Bureau, Derived from Records of the Examination for Military Service in the Armies of the United States during the Late War of the Rebellion, of Over a Million Recruits, Drafted Men, Substitutes, and Enrolled Men. Vol. 1. Washington, DC: Government Printing Office, 1875.

Superintendent's Report to the Board of Trustees of the New York State Inebriate Asylum. Binghamton: Daily Republic Steam Printing Establishment, 1867.

Thirteenth Annual Report of the State Hospital Commission July 1, 1917, to June 30, 1918. Albany: J. B. Lyon, 1919.

United States Commission on Marihuana and Drug Abuse. *Drug Use in America: Problem in Perspective: Second Report.* Vol. 1. Washington, DC: Government Printing Office, 1973.

The War of the Rebellion: A Compilation of the Official Records of the Union and Confederate Armies. 70 vols. in 128. Washington, DC: Government Printing Office, 1894-1922.

Newspapers and Popular Periodicals Consulted

Akron Beacon-Journal
Akron Times-Democrat
The Albany Journal
Alexandria Gazette
Annals of Iowa
The Annals of the American Academy of
   Political and Social Science
Anti-Slavery Reporter (London)
The Arena
Athens Georgian
Atlanta Daily Intelligencer
The Atlantic Monthly
The Baltimore Sun
Banner of Light
Boston Cultivator
Boston Daily Globe
Boston Morning Journal
Brooklyn Daily Eagle
Capitolian Advocate (Baton Rouge)
The Century Illustrated Monthly
   Magazine
The Charleston Daily Courier
The Charleston Mercury
Chicago Daily Tribune
Chicago Tribune
Christian Advocate
The Christian Union
Collier's: The National Weekly
Confederate Veteran
The Congressional Globe
Daily Evening Bulletin (San Francisco)
The Daily Intelligencer (Atlanta)
Daily Morning Union (Grass Valley,
   California)
Days' Doings
De Bow's Review
Druggists' Circular & Chemical Gazette
The Ellijay Courier (Ellijay, Georgia)
The Epitome: A Monthly Retrospect of
   American Practical Medicine
Flag of Our Union
Frank Leslie's Illustrated Newspaper
Frank Leslie's Popular Monthly
The Free Press

The Galaxy: A Magazine of Entertaining
   Reading
The Galveston Journal
Galveston News
The Greenville Democrat (Ohio)
The Guardian
Harper's New Monthly Magazine
Harper's Weekly
Indiana Herald (Huntington)
The Inter Ocean (Chicago)
LaGrange (GA) Reporter
Lippincott's Magazine of Literature, Science
   and Education
Los Angeles Times
Memphis Daily Avalanche
Morning Herald (New York)
The National Police Gazette
National Review
The National Tribune
New England Magazine
The Newnan Herald (Newnan, Georgia)
New-York Daily Tribune
New York Evangelist
The New York Herald
New York Observer and Chronicle
The New-York Times
The North American Review
The Ohio Soldier
The Pantagraph (Bloomington, Illinois)
Penn Monthly
Philadelphia Medical Times
Popular Science Monthly
Practice (Richmond)
Providence (RI) Journal
Press and Messenger (Baltimore)
Puck
Richmond Christian Advocate
Richmond Daily Dispatch
Richmond Daily Whig
Richmond Dispatch
Richmond Indiana Palladium
Richmond Semi-Weekly Examiner
Richmond Times-Dispatch
Sandersville (GA) Herald

Sanitarian
Savannah Morning News
Sentinel (Richmond)
Scientific American
Shenandoah Herald (Woodstock, Virginia)
The Springfield (MA) Weekly Republican
Southern Confederacy (Atlanta)
Star Tribune (Minneapolis)
The State Journal (Lincoln, Nebraska)
Staunton Spectator
Staunton Vindicator
St. Louis Daily Dispatch
St. Louis Daily Globe-Democrat
St. Louis Republican
The Sun (New York)
Sunday Gazette (Atlanta)
Sunny South (Atlanta)
Theriaki: A Magazine Devoted to the Interests of Opium Eaters
Times-Picayune (New Orleans)
Tri-Weekly Telegraph (Houston)
True American (New Orleans)
The Twin-City Daily Sentinel (Winston-Salem, North Carolina)
The United States Army and Navy Journal and Gazette of the Regular and Volunteer Forces
Valley Spirit (Franklin County, Pennsylvania)
Vermont Watchman & State Journal
Voice of the West (Buchanan, Michigan)
The Washington Post
Weston (WV) Democrat
Winchester Times
Worcester Evening Gazette (Worcester, Massachusetts)
Zion's Herald

Books, Journal Articles, and Pamphlets

Adams, J[ames] F[orster] A[lleyne]. "Substitutes for Opium in Chronic Diseases." *Boston Medical and Surgical Journal*, October 10, 1889, 351–56.

Adams, Samuel Hopkins. *The Great American Fraud*. Chicago: American Medical Association, 1912.

Aldrich, Corinna Brown. *Echoes from a Distant Frontier: The Brown Sisters' Correspondence from Antebellum Florida*. Edited by Ellen Brown Anderson, James M. Denham, and Keith L. Huneycutt. Columbia: University of South Carolina Press, 2004.

Allen, J. Adams. *Medical Examinations for Life Insurance*. 3rd ed. Chicago: Clarke, 1866.

American Association for the Cure of Inebriates. *Proceedings of the First Meeting, Held in New York, November 29th & 30th, 1870*. Philadelphia: Henry B. Ashmead, 1871.

———. *Proceedings of the Second Meeting, Held in New York, November 14th & 15th, 1871*. Philadelphia: Henry B. Ashmead, 1872.

American Association for the Study and Cure of Inebriety, *The Disease of Inebriety from Alcohol, Opium, and Other Narcotic Drugs*. New York: E. B. Treat, 1893.

American Eclectic Medical Review 5 (December 1865): 275.

The American Journal of Obstetrics and Diseases of Women and Children 15 (1882): 160.

American Temperance Magazine, and Sons of Temperance Offering. Edited by Samuel F. Cary. New York: R. Van Dien, 1851.

Andrews, E. "Cure of a Confirmed Opium-Eater.—A Record of the Symptoms." *Chicago Medical Examiner*, February 1867, 67–70.

"Annual Meeting of the American Association for the Cure of Inebriates." *Quarterly Journal of Inebriety* 9 (1887): 12–15.

"An Opium-Eater in America." *Knickerbocker, or New York Monthly Magazine* 20 (1842): 47–57.

Armed Forces Information Service. *Drug Abuse: Game without Winners; A Basic Handbook for Commanders*. Washington, DC: Government Printing Office, 1972.

"The Army of the South-West." *Annals of Iowa* 6 (July 1868): 152.

Arnold, Edmund S. F. *"Back from the Mouth of Hell": Or, The Rescue from Drunkenness: The Causes, Progress and Results of Intemperance, with the Possibility and Effectual Methods of Accomplishing Permanent Reform*. Hartford: American, 1878.

———. *On the Uses of Opium in Managing the Shock and Reaction of Severe Surgical Injuries*. New York: M. B. Brown, 1863.

———. "On the Uses of Opium in Shock, Reaction, and Inflammations." *Transactions of the Medical Society of the State of Pennsylvania, Sixteenth Annual Session, Held at Altoona, June 1865*, 4th ser., pt. 1 (1865): 183–206.

Bailey, F. K. "Cases in Toxicology." *Medical and Surgical Reporter* 26 (January 27, 1872): 75–77.

Baltimore Physician and Surgeon 2, no. 9 (September 1874): 71.

Barratt, Joseph. "Case of Successful Treatment by Flagellation, Where a Large Dose of Laudanum Had Been Taken." *Boston Medical and Surgical Journal*, May 4, 1836, 197–99.

Bartholow, Roberts. *A Manual of Instructions for Enlisting and Discharging Soldiers: With Special Reference to the Medical Examination of Recruits, and the Detection of Disqualifying and Feigned Diseases*. Philadelphia: J. B. Lippincott, 1863.

———. *Manual of Hypodermic Medicine*. Philadelphia: J. B. Lippincott, 1869.

———. *The Treatment of Diseases by the Hypodermic Method: A Manual of Hypodermic Medicine*. 3rd ed. Philadelphia: J. B. Lippincott, 1879.

Bates, James. "Successful Treatment of Opium Eaters." *Boston Medical and Surgical Journal*, February 23, 1853, 77.

Beach, W. *The American Practice Condensed, or the Family Physician: Being the Scientific System of Medicine: On Vegetable Principles, Designed for All Classes*. Vol. 1. New York: James M'Alister, 1851.

Beard, Charles M. *Stimulants and Narcotics Medically, Philosophically, and Morally Considered*. New York: G. P. Putnam & Sons, 1871.

Beecher, Lyman. *Six Sermons on the Nature, Occasions, Signs, Evils, and Remedies of Intemperance*. 10th ed. New York: American Tract Society, 1833.

Bierce, Ambrose. "What I Saw at Shiloh." In *The Collected Works of Ambrose Bierce*. Vol. 1. New York: Neale Publishing Company, 1909.

Billings, John S. "Medical Reminisces of the Civil War." National Library of Medicine Digital Collections. https://collections.nlm.nih.gov/bookviewer?PID=nlm:nlm uid-101718577-bk.

A Biographical Dictionary of Contemporary American Physicians and Surgeons. Edited by William B. Atkinson. 2nd ed. Philadelphia: D. G. Brinton, 1880.

Bishop, Ernest Simons. *The Narcotic Drug Problem*. New York: Macmillan, 1921.

Brewster, Charles Harvey. *When This Cruel War Is Over: The Civil War Letters of Charles Harvey Brewster*. Edited by David W. Blight. Amherst: University of Massachusetts Press, 1992.

Brigham, Amariah. *Inquiry concerning the Diseases and Functions of the Brain*. New York: George Adlard, 1840.

Brobst, John F. *Well Mary: Civil War Letters of a Wisconsin Volunteer*. Edited by Margaret Brobst Roth. Madison: University of Wisconsin Press, 1960.

Brock, Robert Alonzo. *Virginia and Virginians*. Vol. 2. Richmond: H. H. Hardesty, 1888.

Brown, H. James. *An Opium Cure: Based upon Science, Skill and Matured Experience; Not an Invariable Nostrum, but an Enlightened Treatment, Constituting a Sovereign Antidote and Restorative for the Opium Disease*. 2nd ed. New York: Fred. M. Brown, 1872.

Browne, W. A. F. *Opiophagism, or, Psychology of Opium Eating*. London: Smith, Elder, [1875].

Buck, Marcus C. "On the Use and Abuse of Medicine." *Boston Medical and Surgical Journal*, April 23, 1845, 229–33.

Buffalo Medical and Surgical Journal 2 (1862–63): 274.

Buffalo Medical and Surgical Journal 5 (1865–66): 34.

Buffalo Medical and Surgical Journal 6 (1866–67): 421.

Buffalo Medical and Surgical Journal 7 (1867–68): 108.

Calkins, Alonzo. *Opium and the Opium Appetite*. Philadelphia: J. B. Lippincott, 1871.

Campbell, Henry Fraser. *Caffeine as an Antidote in the Poisoning Narcotism of Opium*. Augusta, GA: Steam Power Press of the Chronicle & Sentinel, 1860.

Carpenter, George W. *Carpenter's Family Medicine Chest Dispensatory*. Philadelphia: George W. Carpenter's Chemical Warehouse, 1835.

Carter, Robert. *An Inaugural Essay, Being a Comparative Inquiry into the Properties and Uses of Opium*. Philadelphia: Printed at the office of the Gazette of the United States, 1803.

Cartwright, Samuel A. "Diseases and Peculiarities of the Negro Race." *De Bow's Review* 2 (September 1851): 331–32.

Ceremonies, Etc.: New York State Inebriate Asylum, Binghamton, New York. New York: Wynkoop, Hallenbeck & Thomas, 1859.

Chassaignac, Charles. "Case of Opium Habit Cures by Sudden Deprivation." *New Orleans Medical and Surgical Journal* 34 [n.s., vol. 9] (1881–82): 256–59.

Child, Lydia Maria. *The Family Nurse; or, Companion of the Frugal Housewife*. Boston: Charles J. Hendee, 1837.

Chesnut, Mary Boykin. *A Diary from Dixie*. Edited by Isabella D. Martin and Myrta Lockett Avary. New York: D. Appleton, 1905.

Chicago Medical Examiner 26 (1869): 29.

Clarke, Edward H., Samuel D. Gross, T. Gaillard Thomas, and J. S. Billings. *A Century of American Medicine, 1776–1876*. Philadelphia: Henry C. Lea, 1876.

———. "Hydrate of Chloral, with Cases Illustrating Its Action." *Boston Medical and Surgical Journal*, June 16, 1870, 449–57.

"The Classification of Inebriety." *Quarterly Journal of Inebriety* 8 (1886): 114–16.

"Clinic of the Month." *American Practitioner: A Monthly Journal of Medicine and Surgery* 1 (1870): 123.

Cobbe, William Rosser. *Doctor Judas: A Portrayal of the Opium Habit*. Chicago: S. C. Griggs, 1895.

"Cocaine in Inebriety." *Quarterly Journal of Inebriety* 8 (1886): 127.

"Coca in the Opium Habit." *Students Medical Journal and Hospital Gazette*, October 9, 1880, 246. "Cocaine Dosage and Cocaine Addiction." *Quarterly Journal of Inebriety* 9 (1887): 123–24.

Coggeshall, William H. "The Hypodermic Use of Sulphate of Morphia." *Virginia Medical Monthly* 10 (1883–84): 151–70.

Cole, Henry G. *Confessions of an American Opium Eater: From Bondage to Freedom.* Boston: James H. Earle, 1895.

Collins, S[amuel] B. *Positive Cure for the Opium Habit.* San Francisco: Alta California Book and Job Printing House, 1874.

———. *Theriaki: An Annual Devoted to the Interests of Opium Eaters.* La Porte, IN: La Porte Chronicle Steam Print, 1878.

———. *Theriaki and Their Last Dose.* Chicago: Evening Journal Print, 1870.

———. *Theriaki: A Treatise on the Habitual Use of Narcotic Poison.* [La Porte, IN], 1887[?].

Commissioner of Pensions. *A Treatise on the Practice of the Pension Bureau Governing the Adjudication of Army and Navy Pensions.* Washington, DC: Government Printing Office, 1898.

A Compilation of the Messages and Papers of the Presidents. Vol. 14. Edited by James D. Richardson. New York: Bureau of National Literature, 1897.

The Congressional Globe: Containing the Debates and Proceedings of the Second Session Forty-Second Congress; An Appendix, Embracing the Laws Passed at that Session. Washington, DC: Government Printing Office, 1872.

Congressional Record, January 19, 1875, 590.

Conklin, W. J. "ART. V.—Climacteric Insanity." *American Journal of the Medical Sciences*, n.s., vol. 62 (October 1871): 365–73.

Copland, James. *A Dictionary of Practical Medicine.* Vol. 7. New York: Harper & Brothers, 1852.

Cornell, W[illiam] M[ason]. "Muriate of Opium." *Boston Medical and Surgical Journal*, November 6, 1850, 279–80.

———. *Observations on Epilepsy, Its Pathology, and Treatment.* Boston: Fetridge, 1854.

———. *The Sabbath, Or Lord's Day: Its Sanctification and Profanation.* Philadelphia, 1866.

Crothers, T[homas] D[avison]. "Cocaine Inebriety." *Quarterly Journal of Inebriety* 9 (1887): 16–22.

———. *Drug Habits and Their Treatments: A Clinical Summary of Some of the General Facts Recorded in Practice.* Chicago: G. P. Engelhard, 1902.

———. "Inebriety and Its Symptomology." *Quarterly Journal of Inebriety* 2, no. 4 (September 1878): 193–98.

———. "Inebriety Caused by Psychical Traumatism" *Quarterly Journal of Inebriety* 4, no. 4 (October 1882): 219–30.

———. "The Late Dr. Albert Day—A Biographical Sketch." *Quarterly Journal of Inebriety* 18 (1896): 51–55.

———. "The Medical Treatment of Inebriety." *Journal of the American Medical Association* 27, no. 19 (1896): 993–95.

———. "New Sources of Danger in the Use of Opium." *Journal of the American Medical Association* 35, no. 6 (August 11, 1900): 338–42.

———. "Some New Studies of the Opium Disease," *Quarterly Journal of Inebriety* 14, no. 2 (April 1892): 102–12.

Cullen, William. *First Lines of the Practice of Physic.* Vol. 2. Edinburgh: Bell & Bradfute and Adam Black, 1816.

Cummings, Charles. "Letters of Charles Cummings, Provost-Marshall of Fairfax Courthouse, Winter 1862–1863." *Yearbook: The Historical Society of Fairfax County, Virginia* 22, no. 51 (1989/1990): 45–69.

Cutter, Calvin. *The Physiological Family Physician, Designed for Families and Individuals.* West Brookfield, MA: Merriam and Cooke, 1845.

Da Costa, J[acob] M[endes]. *Medical Diagnosis, with Special Reference to Practical Medicine: A Guide to the Knowledge and Discrimination of Diseases.* 9th ed. Philadelphia: J. B. Lippincott, 1900.

———. "On Irritable Heart: A Clinical Study of a Form of Functional Cardiac Disorder and Its Consequences." *American Journal of Medical Sciences* 121, no. 1 (January 1871): 2–52.

———. "Some Observations on the Use of the Hydrochlorate of Cocaine, Especially Its Hypodermic Use." *Transactions of the College of Physicians of Philadelphia*, [3rd ser.], vol. 7 (1884): 39–48.

Dai, Bingham. *Opium Addiction in Chicago.* Montclair, NJ: Paterson Smith, 1970.

"Dangerous Drugs: How to Control Effectually All Such Horrible Habits." *Southern Cultivator and Dixie Farmer* 45 (1887): 70.

"Dangers of Giving Opiates to Children." *Boston Medical and Surgical Journal*, April 23, 1834, 174.

Daniels, E. D. *A Twentieth Century History and Biographical Record of La Porte County, Indiana.* New York: Lewis, 1904.

Day, Albert. *Inebriety and Its Cure: A Paper Read before the Suffolk District Medical Society, December 30, 1876.* Boston: C. W. Calkins, 1876.

———. *The Journal of Inebriety—Extra: The Curability of Inebriety. A Paper Read before the American Association for the Cure of Inebriety, at Chicago, September 12, 1878.* Hartford, CT: Case, Lockwood & Brainard, 1878.

Day, Horace B. *The Opium Habit: With Suggestions as to the Remedy.* New York: Harper & Brothers, 1868.

"The Death of Dr. Albert Day." *Journal of the American Medical Association* 22, no. 21 (May 26, 1894): 815.

De Forest, John William. *Miss Ravenel's Conversion from Secession to Loyalty.* New York: Harper & Brothers, 1867.

Delavan, Edward C. *To the Army of the United States.* Albany: C. Van Benthuysen, December 1, 1862.

De Quincey, Thomas. *Confessions of an English Opium-Eater.* Edited by Richard Garnett. London: Kegan Paul, Trench, 1885.

"Disorderly House." In *The Laws of Texas, 1822–1897.* Vol. 9, compiled and arranged by H. P. N. Gammel. Austin: Gammel, 1898.

Doggett's New York City Directory for 1845 & 1846. New York: John Doggett Jr., 1845.

"Domestic Intelligence-Medical Society of the State of Pennsylvania." *Medical News and Library* 26, no. 308 (July 1868): 104.

Douglass, Frederick. *Narrative of the Life of Frederick Douglass, an American Slave.* Boston: Anti-Slavery Office, 1845.

Downs, Henry S. "On the Mutually Antidotal Properties of Opium and Belladonna, with Cases." In *Transactions of the Medical Society of the State of New York for the Year 1865*, 157–61. Albany: C. Wendell, Printer, 1865.

Dunglison, Robley. *Medical Lexicon: a Dictionary of Medical Science, Containing a Concise Account of the Various Subjects and Terms, with the French and Other Synonymes, Notices of Climate, and of Celebrated Mineral Waters, Formulae for Various Officinal and Empirical Preparations, Etc.* 5th ed. Philadelphia: Lea and Blanchard, 1845.

Eaton, Harriet. *This Birth Place of Souls: The Civil War Nursing Diary of Harriet Eaton.* Edited by Jane E. Schultz. New York: Oxford University Press, 2011.

"Editorial Department." *Buffalo Medical and Surgical Journal* 3 (1863–64): 37–38.

"Effects of Opium Eating." *Boston Medical and Surgical Journal,* April 4, 1832, 128.

"The Effects of the Hypodermic Application of Morphine." *Bulletin of the New York Academy of Medicine,* October 1864, 318–21.

The Epitome: A Monthly Retrospect of American Practical Medicine 6 (1885): 14–15.

Ewell, James. *The Medical Companion, or Family Physician.* 6th ed. Baltimore: B. Edes, 1822.

———. *The Medical Companion, or Family Physician.* 10th ed. Philadelphia: Thomas, Cowperthwait, 1847.

———. *The Medical Companion, or Family Physician* [. . .], 11th ed. Philadelphia: Charles DeSilver, 1859.

"Excessive Opium Eating." *Boston Medical and Surgical Journal,* January 20, 1870, 56.

"Experience with Morphine." *Medical Review: A Weekly Journal of Medicine and Surgery,* January 5, 1895, 10–11.

Fisher, Theodore W. "Habitual Drunkenness." *Boston Medical and Surgical Journal,* January 6, 1881, 8–11.

Fleming, Alexander. "Lecture on the Treatment of the Habit of Opium-Eating." *Richmond Medical Journal,* May 1868, 368–75.

Formento, F[elix], Jr. *Notes and Observations on Army Surgery.* New Orleans: L. E. Marchand, 1863.

Foote, George F. *Inebriety and Opium Eating: In Both Cases a Disease. Method of Treatment, and Conditions of Success.* Portland, ME: Tucker Printing House, 1877.

Frost, C[arleton] P. "Opium; Its Uses and Abuses." In *Transactions of the Vermont Medical Society for the Years 1869 and 1870.* Burlington: R. S. Styles, 1870.

Galen. "On Antidotes." In *Greek Medicine: Being Extracts Illustrative of Medical Writers from Hippocrates to Galen,* trans. Arthur J. Brock, 196–97. London: J. M. Dent & Sons, 1929.

Goldsmith, M. "Of the Duties of Surgeons" [Louisville: Medical Director's Office, Army of Kentucky, 1862], US National Library of Medicine Digital Collections, http://resource.nlm.nih.gov/101533420.

Goolrick, John T. *Historical Fredericksburg: The Story of an Old Town.* Richmond: Whittet & Shepperson, 1922.

Gould, S. W. "The Opium Habit." *Medical and Surgical Reporter* 38 (June 22, 1878): 496–97.

Gunn, John C. *Gunn's Domestic Medicine, or Poor Man's Friend.* 2nd ed. Knoxville, TN: F. S. Heiskell, 1833.

———. *Gunn's Domestic Medicine, or Poor Man's Friend.* Rev. ed. New York: Charles M. Saxton, 1847.

Hammond, William A., ed. *Military Medical and Surgical Essays Prepared for the United States Sanitary Commission.* Philadelphia: J. B. Lippincott, 1864.

———. *On Certain Conditions of Nervous Derangement, Somnambulism—Hypnotism—Hysteria—Hysteriod Affections, Etc.* New York: G. P. Putnam's Sons, 1881.

———. *On Wakefulness: With an Introductory Chapter on the Physiology of Sleep.* Philadelphia: J. B. Lippincott, 1866.

———. "Remarks on Cocaine and the So-called Cocaine Habit." *Journal of Nervous and Mental Disease* 13 (1886): 754–58.

———. *A Treatise on Diseases of the Nervous System*. New York: D. Appleton, 1871.
Happel, T. J. "Morphinism from the Standpoint of the General Practitioner." *Journal of the American Medical Association* 35 (1900): 407.
Harnan, William, "A Case of Morphine Narcosis." *New Orleans Medical and Surgical Journal*, n.s., vol. 13 (1885–86): 701–2.
Harrison, George L. *A Collection of All the Lunacy Laws of the States and Territories of the United States to the Year 1883, Inclusive. Also the Laws of England on Insanity, Legislation in Canada on Private Houses, and Important Portions of the Lunacy Laws of Germany, France, etc.* Philadelphia: Privately printed, 1884.
Harrison, James Bower. "The Psychology of Opium Eating." *Littell's Living Age*, June 24, 1854, 579–88.
Hartsock, Andrew Jackson. *Soldier of the Cross: The Civil War Diary and Correspondence of Rev. Andrew Jackson Hartsock*. Edited by James C. and Eleanor A. Duram. Manhattan, KA: Military Affairs/Aerospace Historian, 1979.
Hening, William Waller. *The Statutes at Large: Being a Collection of All the Laws of Virginia, from the First Session of the Legislature in the Year 1619*. Vol. 6. Richmond, 1819.
Hinsdale, Guy. "S. Weir Mitchell, M.D., L.L.D." *International Clinics*, 12th ser., vol. 1. Philadelphia: J. B. Lippincott, 1902.
The History of Warren County, Ohio. Chicago: W. H. Beers, 1882.
Hitchcock, Edward. *An Essay on Temperance, Addressed Particularly to Students and the Young Men of America*. 2nd ed. Amherst, MA: J. S. & C. Adams, 1830.
Holston, John G. F. "Surgical Reminiscences of an Old Practitioner." *Medical and Surgical Reporter* 20, no. 9 (February 27, 1869): 161–63.
Holt, Daniel M. *A Surgeon's Civil War: The Letters and Diary of Daniel M. Holt, M.D.* Edited by James M. Greiner, Janet L. Coryell, and James R. Smither. Kent: Kent State University Press, 1994.
Hon, Benton J. "Coca in the Opium Habit." *Louisville Medical News: A Weekly Journal of Medicine and Surgery* 9–10 (August 7, 1880): 63–64.
Hopkins, H. R. "The Intoxicant Habit." *Transactions of the Medical Society of the State of New York* (1887): 193–207.
"How the Opium Habit Is Acquired." *Journal of the American Medical Association* 11, no. 12 (1888): 419–20.
Howison, William. "Precautions in Prescribing Medicine." *Boston Medical and Surgical Journal*, June 6, 1832, 261–66.
Hubbard, Frederick Heman. *The Opium Habit and Alcoholism: A Treatise on the Habits of Opium and Its Compounds; Alcohol; Chloral-Hydrate; Chloroform; Bromide Potassium; and Cannabis Indica: Including Their Therapeutical Indications: With Suggestions for Treating Various Painful Complications*. New York: A. A. Barnes, 1881.
Hughes, C. H. "Hydrate of Chloral in Trismus and Tetanus of Newborn Children." *American Practitioner: A Monthly Journal of Medicine and Surgery*, September 1874, 190.
———. "The Opium Psycho-Neurosis—Chronic Meconism or Papaverism." *Alienist and Neurologist* 5, no. 1 (January 1, 1884): 123–45.
"Inebriates Home for Kings Co. Near Bay Ridge, New York." In *Proceedings of the Sixth Meeting, American Association for the Cure of Inebriates*, 102–3. Baltimore: William K. Boyle & Son's Steam Book Press, 1875.

"The Inebriates Home Fort Hamilton, N.Y." *Quarterly Journal of Inebriety* 4, no. 2 (April 1881): 13.

Jameson, Horatio Gates. *American Domestic Medicine; or, Medical Admonisher.* Baltimore: F. Lucas, 1817.

Jarvis, Edward. *On the Comparative Liability of Males and Females to Insanity and their Comparative Curability and Mortality when Insane.* Utica: New York State Lunatic Asylum, 1850.

Johnson, Charles Beneulyn. *Muskets and Medicine or Army Life in the Sixties.* Philadelphia: F. A. Davis, 1917.

Jones, John. *Plain Concise Practical Remarks on the Treatment of Wounds and Fractures.* New York: John Holt, 1775.

Journal of Health 1, no. 5 (November 11, 1829): 66.

Journal of Insanity 18 (1861–62): 318.

Journal of Insanity 19 (1862–63): 309.

Journal of Insanity 19 (1862–63): 368.

Journal of Insanity 20 (1863–64): 477.

Journal of Insanity 21 (1864–65): 566.

Journal of Insanity 22 (1865–66): 566–68.

Journal of Insanity 23 (1866–67): 572–73.

Journal of Insanity 25 (1868–69): 105.

Journal of Insanity 26 (1869–70): 363.

Journal of Insanity 29 (1872–73): 116.

Journal of Insanity 31 (1874–75): 231.

Journal of Insanity 28 (1871–72): 50.

Kane, H. H. *Drugs that Enslave: The Opium, Morphine, Chloral and Hashisch Habits.* Philadelphia: Presley Blakiston, 1881.

———. *The Hypodermic Injection of Morphia: Its History, Advantages and Dangers.* New York: Chas. L. Bermingham, 1880.

The Keeley Institutes of the United States, Canada, and Other Countries. [Dwight(?), IL]: Leslie E. Keeley, [1895?].

Keeley, Leslie E. *The Morphine Eater, or, From Bondage to Freedom.* Dwight, IL: C. L. Palmer, 1881.

Keen, W. W. "Military Surgery in 1861 and in 1918." *Annals of the American Academy of Political and Social Science* 80 (November 1918): 11–22.

Kolb, Lawrence, and A. G. Du Mez. "The Prevalence and Trend of Drug Addiction in the United States and Factors Influencing It." *Public Health Reports* 39, no. 21 (May 23, 1924): 1179–1204.

Letterman, Jonathan. *Medical Recollections of the Army of the Potomac.* New York: D. Appleton, 1866.

Lindesmith, Alfred R. *Addiction and Opiates.* Chicago: Aldine, 1968.

Lineberger, Walter F. *Milestones in the War against the Narcotic Peril.* Washington, DC: Government Printing Office, 1925.

List of Pensioners on the Roll January 1, 1883. Vols. 1–5. Washington, DC: Government Printing Office, 1883.

Lowell, Maria. "An Opium Fantasy." In *The Poems of Maria Lowell.* Cambridge, MA: Riverside Press, 1907.

Ludlow, Fitz Hugh. *The Hasheesh Eater: Being Passages from the Life of a Pythagorean.* 4th ed. New York: Harper & Brothers, 1857.

Mann, Edward C. "Cases Illustrative of the Treatment of Alcoholic and Opium Inebriety." *Practice* 1, no. 12 (December 15, 1887): 393–401.

———. "A Plea for Medical Jurisprudence to Keep Pace with the Conclusions of Science Respecting the Disease." *Quarterly Journal of Inebriety* 6, no. 2 (April 1884): 65–74.

Manual of Military Surgery Prepared for the Use of the Confederate States Army Illustrated by Order the Surgeon-General. Richmond, VA: Ayers & Wade, 1863.

Marcy, E. E. "Electro-Magnetism a Remedy for Opium Poisoning." *Boston Medical and Surgical Journal,* July 12, 1843, 463.

Marks, Jeannette. "The Curse of Narcotism in America—A Reveille." *American Journal of Public Health* (April 1915): 314–22.

———. *Leviathan: The Record of a Struggle and a Triumph.* New York: Hodder & Stoughton, 1913.

Marsh, John. *Temperance Recollections. Labors, Defeats, Triumphs. An Autobiography.* New York: C. Scribner, 1866.

Maryland Medical Journal: A Weekly Journal of Medicine and Surgery, November 2, 1889, 3.

Mattison, J. B. "The Curability of Opium Addiction." *Quarterly Journal of Inebriety* 5, no. 4 (October 1883): 252–57.

———. "A Curious Case of Opium Addiction." *Maryland Medical Journal* 10 (1884): 849–51.

———. "The Ethics of Opium Habitués." *Brooklyn Medical Journal* 2 (July–December 1888): 125–30.

———. "Opium Addiction among Medical Men." *Medical Record* 23 (June 9, 1883): 621–23.

———. "'Opium Antidotes,' and Their Vendors." *Journal of the American Medical Association* 7, no. 21 (November 20, 1886): 568–70.

———. "Prevention and Treatment of Opium Addiction." *Louisville Medical News,* February 23, 1884, 113–15.

———. "The Remedy for the Diminution of Opium Inebriety." *Quarterly Journal of Inebriety* 2, no. 4 (September 1878): 207–8.

McGown, Thompson. *A Practical Treatise on the Most Common Diseases of the South.* Philadelphia: Grigg, Elliot, 1849.

McGuire, Hunter. "Last Wound of the Late Gen. Jackson (Stonewall)—The Amputation of the Arm—His Last Moments and Death." *Richmond Medical Journal* 1 (May 1866): 403–12.

M'Dowell, A. W. "Hospital Observations upon Negro Soldiers." *American Practitioner,* September 1874, 155–68.

"Medical and Surgical Cases at Port Royal, S.C." *Boston Medical and Surgical Journal,* November 6, 1862, 260–76.

Medical Council [Philadelphia] 19 (1914): 280.

The Medical Gazette: A Weekly Review of the Medical Sciences 4 (1870): 44.

The Medical News 31–32 (1873): 124.

"Memoir of the Milford Bard." In *The Poetical and Prose Writings of Dr. John Lofland, the Milford Bard [. . .].* Baltimore: John Murphy, 1853.

Merwin, Samuel. *Drugging a Nation: The Story of China and the Opium Curse.* New York: Fleming H. Revell, 1908.

Mitchell, John K. *Remote Consequences of Injuries of Nerves and Their Treatment:*

An Examination of the Present Condition of Wounds Received 1863–65, with Additional Illustrative Cases. Philadelphia: Lea Brothers, 1895.

Mitchell, S[ilas] Weir. *Doctor and Patient*. Philadelphia: J. B. Lippincott, 1888.

———. *Injuries of Nerves and Their Consequences*. Philadelphia: J. B. Lippencott, 1872.

———. "The Medical Department in the Civil War." *Journal of the American Medical Association* 62, no. 19 (May 9, 1914): 1145–450.

———. *On the Effect of Opium and Its Derivative Alkaloids*. [Philadelphia?], [1870?].

Mitchell, S[ilas] Weir, George R. Morehouse, and William W. Keen, *Gunshot Wounds, and Other Injuries of Nerves*. Philadelphia: J. B. Lippincott, 1864.

Mitchell, S[ilas] Weir, William W. Keen, and George R. Morehouse. "The Antagonism of Atropia and Morphia, Founded upon Observations and Experiments Made at the USA Hospital for Injuries and Diseases of the Nervous System." *Galveston Medical and Surgical Journal* 2, no. 1 (January 1867): 721–29.

———. "Morphiomania." *Boston Medical and Surgical Journal*, March 14, 1889, 271–72.

———. "On the Antagonism of Atropia and Morphia, Founded upon Observations and Experiments Made at the U.S.A. Hospital for Injuries and Diseases of the Nervous System." *Boston Medical and Surgical Journal*, August 31, 1865, 118–21.

Morris, F. Baldwin. "The Panorama of a Life, and Experience in Association and Battling with Opium and Alcoholic Stimulants." In *American Perceptions of Drug Addiction: Five Studies, 1872–1912*, edited by Gerald Grob. New York: Arno Press, 1981.

Morris, J. Cheston. "Obituary Notices of Members Deceased. Henry Hartshorne." *Proceedings of the American Philosophical Society* 39, no. 164 (October–December 1900): i–xii.

Murray, J., and Nathaniel Chapman. *A System of Materia Medica and Pharmacy*. Vol. 1. Philadelphia: Thomas Dobson, 1815.

Murray, John. *A System of Materia Medica and Pharmacy*. New York: Collins and Hannay, and J. B. Collins, 1834.

National Institute on Drug Abuse. *Research Issues 26: Guide to Drug Abuse Research Terminology*. Edited by Jack E. Nelson, Helen Wallenstein Pearson, Mollie Sayers, and Thomas J. Glynn. US Department of Health and Human Services, 1982.

The National Tribune Soldier's Handbook. Washington, DC: National Tribune, 1898.

New Charlotte Medical Journal 69–70 (1914): 246.

"No. 80: Appendix." *Documents of the US Sanitary Commission*. Vol. 2: Numbers 61 to 95. New York, 1866, [69–70].

Notes and Queries." *American Practitioner: A Monthly Journal of Medicine and Surgery* 1 (1870): 249–50.

The Ohio Medical Journal 1 (1881–82): 562.

"On the Influence of Opium-Eating on Health and Longevity." *American Journal of the Medical Sciences* 10, no. 19 (May 1832): 252–55.

"On the Use of Opium." *Boston Medical and Surgical Journal*, April 18, 1832, 156.

"'Opiokapnism,' or Opium Smoking." *Journal of the American Medical Association* 18, no. 24 (June 4, 1892): 719–20.

"Opium." *Boston Medical and Surgical Journal*, May 10, 1837, 221.

"'Opium Antidotes' Exposed." *Boston Medical and Surgical Journal*, October 26, 1876, 500–501.

"Opium-Eaters and Snuff-Chewers." *Journal of Health* 1, no. 19 (June 9, 1830): 297–99.

Opium Eating: An Autobiographical Sketch by an Habituate. Philadelphia: Claxton, Remsen & Haffelfinger, 1876.
"Opium Eating." *Boston Medical and Surgical Journal*, September 4, 1833, 66.
"Opium Eating." *Boston Medical and Surgical Journal*, June 20, 1872, 412.
"Opium Eating." *Boston Medical and Surgical Journal*, December 9, 1875, 679.
"Opium Eating." *Druggists' Circular & Chemical Gazette*, March 1, 1873, 1.
"Opium Eating in Siam." *Boston Medical and Surgical Journal*, April 26, 1837, 193.
"Opium Habit." *The Bistoury: A Quarterly Medical Journal, Devoted to the Exposition of Charlatanism in Medicine*, January 1, 1879, 94.
Otis, George A. *Photographs of Surgical Cases and Specimens*. Vol. 2. Washington, DC: Surgeon General's Office, 1865.
Packard, Jasper. *History of La Porte County, Indiana, and Its Townships, Towns and Cities*. La Porte, IN, 1876.
The Papers of Jefferson Davis. Vol. 13, 1871–79. Edited by Lynda L. Crist and Suzanne Scott Gibbs. Baton Rouge: Louisiana State University Press, 2012.
Parker, George F. *Recollections of Grover Cleveland*. New York: The Century Co., 1909.
Parrish, Joseph. *The Probe: An Inquiry into the Use of Stimulants and Narcotics: The Social Evils Resulting Therefrom: and Methods of Reform and Cure*. Philadelphia: J. Moore & Sons, [1869].
"Perkins and Company, Canton 1803–1827." *Bulletin of the Business Historical Society* 6, no. 2 (March 1932): 1–5.
Perry, M. S. "Autopsy of an Opium Eater." *Boston Medical and Surgical Journal*, December 23, 1835, 319–20.
The Pharmacology of the Newer Materia Medica: Embracing the Botany, Chemistry, Pharmacy and Therapeutics of New Remedies. Edited by George S. Davis. Detroit: George S. Davis, 1889.
The Pharmacopoeia of the United States of America. 4th decennial rev. Philadelphia: J. B. Lippincott, 1864.
The Physicians and Surgeons of the United States. Edited by William B. Atkinson. Philadelphia: Charles Robson, 1878.
The Physician's Visiting List, Diary, and Book of Engagements, for 1852. Philadelphia: Lindsay & Blakiston, 1851.
Pickett, N. B. "Tartar-Emetic and Opium to Infants." *Boston Medical and Surgical Journal*, February 7, 1849, 117–18.
"The Pinel Hospital." *Virginia Medical Monthly* 3 (1877): 303.
"Poisoning by Opium and Belladonna, Used as an Injection." *Boston Medical and Surgical Journal*, December 6, 1830, 682.
Polley, J. B. *A Soldier's Letters to Charming Nellie*. New York: Neale, 1908.
Porcher, Francis Peyre. *Resources of the Southern Fields and Forests, Medical, Economical, and Agricultural: Being Also a Medical Botany of the Confederate States, with Practical Information on the Properties of the Trees, Plants, and Shrubs*. Charleston: Steam-Power Press of Evans & Cogswell, 1863.
"Proceedings of the Association of Medical Superintendents." *Journal of Insanity* 31 (1874–75): 129–240.
Proceedings of the Twenty-Seventh National Encampment of the Grand Army of the Republic at, Indianapolis, Indiana. Milwaukee: Swain & Tate, 1893.

The Public Papers of Grover Cleveland. Washington, DC: Government Printing Office, 1889.

Quarterly Journal of Inebriety 11 (1889): 295.

Quarterly Journal of Inebriety 4, no. 4 (October 1882): 4.

Ramsey, H. A. *The Necrological Appearance of Southern Typhoid Fever in the Negro: With Hints upon It Proplylaxis [sic] and Therapeutic Management [. . .].* Columbia Co., GA: Printed at the Office of the Constitutionalist and Republic, 1852.

"Recent Deaths." *Boston Medical and Surgical Journal,* May 3, 1894, 456.

"Recognition of Inebriety." *Quarterly Journal of Inebriety* 8 (1886): 36–37.

Register of Commissioned and Warrant Officers of the United States Navy and Marine Corps and Reserve Officers on Active Duty. Washington, DC: Government Printing Office, 1865.

Register of Prescriptions, July–August 1865, Freedman's Hospital New Orleans. www.familysearch.org/ark:/61903/3:1:3QS7-99GF-5J7B?cc=2333781&wc=STRY-&lang=en&i=0. Accessed July 21, 2022.

"Remarks on the Opium Habit." *Medical and Surgical Reporter* 17, no. 22 (December 1, 1877): 436–37.

Report of the Committee on Intemperance as a Disease (Philadelphia: Collins, 1869).

Richardson, Benjamin Ward. *The Field of Disease: A Book of Preventive Medicine.* Philadelphia: Henry C. Lea's Son, 1884.

Roberts, J. D. "Opium Habit in the Negro." *North Carolina Medical Journal* 15–16 (1885): 206–7.

Roe, Edward Payson. *Without a Home.* New York: Dodd, Mead, 1898.

Rogers, Lewis. "Facts and Reminiscences of the Medical History of Kentucky." *American Practitioner: A Monthly Journal of Medicine and Surgery* 7 (1873): 193–222.

Seeger, C. L. "Opium Eating," *Boston Medical and Surgical Journal,* October 2, 1833, 117–20.

Sell, E. H. M. *The Opium Habit: Its Successful Treatment by the Avena Sativa.* Jersey City, NJ: Evening Journal Print, 1883.

Sewall, J. G. "Opium-Eating and Hypodermic Injection." *Boston Medical and Surgical Journal,* June 2, 1870, 422.

Shaw, William A. *Lectures on the Utility of Temperance Societies.* Washington, NC: 1832.

Sims, J. Marion. *The Bromide of Ethyl as an Anaesthetic.* [New York?]: [Compliments of the author], 1880.

———. *On Ovariotomy.* New York: Appleton, 1873.

———. *On the Treatment of Vesico-Vaginal Fistula.* Philadelphia: Blanchard & Lea, 1853.

———. *The Treatment of Epithelioma of the Cervix Uteri.* New York: William Wood, 1879.

Slack, David B. "Opium in Cholera, Dysentery and Diarrhea." *Boston Medical and Surgical Journal,* September 28, 1830, 530.

Smith, Stephen. *Handbook of Surgical Operations.* 3rd ed. New York: Bailliere Brothers, 1863.

"Some Observations on the Deep Injection of Morphia." *Pacific Medical and Surgical Journal,* October 1878, 212–14.

"Some Private Asylums and Homes." *Quarterly Journal of Inebriety* 11 (1889): 98–100.

"Spurious Opium." *Boston Medical and Surgical Journal,* July 15, 1846, 483–84.

Stevens, C. A. *Berdan's United States Sharpshooters in the Army of the Potomac, 1861–1865.* St. Paul: Price-McGill, 1892.

Stillman, Charles F. *The Life Insurance Examiner: A Practical Treatise upon Medical Examinations for Life Insurance.* New York: Spectator, 1888.

Stout, Arthur B. *Chinese Immigration and the Physiological Causes of the Decay of a Nation.* San Francisco: Agnew & Deffebach, 1862.

Straight, N. A. *Roster of All Regimental Surgeons and Assistant Surgeons in the Late War, with Their Service, and Last-Known Post-Office Address.* [Washington, DC?]: N. A. Straight, 1882.

"Suicidal Death from Opium, With Some Unusual Symptoms." *Boston Medical and Surgical Journal*, December 10, 1834, 284–86.

"A Symposium on Drugs." *Medical Review of Reviews: A Monthly Magazine of the Medical Sciences* 22, no 1 (January 1916): 15–26.

A System of Medicine. Vol. 8. Edited by Thomas Clifford Albutt. New York, Macmillan, 1899.

Thacher, James. *American Modern Practice; or, a Simple Method of Prevention and Cure of Diseases.* Boston: Ezra Read, 1817.

———. *American Modern Practice; or, a Simple Method of Prevention and Cure of Diseases.* New and improved ed. Boston: Cottons & Barnard, 1826.

———. *The American New Dispensatory.* 4th ed. Boston: Thomas B. Wait, 1821.

Tipton, F. "The Negro Problem from a Medical Standpoint." *New York Medical Journal* (1886): 569–74.

"Treatment of Diarrhea and Dysentery." *American Journal of the Medical Sciences*, n.s., vol. 47 (January 1864): 238–39.

"Treatment of Opiamania and Morphiamania." *Quarterly Journal of Inebriety* 1, no. 2 (March 1877): 113–16.

Tully, William. "Experiments with Narcotine: Results of Experiments and Observations." *Boston Medical and Surgical Journal*, August 15, 1832, 5–12.

Turner, J. Edward. *The History of the First Inebriate Asylum in the World: By its Founder; an Account of His Indictment, Also a Sketch of the Woman's National Hospital, by its Projector.* New York: J. Edward Turner, 1888.

United States Pension Bureau. *General Instructions to Special Examiners of the United States Pension Office.* Washington, DC: Government Printing Office, 1881.

US Statutes at Large. Vol. 13. Boston: Little, Brown, 1866.

Watson, I. A. "Caution in the Use of Chloral Hydrate." *Medical and Surgical Reporter*, January 27, 1872, 77.

Webster, E. M. "Opium Eating Cured by Belladonna Poisoning." *Boston Medical and Surgical Journal*, January 13, 1870, 23–24.

Whitney, Daniel H. *The Family Physician and Guide to Health.* Penn-Yan: H. Gilbert, 1833.

———. *The Family Physician, or Every Man His Own Doctor.* New York: N. and J. White, 1834.

Williams, Edward Huntington. *Opiate Addiction: Its Handling and Treatment.* New York: Macmillan, 1922.

Wilson, Daniel. *An Inaugural Dissertation on the Morbid Effects of Opium upon the Human Body [. . .].* Philadelphia: Printed for the Author, by Solomon W. Condrad, 1803.

Wilson, J. C. "The Causes and Prevention of the Opium Habit and Kindred Affections." *Boston Medical and Surgical Journal*, November 22, 1888, 505–6.

Wood, George B., and Franklin Bache. *The Dispensatory of the United States of America.* Philadelphia: Grigg and Elliot, 1833.

———. *The Dispensatory of the United States of America.* 6th ed. Philadelphia: Grigg and Elliot, 1845.

Wood, Thomas Fanning. *Doctor to the Front: The Recollections of Confederate Surgeon Thomas Fanning Wood*. Edited by Donald B. Koonce. Knoxville: University of Tennessee Press, 2000.

Woodbury, Frank. "Physic-Tippling and Medicine-Bibbling." *Annals of Hygiene* 1 (1884–86): 195.

Woodward, Joseph Janvier. *The Hospital Steward's Manual: For the Instruction of Hospital Stewards, Ward-Masters, and Attendants, in their Several Duties*. Philadelphia: J. B. Lippincott, 1862.

———. *Outlines of the Chief Camp Diseases of the United States Armies as Observed during the Present War*. Philadelphia: J. B. Lippincott, 1863.

Woodward, Samuel Bayard. *Essays on Asylums for Inebriates*. Worcester, MA: n.p., 1838.

Woolley, B[asil] M. *The Opium Habit and Its Cure*. [Atlanta]: Atlanta Constitution Print, [1879].

Wright, Isaac. *Wright's Family Medicine, or System of Domestic Practice*. Madisonville, TN: J. F. Grant, 1833.

Wright, M. B. *Drunkenness, Its Nature and Cure; Or Asylums for Inebriates. An Address Delivered before the Ohio State Medical Society at Its Annual Session, June 1859*. Columbus: Follett, Foster, 1859.

Yandell, Lunsford P. "On the Origin and Treatment of Epidemic Cholera." *American Practitioner: A Monthly Journal of Medicine and Surgery* 4 (1871): 209–25.

Secondary Sources

Abrams, Jeanne E. *Revolutionary Medicine: The Founding Fathers and Mothers in Sickness and in Health*. New York: New York University Press, 2013.

Acker, Caroline Jean. *Creating the American Junkie: Addiction Research in the Classic Era of Narcotic Control*. Baltimore: Johns Hopkins University Press, 2002.

Adams, George Worthington. *Doctors in Blue: The Medical History of the Union Army in the Civil War*. New York: Henry Schuman, 1952.

Adams, Michael C. C. *Living Hell: The Dark Side of the Civil War*. Baltimore: Johns Hopkins University Press, 2014.

Ahmad, Diana L. *The Opium Debate and Chinese Exclusion Laws in the Nineteenth-Century American West*. Reno: University of Nevada Press, 2011.

———. "Opium Smoking, Anti-Chinese Attitudes, and the American Medical Community, 1850–1890." *American Nineteenth Century History* 1, no. 2 (2000): 53–68.

Anderson, David. "Dying of Nostalgia: Homesickness in the Union Army during the Civil War." *Civil War History* 56, no. 3 (September 2010): 247–82.

Andreas, Peter. *Killer High: A History of War in Six Drugs*. New York: Oxford University Press, 2020.

Ash, Stephen V. *Rebel Richmond: Life and Death in the Confederate Capital*. Chapel Hill: University of North Carolina Press, 2019.

Astyrakaki, Elisabeth, Alexandra Papaioannou, and Helen Askitopoulou. "References to Anesthesia, Pain, and Analgesia in the Hippocratic Collection." *Anesthesia and Analgesia* 110, no. 1 (2010): 188–94.

Axelson, Diana. "Women as Victims of Medical Experimentation: J. Marion Sims' Surgery on Slave Women, 1845–1850." *SAGE* 2, no. 2 (Fall 1985): 10–13.

Ayers, Edward L. *In the Presence of Mine Enemies: The Civil War in the Heart of America.* New York: W. W. Norton, 2003.

———. *Thin Light of Freedom: The Civil War and Emancipation in the Heart of America.* New York: W. W. Norton, 2017.

Baldini, AnGee, Michael Von Korff, and Elizabeth H. B. Lin. "A Review of Potential Adverse Effects of Long-Term Opioid Therapy: A Practitioner's Guide." *Primary Care Companion for CNS Disorders* 14, no. 3 (2012). DOI: 10.4088/PCC.11m01326.

Ball, John C., William O. Thompson, and David M. Allen. "Readmission Rates at Lexington Hospital for 43,215 Narcotic Drug Addicts." *Public Health Reports* 85, no. 7 (July 1970): 610–16.

Barclay, Jenifer L. *The Mark of Slavery: Disability, Race, and Gender in Antebellum America.* Champaign: University of Illinois Press, 2021.

Baumohl, Jim. "Inebriate Institutions in North America, 1840–1920." *British Journal of Addiction* 85 (1990): 1185–1204.

Bederman, Gail. *Manliness and Civilization: A Cultural History of Gender and Race in the United States, 1880–1917.* Chicago: University of Chicago Press, 1995.

Bell, Andrew McIlwaine. *Mosquito Soldiers: Malaria, Yellow Fever, and the Course of the American Civil War.* Baton Rouge: Louisiana State University Press, 2010.

Berridge, Virginia. *Opium and the People: Opiate Use and Drug Control Policy in Nineteenth and Early Twentieth Century England.* Rev. ed. London: Free Association, 1999.

Berry, Stephen W. *All that Makes a Man: Love and Ambition in the Civil War South.* Oxford: Oxford University Press, 2003.

———. "The Historian as Death Investigator." In *Weirding the War: Stories from the Civil War's Ragged Edges*, edited by Stephen Berry, 176–88. Athens: University of Georgia Press, 2011.

———. "Origins of the Coroner's Office." *CSI: Dixie.* https://csidixie.org/genesis/origins-coroners-office. Accessed June 16, 2021.

———, ed. *Weirding the War: Stories from the Civil War's Ragged Edges.* Athens: University of Georgia Press, 2011.

Bever, Megan L. *At War with King Alcohol: Debating Drinking and Masculinity in the Civil War.* Chapel Hill: University of North Carolina Press, 2022.

Blackmon, Douglas A. *Slavery by Another Name: The Re-Enslavement of Black Americans from the Civil War to World War II.* New York: Doubleday, 2008.

Blight, David W. *Frederick Douglass: Prophet of Freedom.* New York: Simon & Schuster, 2018.

———. *Race and Reunion: The Civil War in American Memory.* Cambridge, MA: Belknap Press of Harvard University Press, 2001.

Blumberg, Leonard. "American Association for the Study and Cure of Inebriety." *Alcoholism: Clinical and Experimental Research* 2, no. 3 (July 1978): 235–40.

Blustein, Bonnie Ellen. *Preserve Your Love for Science: Life of William A. Hammond, American Neurologist.* New York: Cambridge University Press, 2002.

Bollet, Alfred Jay. *Civil War Medicine: Challenges and Triumphs.* Tucson: Galen Press, 2002.

Bonner, Thomas Neville. *Becoming a Physician: Medical Education in Great Britain, France, Germany, and the United States, 1750–1945.* New York: Oxford University Press, 1995.

Booth, Martin. *Opium: A History.* New York: St. Martin's Griffin, 1999.

Bowen-Murphy, Ashley Elizabeth. "'All Broke Down': Negotiating the Meaning and Management of Civil War Trauma." PhD diss., Brown University, 2017.

Boydston, Jeanne. *Home and Work: Housework, Wages, and the Ideology of Labor in the Early Republic*. New York: Oxford University Press, 1990.

Boyer, Edward W. "Management of Opioid Analgesic Overdose." *New England Journal of Medicine* 367, no. 2 (July 12, 2012): 146–55. www.nejm.org/doi/full/10.1056/NEJMra1202561.

Breen, Benjamin. *The Age of Intoxication: Origins of the Global Drug Trade*. Philadelphia: University of Pennsylvania Press, 2019.

Breslaw, Elaine G. *Lotions, Potions, Pills, and Magic: Health Care in Early America*. New York: New York University Press, 2012.

Brown, Edward M. "'What Shall We Do with the Inebriate?': Asylum Treatment and the Disease Concept of Alcoholism in the Late Nineteenth Century." *Journal of the History of Behavioral Sciences* 21 (January 1985): 48–59.

Browning, Judkin, and Timothy Silver. *An Environmental History of the Civil War*. Chapel Hill: University of North Carolina Press, 2020.

Brumberg, Joan Jacobs. *Fasting Girls: The History of Anorexia Nervosa*. New York: Vintage, 2000.

Burnham, John C. *Health Care in America: A History*. Baltimore: Johns Hopkins University Press, 2015.

Campbell, Nancy D. *Discovering Addiction: The Science and Politics of Substance Abuse Research*. Ann Arbor: University of Michigan Press, 2007.

———. *OD: Naloxone and the Politics of Overdose*. Cambridge, MA: MIT Press, 2020.

Campbell, Nancy D., and David Herzberg. "Gender and Critical Drug Studies: An Introduction and An Invitation." *Contemporary Drug Problems* 44, no. 4 (December 2017): 251–64.

Canaday, Margot. *The Straight State: Sexuality and Citizenship in Twentieth-Century America*. Princeton, NJ: Princeton University Press, 2009.

Carmichael, Peter. *The War for the Common Soldier: How Men Thought, Fought, and Survived in Civil War Armies*. Chapel Hill: The University of North Carolina Press, 2018.

Carroll, Dillon J. "'The God Who Shielded Me Before, Yet Watches Over Us All': Confederate Soldiers, Mental Illness, and Religion." *Civil War History* 61, no. 3 (September 2015): 252–80.

———. *Invisible Wounds: Mental Illness and Civil War Soldiers*. Baton Rouge: Louisiana State University Press, 2021.

Casey, John A., Jr. *New Men: Reconstructing the Image of the Veteran in Late-Nineteenth-Century American Literature and Culture*. New York: Fordham University Press, 2015.

Cashin, Joan E. *A Family Venture: Men and Women on the Southern Frontier*. New York: Oxford University Press, 1991.

———. *War Stuff: The Struggle for Human and Environmental Resources in the American Civil War*. New York: Cambridge University Press, 2018.

Cassedy, James H. *Medicine in America*. Baltimore: Johns Hopkins University Press, 1991.

Chen, Constance "'Seeds for a New Life': Modernity and the Pacific Turn in the Progressive Era." *Journal of the Gilded Age and Progressive Era* 19, no. 3 (July 2020): 447–72.

Chouvy, Pierre-Arnaud. *Opium: Uncovering the Politics of the Poppy*. Cambridge, MA: Harvard University Press, 2010.

Clark, Claire D. *The Recovery Revolution: The Battle over Addiction Treatment in the United States*. New York: Columbia University Press, 2017.

Clark, Elizabeth B. "'The Sacred Rights of the Weak': Pain, Sympathy, and the Culture of Individual Rights in Antebellum America." *Journal of American History* 82, no. 2 (September 1995): 463–93.
Clarke, Frances. "So Lonesome I Could Die: Nostalgia and Debates over Emotional Control in the Civil War North." *Journal of Social History* 41, no. 2 (Winter 2007): 253–82.
———. *War Stories: Suffering and Sacrifice in the Civil War North*. Chicago: University of Chicago Press, 2011.
Clinton, Catherine. *The Plantation Mistress: Women's World in the Old South*. New York: Pantheon, 1982.
Coddington, Ronald S. *Faces of the Civil War Navies: An Album of Union and Confederate Sailors*. Baltimore: Johns Hopkins University Press, 2016.
Cohan, Andrew Wender. *Contraband: Smuggling and the Birth of the American Century*. New York: W. W. Norton, 2015.
Cohen, Michael M. "Jim Crow's Drug War: Race, Coca Cola, and the Southern Origins of Drug Prohibition." *Southern Cultures* 12, no. 3 (Fall 2006): 55–79.
Collett, Beverly-Jane. "Opioid Tolerance: The Clinical Perspective." *British Journal of Anaesthesia* 81 (1998): 58–68.
Conrad, Peter. *The Medicalization of Society: On the Transformation of Human Conditions into Treatable Disorders*. Baltimore: Johns Hopkins University Press, 2007.
Conrad, Peter, and Kristin K. Barker. "The Social Construction of Illness: Key Insights and Policy Implications." *Journal of Health and Social Behavior* 51, no. 1, supp. (March 2010): S67–79.
Cooper Owens, Deirdre. *Medical Bondage: Race, Gender, and the Origins of American Gynecology*. Athens: University of Georgia Press, 2017.
Costa, Dora L., Noelle Yetter, and Heather DeSomer. "Intergenerational Transmission of Paternal Trauma among US Civil War Ex-POWs." *Proceedings of the National Academy of Sciences* 115, no. 44 (October 30, 2018): 11215–220.
———. "Wartime Health Shocks and Postwar Socioeconomic Status and Mortality of Union Army Veterans and Their Children." *Journal of Health Economics* 70 (March 2020). https://doi.org/10.1016/j.jhealeco.2019.102281.
Courtwright, David T. "Addiction and the Science of History." *Addiction* 107, no. 3 (2012): 486–92.
———. *Dark Paradise: A History of Opiate Addiction in America*. 1982. Reprint, Cambridge, MA: Harvard University Press, 2001.
———. *Forces of Habit: Drugs and the Making of the Modern World*. Cambridge, MA: Harvard University Press, 2001.
———. "The Hidden Epidemic: Opiate Addiction and Cocaine Use in the South, 1860–1920." *Journal of Southern History* 49, no. 1 (February 1983): 57–72.
———. "Opiate Addiction as a Consequence of the Civil War." *Civil War History* 24, no. 2 (June 1978): 110–11.
———. "Opiate Addiction in the American West, 1850–1920." *Journal of the West* 21, no. 3 (July 1982): 23–31.
———. "Preventing and Treating Narcotic Addiction—A Century of Federal Drug Control." *New England Journal of Medicine* 373, no. 22 (November 26, 2015): 2095–97.
Cowen, David L., and Donald F. Kent. "Medical and Pharmaceutical Practice in 1854." *Pharmacy in History* 39, no. 3 (1997): 91–100.

Cowen, David L., Louis D. King, and Nicholas G. Lordi. "Nineteenth Century Drug Therapy: Computer Analysis of the 1854 Prescription File of a Burlington Pharmacy." *Journal of the Medical Society of New Jersey* 78, no. 11 (October 1981): 758–61.

Crowley, John W. "Slaves to the Bottle: Gough's *Autobiography* and Douglass's *Narrative*." In *The Serpent in the Cup: Temperance in American Literature*, edited by David S. Reynolds and Debra J. Rosenthal, 115–35. Amherst: University of Massachusetts Press, 1997.

Crowley, John W., and William L. White. *Drunkard's Refuge: The Lessons of the New York State Inebriate Asylum*. Amherst: University of Massachusetts Press, 2004.

Cunningham, H. H. *Doctors in Gray: The Confederate Medical Service*. Baton Rouge: Louisiana State University Press, 1998.

Cypel, Yasmin S., D. DePhilippis, and V. J. Davey. "Substance Use in US Vietnam War Era Veterans and Nonveterans: Results from the Vietnam Era Health Retrospective Observational Study." *Substance Use & Misuse* 58, no. 7 (2023): 858–70.

Dark, Shane, Sarah Larney, and Michael Farrell. "Yes, People Can Die from Opiate Withdrawal." *Addiction* 112, no. 2 (February 2017): 199–200.

Davenport-Hines, Richard. *The Pursuit of Oblivion: A Global History of Narcotics*. New York: W. W. Norton, 2003.

Dean, Eric T., Jr. *Shook over Hell: Post-Traumatic Stress, Vietnam, and the Civil War*. Cambridge, MA: Harvard University Press, 1997.

"Definition of Addiction." American Society of Addiction Medicine. Updated September 15, 2019. www.asam.org/quality-care/definition-of-addiction.

Devine, Shauna. "Civil War Health and Medicine." In *Cambridge History of the Civil War*. Vol. 2, *Affairs of the State*, edited by Aaron Sheehan-Dean, 278–84. New York: Cambridge University Press, 2019.

———. *Learning from the Wounded: The Civil War and the Rise of American Medical Science*. Chapel Hill: University of North Carolina Press, 2014.

Dewey, Joseph. "American Association for the Study and Cure of Inebriety." In *The SAGE Encyclopedia of Alcohol: Social, Cultural, and Historical Perspectives*, edited by Scott C. Martin, 122–24. Los Angeles: SAGE, 2014.

Dormandy, Thomas. *Opium: Reality's Dark Dream*. New Haven, CT: Yale University Press, 2012.

Downs, Gregory P. *After Appomattox: Military Occupation and the Ends of the War*. Cambridge, MA: Harvard University Press, 2015.

Downs, Jim. *Sick from Freedom: African-American Illness and Suffering during the Civil War and Reconstruction*. Oxford: Oxford University Press, 2012.

Duffy, John. "Medical Practice in the Ante Bellum South." *Journal of Southern History* 25, no. 1 (February 1959): 53–72.

Dwyer, Ellen. "Civil Commitment Laws in Nineteenth-Century New York." *Behavioral Sciences & the Law* 6, no. 1 (1988): 79–98.

———. *Homes for the Mad: Life Inside Two Nineteenth-Century Asylums*. New Brunswick, NJ: Rutgers University Press, 1987.

Ebert, Myrl. "The Rise and Development of the American Medical Periodical, 1797–1850." *Bulletin of the Medical Library Association* 40, no. 3 (1952): 243–76.

Edwards-Grossi, Élodie. *Mad with Freedom: The Political Economy of Blackness, Insanity, and Civil Rights in the US South, 1840–1940*. Baton Rouge: Louisiana State University Press, 2023.

Egerton, Douglas R. *Heirs of an Honorable Name: The Decline of the Adams Family and the Rise of Modern America*. New York: Basic Books, 2019.

Emberton, Carole. "Unwriting the Freedom Narrative: A Review Essay." *Journal of Southern History* 82, no. 2 (May 2016): 377–94.

Farber, David. *Crack: Rock Cocaine, Street Capitalism, and the Decade of Greed*. New York: Cambridge University Press, 2019.

Faust, Drew Gilpin. *This Republic of Suffering: Death and the American Civil War*. New York: Vintage, 2009.

———. "'We Should Grow Too Fond of It': Why We Love the Civil War." *Civil War History* 50, no. 4 (December 2004): 368–83.

Fett, Sharla. *Working Cures: Healing, Health, and Power on Southern Slave Plantations*. Chapel Hill: University of North Carolina Press, 2002.

Fialka, Andrew. *Hope to Never See It: A Graphic History of Guerrilla Violence during the American Civil War*. Illustrated by Anderson Carman. Athens: University of Georgia Press, 2025.

Fink, David S., Suzanne P. Lindsay, Donald J. Slymen, Alex H. Kral, and Ricky N. Bluthenthal. "Abscess and Self-Treatment among Injection Drug Users at Four California Syringe Exchanges and Their Surrounding Communities." *Substance Use & Misuse* 48, no. 7 (2013): 523–31.

Flannery, Michael A. *Civil War Pharmacy: A History of Drugs, Drug Supply and Provision, and Therapeutics for the Union and Confederacy*. New York: Pharmaceutical Products Press, 2004.

———. "The Life of a Hospital Steward: The Civil War Journal of Spencer Bonsall." *Pharmacy in History* 42, no. 3/4 (January 1, 2000): 87–98.

———. "Medicine and Health Care." In *Blackwell Companion to the Civil War Era*, edited by Aaron Sheehan-Dean, 590–607. West Sussex, UK: John Wiley & Sons, 2014.

Foner, Eric. *Reconstruction: America's Unfinished Revolution, 1863–1877*. New York: Harper & Row, 1989.

Foote, Lorien. *The Gentlemen and the Roughs: Violence, Honor, and Manhood in the Union Army*. New York: New York University Press, 2010.

Foster, Anne L. *The Long War on Drugs*. Durham, NC: Duke University Press, 2023.

———. "Opium, the United States, and the Civilizing Mission in Colonial Southeast Asia." *Social History of Alcohol and Drugs* 24, no. 1 (2010): 6–19.

———. "The Philippines, the United States, and the Origins of Global Narcotics Prohibition." *Social History of Alcohol and Drugs* 33, no. 1 (Spring 2019): 13–36.

Franke, Norman H. "Official and Industrial Aspects of Pharmacy in the Confederacy." *Georgia Historical Quarterly* 37, no. 3 (September 1953): 175–87.

Freemon, Frank R. "The First Neurological Research Center: Turner's Lane Hospital during the American Civil War." *Journal of the History of the Neurosciences* 2, no. 2 (1993): 135–42.

———. *Gangrene and Glory: Medical Care during the American Civil War*. Urbana: Illinois University Press, 2001.

Fuentes, Marisa J. *Dispossessed Lives: Enslaved Women, Violence, and the Archive*. Philadelphia: University of Pennsylvania Press, 2016.

Gabriel, Joseph M. "Restricting the Sale of 'Deadly Poisons': Pharmacists, Drug Regulation, and Narratives of Suffering in the Gilded Age." *Journal of the Gilded Age and Progressive Era* 9, no. 3 (July 2010): 313–36.

Gannon, Barbara A. *The Won Cause: Black and White Comradeship in the Grand Army of the Republic*. Chapel Hill: University of North Carolina Press, 2011.

Garg, Piyush, Asif Ali Hitawala, and Manoj Agarwal. "Cardiotoxic Effects of Raw Opium." *Indian Journal of Critical Care Medicine* 22, no. 1 (January 2018): 46–48.

Genovese, Eugene. *The Sweetness of Life: Southern Planters at Home*. Edited by Douglas Ambrose. New York: Cambridge University Press, 2017.

Gerstle, Gary. "The Civil War and State-Building: A Reconsideration." *Journal of the Civil War Era*. www.journalofthecivilwarera.org/forum-the-future-of-reconstruction-studies/the-civil-war-and-state-building/. Accessed June 4, 2025.

Giesberg, Judith Ann. *Army at Home: Women and the Civil War on the Northern Home Front*. Chapel Hill: University of North Carolina Press, 2009.

———. *Civil War Sisterhood: The U.S. Sanitary Commission and Women's Politics in Transition*. Boston: Northeastern University Press, 2000.

———. *Sex and the Civil War: Soldiers, Pornography, and the Making of American Morality*. Chapel Hill: University of North Carolina Press, 2017.

Ginzberg, Lori D. *Women and the Work of Benevolence: Morality, Politics, and Class in the Nineteenth-Century United States*. New Haven, CT: Yale University Press, 1990.

Glymph, Thavolia. *The Women's Fight: The Civil War's Battles for Home, Freedom, and Nation*. Chapel Hill: University of North Carolina Press, 2020.

Gonaver, Wendy. *The Peculiar Institution and the Making of Modern Psychiatry, 1840–1880*. Chapel Hill: University of North Carolina Press, 2019.

Gordon, Lesley J. *A Broken Regiment: The 16th Connecticut's Civil War*. Baton Rouge: Louisiana State University Press, 2014.

———. *Dread Danger: Cowardice and Combat in the American Civil War*. New York: Cambridge University Press, 2024.

Gorman, Kathleen. "Confederate Pensions as Southern Social Welfare." In *Before the New Deal: Social Welfare in the South, 1830–1930*, edited by Elna C. Green, 24–39. Athens: University of Georgia Press, 1999.

Gray, Elizabeth Kelly. *Habit Forming: Drug Addiction in America, 1776–1914*. New York: Oxford University Press, 2023.

———. "The Trade Off: Chinese Opium Traders and Antebellum Reform in the United States, 1815–1860." In *Drugs and Empires: Essays in Modern Imperialism and Intoxication*, edited by James H. Mills and Patricia Barton, 220–42. London: Palgrave Macmillan, 2007.

Greenberg, Amy S. *Manifest Manhood and the Antebellum American Empire*. New York: Cambridge University Press, 2005.

Grob, Gerald N. *The Inner World of American Psychiatry, 1890–1940*. New Brunswick, NJ: Rutgers University Press, 1985.

———. *Mental Illness and American Society, 1875–1940*. Princeton: Princeton University Press, 1983.

———. *Mental Institutions in America: Social Policy to 1875*. New York: Free Press, 1973.

Hacker, J. David. "A Census-Based Count of the Civil War Dead." *Civil War History* 57, no. 4 (December 2011): 307–48.

Haller, John S. "Hypodermic Medication: Early History." *New York State Journal of Medicine* 81, no. 11 (October 1981): 1671–79.

Halttunen, Karen. *Confidence Men and Painted Women: A Study of Middle-Class Culture in America, 1830–1870*. New Haven, CT: Yale University Press, 1982.

Handley-Cousins, Sarah. *Bodies in Blue: Disability in the Civil War North*. Athens: University of Georgia Press, 2019.

———. "'Wrestling at the Gates of Death': Joshua Lawrence Chamberlain and Nonvisible Disability in the Post–Civil War North." *Journal of the Civil War Era* 6, no. 2 (June 2016): 220–42.

Handley-Cousins, Sarah, Jenifer L. Barclay, Moyra Williams Eaton, Jean Franzino, Allison M. Johnson, Fred Pelka. "Disability in the Civil War Era." *Journal of the Civil War Era* 14, no. 2 (June 2024): 194–224.

Hedrick, Joan D. *Harriet Beecher Stowe: A Life*. New York: Oxford University Press, 1995.

Herbert, Christopher. *Gold Rush Manliness: Race and Gender on the Pacific Slope*. Seattle: University of Washington Press, 2018.

Herzberg, David. *White Market Drugs: Big Pharma and the Hidden History of Addiction in America*. Chicago: University of Chicago Press, 2020.

Hickman, Timothy A. "Leslie E. Keeley, the Gold Cure and the 19th-Century Neuroscience of Addiction." *Addiction* 113 (2018): 1739–49.

———. "'Mania Americana': Narcotic Addiction and Modernity in the United States, 1870–1920." *Journal of American History* 90, no. 4 (March 2004): 1269–94.

———. *The Secret Leprosy of Modern Days: Narcotic Addiction and Cultural Crisis in the United States, 1870–1920*. Amherst: University of Massachusetts Press, 2007.

Higby, Greg, and Nydia M. King. "Occasional Bibliographic Note: Primary Sources in the History of American Pharmacy Available Online, no. 3: The Dispensatory of the United States of America, 2nd ed., 1834." *Pharmacy in History* 55, no. 1 (2013): 31–32.

Historic Architecture of La Porte, Indiana: The First 20 Years of the Candlelight Tour. La Porte, IN: People Engaged in Preservation, 2017.

Hoffman, Kelly M., Sophie Trawalter, Jordan R. Axt, and M. Norman Oliver. "Racial Bias in Pain Assessment and Treatment Recommendations, and False Beliefs about Biological Differences between Blacks and Whites." *PNAS* 113, no. 6 (April 19, 2016): 4296–4301.

Hsieh, Wayne Wei-Siang. "'Go to Your Gawd Like a Soldier': Transnational Reflections on Veteranhood." *Journal of the Civil War Era* 5, no. 4 (December 2015): 551–77.

Humphreys, Margaret. *Intensely Human: The Health of the Black Soldier in the American Civil War*. Baltimore: Johns Hopkins University Press, 2008.

———. *Marrow of Tragedy: The Health Crisis of the American Civil War*. Baltimore: Johns Hopkins University Press, 2013.

———. *Yellow Fever and the South*. Baltimore: Johns Hopkins University Press, 1992.

Immerwahr, Daniel. "Burning Down the House: Slavery and Arson in America." *Journal of American History* 110, no. 3 (December 2023): 449–473.

Jacobson, Matthew Frye. *Barbarian Virtues: The United States Encounters Foreign Peoples at Home and Abroad, 1876–1917*. New York: Hill and Wang, 2001.

———. *Whiteness of a Different Color: European Immigrants and the Alchemy of Race*. Cambridge, MA: Harvard University Press, 1999.

Jacomet, Stefanie. "Plant Economy and Village Life in Neolithic Lake Dwellings at the Time of the Alpine Iceman." *Vegetation History and Archaeobotany* 18 (2009): 47–59.

Jaffe, Arnold. *Addiction Reform in the Progressive Age: Scientific and Social Responses to Drug Dependence in the United States, 1870–1930*. New York: Arno Press, 1981.

Jones, Jonathan S. "'Died from Eating Too Much Morphine': Researching Opioid Addiction in Civil War–Era Kentucky." *Register of the Kentucky Historical Society* 122, no. 3–4 (Summer/Autumn 2024): 341–74.

———. "The Life and Death of Frank Clewell, Confederate Veteran: Microhistory and the Civil War–Era South." *North Carolina Historical Review* 98, no. 3 (July 2021): 249–82.

———. "The 'Right' and 'Wrong' Kind of Addict: Iatrogenic Opioid Addiction in Historical Context." *Nursing Clio*, July 25, 2017. https://nursingclio.org/2017/07/25/the-right-and-wrong-kind-of-addict-iatrogenic-opioid-addiction-in-historical-context/.

Jordan, Brian Matthew. *Marching Home: Union Veterans and Their Unending Civil War*. New York: Liveright, 2014.

———. "Veterans in New Fields: Directions for Future Scholarship on Civil War Veterans." In *The War Went On: Reconsidering the Lives of Civil War Veterans*, edited by Brian Matthew Jordan and Evan C. Rothera, 307–20. Baton Rouge: Louisiana University Press, 2020.

Journet, Debra. "Phantom Limbs and 'Body-Ego': S. Weir Mitchell's 'George Dedlow.'" *Mosaic: An Interdisciplinary Critical Journal* 23, no. 1 (Winter 1990): 87–99.

Kalant, H. "Opium Revisited: A Brief Review of Its Nature, Composition, Non-Medical Use, and Relative Risks." *Addiction* 92, no. 3 (March 1997): 267–78.

Kamienski, Lukasz. *Shooting Up: A Short History of Drugs and War*. New York: Oxford University Press, 2016.

Kasson, John F. *Houdini, Tarzan, and the Perfect Man: The White Male Body and the Challenge of Modernity in America*. New York: Hill and Wang, 2001.

Keire, Mara L. "Dope Fiends and Degenerates: The Gendering of Addiction in the Early Twentieth Century." *Journal of Social History* 31, no. 4 (Summer 1999): 809–22.

Kelly, Patrick J. *Creating a National Home: Building the Veterans' Welfare State, 1860–1900*. Cambridge, MA: Harvard University Press, 1997.

Kesten, Joanna May, Ed Holder, Rachel Ayres, Pete Ellis, Steve Taylor, Matthew Hickman, and Graeme Henderson. "Changes in the Development of Opioid Tolerance on Re-Exposure among People Who Use Heroin: A Qualitative Study." *PLoS ONE* 17, no. 6 (June 23, 2022), e0269379. https://doi.org/10.1371/journal.pone.0269379.

Kiechle, Melanie A. *Smell Detectives: An Olfactory History of Nineteenth-Century Urban America*. Seattle: University of Washington Press, 2017.

Kim, Diane S. *The Rise of Opium Prohibition Across Southeast Asia*. Princeton, NJ: Princeton University Press, 2020.

King, Monroe Martin. "Dr. John S. Pemberton: Originator of Coca-Cola." *Pharmacy in History* 29, no. 2 (1987): 85–89.

Kinlock, Timothy W., and Michael S. Gordon. "Heroin and Other Opiates." In *The Handbook of Drugs and Society*, edited by Henry H. Brownstein. London: John Wiley & Sons, 2016.

Kolchin, Peter. *American Slavery: 1619–1877*. First rev. ed. New York: Hill and Wang, 2003.

Kraut, Alan M. *Silent Travelers: Germs, Genes, and the "Immigrant Menace."* Baltimore: Johns Hopkins University Press, 1995.

Kushner, Howard L. "Taking Biology Seriously: The Next Task for Historians of Addiction?" *Bulletin of the History of Medicine* 80, no. 1 (Spring 2006): 115–43.

Lassiter, Matthew D. *The Suburban Crisis: White America and the War on Drugs*. Princeton: Princeton University Press, 2023.

Lazich, Michael C. "American Missionaries and the Opium Trade in Nineteenth-Century China." *Journal of World History* 17, no. 2 (June 2006): 197–223.

Lears, T. J. Jackson. *Fables of Abundance: A Cultural History of Advertising in America*. New York: Basic Books, 1994.

Legan, M. Scott. "Drugs for Louisiana: The Louisiana State Laboratory, 1864–1865." *Louisiana History* 28, no. 2 (Spring 2007): 193–202.

Lemon, Rebecca. *Addiction and Devotion in Early Modern England*. Philadelphia: University of Pennsylvania Press, 2018.

Levine, Harry Gene. "The Discovery of Addiction: Changing Conceptions of Habitual Drunkenness in America." *Journal on Studies of Alcohol* 39, no. 1 (1978): 143–74.

Levine, Lawrence W. *Black Culture and Black Consciousness: Afro-American Folk Thought from Slavery to Freedom*. New York: Oxford University Press, 1977.

Levy, Jonathan. *Freaks of Fortune: The Emerging World of Capitalism and Risk in America*. Cambridge, MA: Harvard University Press, 2012.

Lew-Williams, Beth. *The Chinese Must Go: Violence, Exclusion, and the Making of the Alien in America*. Cambridge, MA: Harvard University Press, 2018.

Lewy, Jonathan. "The Army Disease: Drug Addiction and the Civil War." *War in History* 21, no. 1 (2013): 102–19.

Linderman, Gerald F. *Embattled Courage: The Experience of Combat in the American Civil War*. New York: Free Press, 1987.

Link, William A. *Atlanta, Cradle of the New South: Race and Remembering in the Civil War's Aftermath*. Chapel Hill: University of North Carolina Press, 2013.

Loewer, Peter. *Jefferson's Garden*. Mechanicsburg, PA: Stackpole, 2004.

Long, Gretchen. *Doctoring Freedom: The Politics of African American Medical Care in Slavery and Emancipation*. Chapel Hill: University of North Carolina Press, 2012.

Lord, Francis A. *Civil War Sutlers and Their Wares*. New York: Thomas Yoseloff, 1969.

Luther, Kurt. "Photo Sleuth: Reverse Engineering an Image Macro." *Military Images*, last modified March 15, 2018. https://militaryimages.atavist.com/photo-sleuth-spring-2018 (no longer available).

Macy, Beth. *Dopesick: Dealers, Doctors, and the Drug Company That Addicted America*. Boston: Little, Brown, 2018.

Mahoney, Mary. "Prescribing from the Bookshelf: S. Weir Mitchell and the Therapeutic Value of Restricting Reading." *Fugitive Leaves*, April 12, 2016. https://histmed.collegeofphysicians.org/prescribing-from-the-bookshelf/.

Malleck, Daniel. "'A State Bordering on Insanity?': Identifying Drug Addiction in Nineteenth-Century Canadian Asylums." *Canadian Bulletin of Medical History* 16, no. 2 (1999): 247–69.

———. *When Good Drugs Go Bad: Opium, Medicine, and the Origins of Canada's Drug Laws*. Vancouver: University of British Columbia Press, 2015.

Marshall, Nicholas. "The Great Exaggeration: Death and the Civil War." *Journal of the Civil War Era* 4, no. 1 (March 2014): 3–27.

Marten, James. *America's Corporal: James Tanner in War and Peace*. Athens: University of Georgia Press, 2014.

———. "Civil War Veterans." In *A Companion to the US Civil War*, edited by Aaron Sheehan-Dean, 608–28. West Sussex, UK: John Wiley & Sons, 2014.

———. "A Running Fight against Their Fellow Man: Civil War Veterans in Gilded Age Literature." *Journal of the Civil War Era* 5, no. 4 (December 2015): 504–27.
———. *Sing Not War: The Lives of Union and Confederate Veterans in the Gilded Age.* Chapel Hill: University of North Carolina Press, 2011.
Martin, Scott C. "'A Soldier Intoxicated Is Far Worse Than No Soldier At All': Intoxication and the American Civil War." *Social History of Alcohol and Drugs* 25 (2011): 66–87.
Martínez, María Antonia, and Salomé Ballesteros. "Opium Poisoning in Modern Times: An Overview." *Forensic Science International* 302 (2019): 1–10.
Mattingly, Carol. *Well-Tempered Women: Nineteenth-Century Temperance Rhetoric.* Carbondale: Southern Illinois University Press, 1998.
Maurer, David W., and Victor H. Vogel. *Narcotics and Narcotic Addiction.* 2nd ed. Springfield, IL: Charles C. Thomas, 1962.
McCandless, Peter. *Moonlight, Magnolias, and Madness: Insanity in South Carolina from the Colonial Period to the Progressive Era.* Chapel Hill: University of North Carolina Press, 1996.
McClintock, Megan J. "Civil War Pensions and the Reconstruction of Union Families." *Journal of American History* 83, no. 2 (September 1996): 456–80.
McClurken, Jeffrey W. *Take Care of the Living: Reconstructing Confederate Veteran Families in Virginia.* Charlottesville: University of Virginia Press, 2009.
McCurry, Stephanie. *Confederate Reckoning: Power and Politics in the Confederacy.* Cambridge, MA: Harvard University Press, 2010.
McLaren, Angus. *Impotence: A Cultural History.* Chicago: University of Chicago Press, 2007.
McPherson, James M. *Battle Cry of Freedom: The Civil War Era.* New York: Ballantine, 1989.
Meier, Kathryn Shively. *Nature's Civil War: Common Soldiers and the Environment in 1862 Virginia.* Chapel Hill: University of North Carolina Press, 2013.
Middleton, William S. "Turner's Lane Hospital." *Bulletin of the History of Medicine* 40, no. 1 (January–February 1966): 14–42.
Miller, Brian Craig. *Empty Sleeves: Amputation in the Civil War South.* Athens: University of Georgia Press, 2015.
Morgan, H. Wayne. *Drugs in America: A Social History, 1800–1980.* Syracuse: Syracuse University Press, 1981.
———. "'No, Thank You. I've Been to Dwight': Reflections on the Keeley Cure for Alcoholism." *Illinois Journal of History* 82, no. 3 (Autumn 1989): 147–66.
———, ed. *Yesterday's Addicts: American Society and Drug Abuse, 1865–1920.* Norman: University of Oklahoma Press, 1974.
Musto, David F. *The American Disease: Origins of Narcotic Control.* 3rd ed. New York: Oxford University Press, 1999.
———. "Iatrogenic Addiction: The Problem, Its Definition and History." *Bulletin of the New York Academy of Medicine* 61, no. 8 (October 1985): 694–705.
Nelson, Megan Kate. *Ruin Nation: Destruction and the American Civil War.* Athens, GA: University of Georgia Press, 2012.
Netherland, Julie, and Helena Hansen. "White Opioids: Pharmaceutical Race and the War on Drugs That Wasn't." *Biosocieties* 12, no. 2 (June 2017): 217–38.
Ngai, Mae. *The Chinese Question: The Gold Rushes and Global Politics.* New York: W. W. Norton, 2021.

Norwood, Dael A. *Trading Freedom: How Trade with China Defined Early America.* Chicago: University of Chicago Press, 2022.

Novak Gustainis, Emily R. "Ever-Evolving: Introducing the Medical Heritage Library." *Journal of the Medical Library Association* 107, no. 2 (April 2019): 265–69.

O'Donnell, John A., and John Charles Ball. *Narcotic Addiction.* New York: Harper & Row, 1966.

Oliver, F. E. "Why People Used Opium." In *Drugs and Drug Policy in America: A Documentary History,* edited by Steven R. Belenko, 5–6. Westport, CT: Greenwood, 2000.

Padwa, Howard. *Social Poison: The Culture and Politics of Opiate Control in Britain and France, 1821–1926.* Baltimore: Johns Hopkins University Press, 2012.

Paludan, Phillip Shaw. *A People's Contest: The Union and the Civil War, 1861–1865.* New York: Harper & Row, 1989.

———. *Victims: A True Story of the Civil War.* Knoxville: University of Tennessee Press, 1981.

Pappert, Eric J. "Philadelphia Infirmity for Nervous Diseases: America's Original Model of Institutional Neurology." *Neurology* 50, no. 6 (June 1998): 1847–53.

Pappritz, Kathleen, and Sophie Van Linthout. "Opioid-Induced Immunomodulation: Consequences for the Experimental Coxsackievirus B3-Induced Myocarditis Model." *Biology* (Basel, Switzerland) 9, no. 10 (2020): 335. https://doi.org/10.3390/biology9100335.

Parks, D. C. *Narcotics and Narcotics Addiction.* New York: Carleton Press, 1969.

Parsons, Elaine Frantz. *Manhood Lost: Fallen Drunkards and Redeeming Women in the Nineteenth-Century United States.* Baltimore: Johns Hopkins University Press, 2003.

———. "Risky Business: The Uncertain Boundaries of Manhood in the Midwestern Saloon." *Journal of Social History* 34, no. 2 (Winter 2000): 283–307.

Pathan, Hasan, and John Williams. "Basic Opioid Pharmacology: An Update." *British Journal of Pain* 6, no. 1 (February 2012): 11–16.

Pearson, Susan J. "A New Birth of Regulation: The State of the State after the Civil War." *Journal of the Civil War Era* 5, no. 3 (September 2015): 422–39.

Pendergrast, Mark. *For God, Country, and Coca-Cola.* 2nd ed. New York: Basic Books, 2000.

Pergolizzi, Joseph V., Jr., Robert B. Raffa, and Melanie H. Rosenblatt. "Opioid W Symptoms, a Consequence of Chronic Opioid Use and Opioid Use Disorder: Current Understanding and Approaches to Management." *Journal of Clinical Pharmacy and Therapeutics* 45, no. 5 (October 2020): 892–903.

Pernick, Martin S. *A Calculus of Suffering: Pain, Professionalism, and Anesthesia in Nineteenth-Century America.* New York: Columbia University Press, 1985.

Pizarro, Judith, Roxane Cohen Silver, and JoAnne Prause. "Physical and Mental Health Costs of Traumatic War Experiences Among Civil War Veterans." *Archives of General Psychiatry* 63, no. 2 (February 1, 2006): 193–200.

Pliley, Jessica. *Policing Sexuality: The Mann Act and the Making of the FBI.* Cambridge, MA: Harvard University Press, 2014.

Plumb, Robert C. *Your Brother in Arms: A Union Soldier's Odyssey.* Columbia: University of Missouri Press, 2011.

Porter, Roy. *The Greatest Benefit to Mankind: A Medical History of Humanity.* New York: Oxford University Press, 1990.

Porter, Theodore M. *Genetics in the Madhouse: The Unknown History of Human Heredity.* Princeton: Princeton University Press, 2018.

Prechtel-Kluskens, Claire. "'A Reasonable Degree of Promptitude': Civil War Pension Application Processing, 1861–1885." *Prologue Magazine* 42, no. 1 (Spring 2010). www.archives.gov/publications/prologue/2010/spring/civilwarpension.html. Accessed October 2, 2022.

Privette, Lindsay Rae Smith. *The Surgeon's Battle: How Medicine Won the Vicksburg Campaign and Changed the Civil War.* Chapel Hill: University of North Carolina Press, 2025.

Prokopowicz, Gerald. "The Common Soldier of the Civil War: His Rise and Fall." *Journal of the Civil War Era* 11, no. 4 (December 2021): 539–62.

Purcell, Sarah J. *Spectacle of Grief: Public Funerals and Memory in the Civil War Era.* Chapel Hill: University of North Carolina Press, 2022.

Quinones, Mark A. "Drug Abuse during the Civil War (1861–1865)." *International Journal of the Addictions* 10, no. 6 (1975): 1007–20.

Rable, George C. *Fredericksburg, Fredericksburg!* Chapel Hill: University of North Carolina Press, 2002.

Reid, Brian Holden. "The Civil War, 1861–1865." In *A Companion to American Military History*, edited by James C. Bradford, 1:99–122. Malden, MA: Wiley-Blackwell, 2010.

Richenbacher, Wayne E. "The Demise of Stonewall Jackson: A Civil War Medical Case Study." *Journal of Military History* 79, no. 3 (July 2015): 635–55.

Risse, Guenter B., and John Harley Warner. "Reconstructing Patient Records: Patient Records in Medical History." *Social History of Medicine* 5, no. 2 (August 1992): 183–205.

Room, Robin, Matilda Hellman, and Kerstin Stenius. "Addiction: The Dance between Concept and Terms." *International Journal of Alcohol and Drug Research* 4, no. 1 (June 2015): 27–35.

Rorabaugh, W. J. *The Alcoholic Republic: An American Tradition.* New York: Oxford University Press, 1979.

Rosenberg, Charles E. *The Cholera Years: The United States in 1832, 1849, and 1866.* 2nd ed. Chicago: University of Chicago Press, 1987.

———. "The Patients' View: Doing Medical History from Below." *Theory and Society* 14, no. 2 (March 1985): 175–98.

———. "The Therapeutic Revolution: Medicine, Meaning, and Social Change in Nineteenth-Century America." *Perspectives in Biology and Medicine* 20, no. 4 (Summer 1977): 485–506.

———. "What Is an Epidemic? AIDS in Historical Perspective." *Daedalus* 118, no. 2 (Spring 1989): 1–17.

Rosenblum, Andrew, Lisa A. Marsch, Herman Joseph, and Russell K. Portenoy. "Opioids and the Treatment of Chronic Pain: Controversies, Current Status, and Future Directions." *Experimental and Clinical Psychopharmacology* 15, no. 5 (October 2008): 405–16.

Rosenburg, R. B. *Living Monuments: Confederate Soldiers' Homes in the New South.* Chapel Hill: University of North Carolina Press, 1993.

Ross, Macintosh. "The Boxing Boys in Blue: Gloved Sparring and Bare-Knuckle Prizefighting in the Union Army, 1861–1865." *Journal of Sport History* 44, no. 3 (Fall 2017): 438–55.

Rothman, David J. *The Discovery of the Asylum: Social Order and Disorder in the New Republic.* Rev. ed. Boston: Little, Brown, 1990.

Rothstein, William G. *American Medical Schools and the Practice of Medicine: A History.* New York: Oxford University Press, 1987.

———. *American Physicians in the Nineteenth-Century South: From Sects to Science.* Baltimore: Johns Hopkins University Press, 1985.

———. "The Botanical Movements and Orthodox Medicine." In *Other Healers: Unorthodox Medicine in America,* edited by Norman Gevits, 29–51. Baltimore: Johns Hopkins University Press, 1988.

Rotundo, E. Anthony. *American Manhood: Transformations in Masculinity from the Revolution to the Modern Era.* New York: Basic Books, 1993.

Roy, Sabita, Jana Ninkovic, Santanu Banerjee, Richard Gene Charboneau, Subhas Das, Raini Dutta, Varvara A Kirchner et al. "Opioid Drug Abuse and Modulation of Immune Function: Consequences in the Susceptibility to Opportunistic Infections." *Journal of Neuroimmune Pharmacology* 6, no. 4 (December 2011): 442–65.

Rutkow, Ira. *Bleeding Blue and Gray: Civil War Surgery and the Evolution of American Medicine.* Mechanicsburg, PA: Stackpole, 2015.

Saunt, Claudio. *Unworthy Republic: The Dispossession of Native Americans and the Road to Indian Territory.* New York: W. W. Norton, 2020.

Savitt, Todd L. *Medicine and Slavery: The Diseases and Health Care of Blacks in Antebellum Virginia.* Urbana: University of Illinois Press, 1978.

Schantz, Mark S. *Awaiting the Heavenly Country: The Civil War and America's Culture of Death.* Ithaca: Cornell University Press, 2008.

Schivelbusch, Wolfgang. *Tastes of Paradise: A Social History of Spices, Stimulants, and Intoxicants.* New York: Vintage, 1993.

Schroeder-Lein, Glenna R. *The Encyclopedia of Civil War Medicine.* Armonk, NY: M. E. Sharpe, 2008.

Schultz, Jane E. *Women at the Front: Hospital Workers in Civil War America.* Chapel Hill: University of North Carolina Press, 2004.

Schuster, David G. "The Rise of a Modern Concept of 'Health.'" In *A Companion to the Gilded Age and Progressive Era,* edited by Christopher McKnight Nichols and Nancy C. Unger, 255–67. West Sussex, UK: John Wiley & Sons, 2017.

Scott, J. M. *The White Poppy: A History of Opium.* New York: Funk & Wagnalls, 1969.

Scott, Kenneth. *Coroners' Reports, New York City, 1823–1842.* New York: New York Genealogical & Biographical Society, 1989.

———. *Coroners' Reports, New York City, 1843–1849.* New York: New York Genealogical & Biographical Society, 1991.

Shearer, Erin Fiona. "Women of Violence: Challenging Perceptions of Enslaved Women's Resistance in the Antebellum United States, 1808–1861." PhD diss., University of Reading, 2023. https://doi.org/10.48683/1926.00115296.

Sheehan-Dean, Aaron. *Why Confederates Fought: Family and Nation in Civil War Virginia.* Chapel Hill: University of North Carolina Press, 2007.

Shelden, Rachel A. *Washington Brotherhood: Politics, Social Life, and the Coming of the Civil War.* Chapel Hill: University of North Carolina Press, 2013.

Silkenat, David. *Moments of Despair: Suicide, Divorce, and Debt in Civil War Era North Carolina.* Chapel Hill: University of North Carolina Press, 2011.

Skocpol, Theda. *Protecting Soldiers and Mothers: The Political Origins of Social Policy in the United States*. Cambridge, MA: Belknap Press of Harvard University Press, 1995.

Smith, George Winston. *Medicines for the Union Army: The United States Army Laboratories during the Civil War*. Binghamton: Pharmaceutical Products, 2001.

Smith, Stacy L. *Freedom's Frontier: California and the Struggle of Unfree Labor, Emancipation, and Reconstruction*. Chapel Hill: University of North Carolina Press, 2013.

Snelders, Stephen, Charles Kaplan, and Toine Pieters. "On Cannabis, Chloral Hydrate, and Career Cycles of Psychotropic Drugs in Medicine." *Bulletin of the History of Medicine* 80, no. 1 (Spring 2006): 95–114.

Snowden, Frank M. *Epidemics and Society from the Black Death to the Present*. New Haven, CT: Yale University Press, 2019.

Sommerville, Diane Miller. *Aberration of Mind: Suicide and Suffering in the Civil War–Era South*. Chapel Hill: University of North Carolina Press, 2018.

Spillane, Joseph F. *Cocaine: From Medical Marvel to Modern Menace in the United States, 1884–1920*. Baltimore: Johns Hopkins University Press, 2002.

Stanley, Amy Dru. *From Bondage to Contract: Wage Labor, Marriage, and the Market in the Age of Slave Emancipation*. New York: Cambridge University Press, 1998.

Sternhell, Yael A. "Revisionism Reinvented? The Antiwar Turn in Civil War Scholarship." *Journal of the Civil War Era* 3, no. 2 (June 2013): 239–56.

———. *War on Record: The Archive and the Afterlife of the Civil War*. New Haven, CT: Yale University Press, 2023.

Stoler, Ann Laura. *Along the Archival Grain: Epistemic Anxieties and Colonial Common Sense*. Princeton: Princeton University Press, 2010.

Stott, Richard. *Jolly Fellows: Male Milieus in Nineteenth-Century America*. Baltimore: Johns Hopkins University Press, 2009.

Stowe, Steven M. "Seeing Themselves at Work: Physicians and the Case Narrative in the Mid-Nineteenth-Century American South." *American Historical Review* 101, no. 1 (February 1996): 41–79.

Streeter, Edward C. "*The Boston Medical and Surgical Journal*—Beginnings and Development." *New England Journal of Medicine* 198, no. 1 (February 23, 1928): 24–26.

Su, Alastair. "'The Cause of Human Freedom': John Quincy Adams and the Problem of Opium in the Age of Emancipation." *Journal of the Early Republic* 40, no. 3 (Fall 2020): 465–96.

Sullivan, Glenda. "Plantation Medicine and Health Care in the Old South." *Legacy* 10, no. 1 (2010): 17–35. http://opensiuc.lib.siu.edu/legacy/vol10/iss1/3.

Summers, Martin. *Madness in the City of Magnificent Intentions: A History of Race and Mental Illness in the Nation's Capital*. New York: Oxford University Press, 2019.

Swank, Walbrook D. *Confederate Letters and Diaries, 1861–1865*. Mineral, VA: W. D. Swank, 1988.

Swatos, William H. "Opiate Addiction in the Late Nineteenth Century: A Study of the Social Problem, Using Medical Journals of the Period." *International Journal of the Addictions* 7, no. 4 (1972): 739–53.

Taylor, Amy Murrell. *Embattled Freedom: Journeys through the Civil War's Slave Refugee Camps*. Chapel Hill: University of North Carolina Press, 2018.

Taylor, Nikki M. *Brooding over Bloody Revenge: Enslaved Women's Lethal Resistance*. New York: Cambridge University Press, 2023.

Teeters, Jenni B., Cynthia L. Lancaster, Delisa G. Brown, and Sudie E. Back. "Substance Use Disorders in Military Veterans: Prevalence and Treatment Challenges." *Substance Abuse and Rehabilitation* 8 (2017): 69–77.

Terry, Charles E., and Mildred Pellens. *The Opium Problem*. New York: Bureau of Social Hygiene, 1928.

Tomes, Nancy. *A Generous Confidence: Thomas Story Kirkbride and the Art of Asylum-Keeping, 1840–1883*. New York: Cambridge University Press, 1984.

———. *The Gospel of Germs: Men, Women, and the Microbe in American Life*. Cambridge, MA: Harvard University Press, 1998.

Tracy, Sarah W. *Alcoholism in America from Reconstruction to Prohibition*. Baltimore: Johns Hopkins University Press, 2005.

Tyrrell, Ian. *Woman's World/Woman's Empire: The Woman's Christian Temperance Union in International Perspective, 1880–1930*. Chapel Hill: University of North Carolina Press, 1991.

Valenčius, Conevery Bolton. *The Health of the Country: How American Settlers Understood Themselves and Their Land*. New York: Basic Books, 2002.

Versalle, Washington F. *Eagles on Their Buttons: A Black Infantry Regiment in the Civil War*. Columbia: University of Missouri Press, 1999.

Wagner, Margaret E., Gary W. Gallagher, and Paul Finkelman. *The Library of Congress Civil War Desk Reference*. New York: Simon & Schuster, 2002.

Waldorf, Dan, Martin Orlick, and Craig Reinarman. *Morphine Maintenance: The Shreveport Clinic, 1919–1923*. Washington, DC: Drug Abuse Council, 1974.

Wall, L. Lewis. "Did J. Marion Sims Deliberately Addict His First Fistula Patients to Opium?" *Journal of the History of Medicine and Allied Sciences* 62, no. 3 (July 2007): 336–56.

Walters, Ronald G. *American Reformers: 1815–1860*. New York: Hill and Wang, 1978.

Warner, John Harley. *The Therapeutic Perspective: Medical Practice, Knowledge, and Identity in America, 1820–1885*. Cambridge, MA: Harvard University Press, 1986.

Warsh, Cheryl Krasnick. "Adventures in Maritime Quackery: The Leslie E. Keeley Gold Cure Institute of Fredericton, N.B." *Acadiensis* 12, no. 2 (1988): 109–30.

Weiner, Barbara, and William White. "The History of Addiction/Recovery-Related Periodicals in America: Literature as Cultural/Professional Artifact." *Contemporary Drug Problems* 28 (Winter 2001): 531–57.

———. "*The Journal of Inebriety* (1876–1914): History, Topical Analysis, and Photographic Images." *Addiction* 102 (2007): 15–23.

White, William L. "American Institutions Specializing in the Treatment of Alcohol and Drug Addiction 1840–1950." WilliamWhitePapers.com. www.williamwhitepapers.com/pr/AddictionTreatmentPrograms1840-1950.pdf. Accessed April 15, 2020.

Whites, LeeAnn. *The Civil War as a Crisis in Gender: Augusta, Georgia, 1860–1890*. Athens: University of Georgia Press, 1995.

———. *Gender Matters: Civil War, Reconstruction, and the Making of the New South*. New York: Palgrave Macmillan, 2005.

Wilder, Burt Green. *Practicing Medicine in a Black Regiment: The Civil War Diary of Burt G. Wilder, 55th Massachusetts*. Edited by Richard M. Reid. Amherst: University of Massachusetts Press, 2010.

Williams, Kidada E. *I Saw Death Coming: A History of Terror and Survival in the War Against Reconstruction*. New York: Bloomsbury, 2023.

Willoughby, Christopher D. E. "Running Away from Drapetomania: Samuel A. Cartwright, Medicine, and Race in the Antebellum South." *Journal of Southern History* 84, no. 3 (August 2018): 579–614.

Wyatt-Brown, Bertram. "War as Hell: Blasting Survivors' Minds." *Reviews in American History* 25, no. 4 (December 1997): 732–37.

Young, James Harvey. *The Toadstool Millionaires: A Social History of Patent Medicines in America before Federal Regulation*. Princeton: Princeton University Press, 1961.

Zieger, Susan. *Inventing the Addict: Drugs, Race, and Sexuality in Nineteenth-Century British and American Literature*. Amherst: University of Massachusetts Press, 2008.

Ziparo, Jessica. *This Grand Experiment: When Women Entered the Federal Workforce in Civil War–Era Washington, D.C.* Chapel Hill: University of North Carolina Press, 2017.

Index

Page numbers in italics refer to illustrations.

abscesses from injections, 118–20, *119*, 187, 247
acetaminophen, 251
acetanilide, 251
Ackerman, Jessie A., 272–73
Adams, Charles Francis, Jr., 86
Adams, James Forster Alleyne, 73, 235, 251–52
Adams, John, 86
Adams, Michael C. C., 4
Adams, Samuel Hopkins, 233
addiction: as choice, myth of, 114–15; concepts of, 218, 279; dangers of, 79–80, 94–95; inebriety clinics, 261–71; medicalization of, 235–36, 258–60; modern vs. nineteenth-century understandings, 143; negative stereotypes of, 275; physical experience of, 107–10; pre–Civil War examples of, 20–21; "slavery" metaphor for, 53, 110–11; social contagion concepts, 264; use of term, 14, 287n29; and "weakness," 111–12, 115–17, *116*; withdrawal, 168–69. *See also* opiate addiction
addiction narratives, 239; *Opium Eating*, 238, 239–40
Aimar, G. W., 138–39
Alabama: Insane Hospital, Tuscaloosa, 152
alcohol use, 5, 204; alcohol users in inebriety clinics, 264–65
Aldrich, Corinna Brown, 45
Aldrich, Edward, 45
Alexander, Sarah J., 153
alternative medicines. *See* patent medicines
American Academy of Medicine, 244, 250, 275

American Association for the Study and Cure of Inebriety (ASSCI), 255, 260–61, 263, 266–67, 269, 271
American Journal of Insanity, 152, 253
American Journal of Medical Sciences, 248
American Medical Association (AMA), 233, 242
American Opium Antidote, 220, 225
American Psychiatric Association, 271
American Public Health Association, 30
American Society of Addiction Medicine, 287n29
American Temperance Society, 56
amputations, 5, 79, 85, 110, 120, 210, 221–22
Andersonville Prison, Georgia, 72, 113–14, 121, 238
Andreas, Peter, 8
Andrews, Robert B., 158–59, 167, 169, 276
antidiarrheal medicine, 24–25. *See also* diarrhea
antipyrine, 251
appetite, loss of, 120–21
Arkansas: Confederate Home, 199
Armory Square Hospital, Washington, DC, 70
Armstrong, S. D., 99–100
army disease model, 2, 277–78, 280–83, 338n1; challenges to, 282
Army Medical Museum, 78
Association of Medical Superintendents, 253, 271
asylum commitments, 150–55; and carceral state, 169–76; decision-making process for, 155–61; lived experience of, 166–69; and suicide, 164. *See also* asylums

asylums, 43; chloral hydrate use in, 253, 254; custodial care vs. curative care, 168–69; and forced labor, 175; overcrowding, 173–74; population statistics for, 173; records of, as archival information, 148–50, 286n16; screening practices of, 151; violence in, 174–75. *See also* asylum commitments; mental illness, addiction as
Atkinson, William Biddle, 259
Atlantic Monthly, 247, 266

Ball, Tamezen, 197
Banks, Nathaniel, 66, 96
Banner of Light (spiritualist periodical), 237
Barber, George M., 132, 137, 201
Barker, Sarah, 36
Bartholow, Roberts, 78, 80, 110–11, 242–43
Bartlett, Elisha, 24–25
Battle Cry of Freedom (McPherson), 281
Battle of Antietam, 67
Battle of Chickamauga, 90
Battle of Cold Harbor, 79
Battle of Fort Donelson, 86
Battle of Fredericksburg, 64, 91
Battle of Gettysburg, 60–61, 66, 131, 229, 237
Battle of the Wilderness, 65, 76, 127
bayonet wounds, 298n16
Beard, George Miller, 139–40, 168, 243, 262, 263
Beauregard, P. G. T., 131
Beecher, Henry Ward, 57
Beecher, Lyman, 56, 57
Benham, M. C., 219
Bever, Megan L., 4
Bierce, Ambrose, 88
Billings, John Shaw, 77–78
Black Americans: and African medical traditions, 47; "Black superbody" myth, 46–47, 80–81; cocaine use by, 83; opiate addiction, racial disparities in, 82–83; and opiates, 46; segregation in asylums, 154; separate drug protocols for, 7; United States Colored Troops, 81
black markets for drugs, 49, 68
Blalock, W. C., 252

Blanchard, J. A., 255
Blankenbaker, William, 145, 147, 154
blockade-runners, 67–68
Blue, Richard Whiting, 232
Boston Medical and Surgical Journal (*BMSJ*), 119, 231; on alternatives to opiates, 251; on chloral hydrate, 253; on cholera remedies, 25–26; opiate addiction, account of (1833), 40–41, 42–43; on prevalence of opiate addiction, 58; review of *Opium Eating*, 239–40; sympathy for "deserving" addicts, 48–49; women as "typical" opiate addicts, 43–44
Bourne, William Oland, 180
Bowser, Perry B., 145, 177, 184–86, 205, 220–21, 228–29, 232, 276, 323n28
Boyd, James R., 163
Bradley, William H., 111, 125
Bragg, Braxton, 90
Branscomb, Lewis Sylvester, 87–88
Bremen, S. G., 76
Brewster, Charles, 86
British East India Company, 22
Brooklyn Daily Eagle (newspaper), 141
Brown, Edward Andrew, 254
Brown, John, 19
Bruisard, Carlos, 219
Bryce, Peter, 152
Buker, Cyrus F., 197
Buker, Mary A., 197
Bull, John, 22
Butler, Benjamin, 93

cabinet cards, *116*, 117
caffeine for overdose reversal, 36
Caldecott, Augustus F., 197
Caldwell, Robert C., 70
Calhoun, John C., 53
Calkins, Alonzo, 237
Campbell, Nancy D., 14, 15
Camp Curtain, Pennsylvania, 259
Camp Stokes, North Carolina, 69
cannabis, 258
carceral state, 169–76
Carroll, Dillon J., 4

Cartwright, Samuel A., 46, 82
"Case of George Dedlow, The" (Mitchell), 247
Century Illustrated Monthly Magazine, 137
Chaplin, Thomas B., 138–39
Chappell, Alpheus M., 60, 61, 131, 227, 237
Chappell, William H., 221–22, 223, 224
charity, concept of, 50, 132, 180–81
Chesnut, Mary, 46
Child, Lydia Maria, 32
Chimborazo Hospital, Richmond, 68, 70, 127, 147
China: Chinese opium smokers, 53–54; and opium trade in the nineteenth century, 22; and stereotypes of opium abuse, 141–42. *See also* Chinese immigrants
Chinese Exclusion Act (1882), 55, 142
Chinese immigrants, 7, 55; and anti-Asian racism, 41, 54–55, 141–43
chloral hydrate, 168, 235, 252–54, 334n91; overdose of, 254
chloroform, 252
cholera, 25–26, 289n44
Christian Advocate (newspaper), 113, 126
Civil War medicine: and causes of increasing opiate addiction, 152–53; hospital expansion, 70; hypodermic morphine, 76–77, 78; injuries and illnesses, range of, 63–64; medication supplies, 64–65; opiates, reliance on, 62–63; opiate supplies, 65–67; sanitation, 71–72; scientific research and development, 77–78; triage system, 69
Civil War soldiers: cooking and hygiene, 72–73; court-martial proceedings, 92–93; emotional distress, 87–89; intoxication, 91; sanitation, 71–72; suicides, 93
Civil War veterans: and addiction as long health crisis, 143–46; and end-of-life care, 84; fatal overdoses, 95–96; and increasing addiction rates, 94–104; military records in asylum commitment process, 155; morphine for mortal wounds, 76; opiates, tendency to use medically, 74; painkillers, need for, 75; widows' pensions, refused, 126–27

Clark, Claire D., 7
Clarke, Edward Hammond, 253
classist frameworks and economic inequality, 130–33
Cleveland, Grover, 117–18, 175, 183, 193–94, 197–98, 272
Clewell, Francis C., 95, 165–66, 276
Cobb, Sylvanus, 52
Cobbe, William Rosser, 103, 126, 238–39, 240
Coca-Cola, 220
cocaine, 83, 103, 186, 235, 251, 254–56, 334n91; Coca-Cola, 220
Cole, Henry G., 205
Collier's (magazine), 233
Collins, Samuel B., 123–24, 209, 214–17, 216, 221–24, 229–30, 232–33, 240, 266, 272–73
commitments. *See* asylum commitments
Committee on Intemperance as a Disease, 102, 134–35, 258, 260, 266
community-level impact of addiction, 138–39; and asylum commitment decisions, 158–59
Confederate Army: *Manual of Military Surgery*, 94; opium supplies, 66–68; pensions, 192–93; soldiers' homes, 198–200
Confederate Veteran (United Confederate Veterans publication), 220, 239
Confessions of an English Opium-Eater (De Quincey), 44, 90–91, 240
Conklin, W. J., 151
Connecticut: Connecticut Hospital for the Insane, 264; Connecticut Soldiers Home, 202–3; Walnut Hill Asylum, Hartford, 270
Cornell, William Mason, 246
coroners' inquests, 34–36
courage: "hospital courage," 85, 117. *See also* masculinity
court-martial proceedings, 92
Courtwright, David T., 2, 7, 8, 15, 34, 49, 98, 236, 275, 282
Covey, Edward, 46
cowardice, perception of, 89–93
Cowles, Edward, 257

Index 383

Crèvecœur, J. Hector St. John de, 20
criminality and moral failings, 135–36
Crothers, Thomas Davison "T. D.," 74, 100, 180, 189–90, 255, 261–62, 270–71
Cullen, William, 19, 20
"cult of sincerity," 136
Cummings, Charles, 87
Cutter, Calvin, 32

Da Costa, Jacob Mendes, 236, 246, 248–49, 253, 254–55
Dalton, Napoleon, 163
Dark Paradise (Courtwright), 2
Darrow, Joseph C., 110, 112, 215, 225, 226
Davis, Varina, 100
Dawson, Eva, 129, 311n89
Dawson, James, 129, 311n89
Day, Albert, 74, 101, 112, 139–40, 255–56, 263, 265, 271
Day, Horace, 99
Dean, Eric T., Jr., 4, 282, 285nn8–9
De Bow's Review, 46
De Forest, John William, 102–3
Delano, Warren, Jr., 22
Dependent Pension Act (1890), 181, 183, 185, 189, 190, 195
dependents' pensions, 197
Depoy, Joseph D., 131–32
De Quincey, Thomas, 44, 90–91, 240
DeRosset, Marie, 100
Devine, Shauna, 6
Diamond, William, 88
diarrhea, 107, 121; chronic, 71–72, 252; and opiate addiction, 70–74; racial discrimination in treatment of, 81–82; treatment of, 24–25
disability history, 5
Doctor Judas (Cobbe), 103, 238, 240
domestic medicine, 31–32
domestic violence, 160
Dorothea Dix Hospital, Raleigh, 155, 159, 167, 254
Double Chloride of Gold, 217–18
Douglass, Frederick, 46, 224
Dover's powder, 23, 152
Downs, Jim, 6

Dr. M'Munn's Elixir of Opium, 212
Drollinger, J. A., 231
Dr. Tanner's Opium and Morphine Cure, 229–30
Dr. Zell's Temperance Powders, 213–14
DuBois, Samuel, 27
dysentery, 24–25, 70

Earle, Charles, 102
Early, Jubal, 96
Eastern State Lunatic Asylum, Virginia, 157, 170–71
Eaton, Harriet, 94
Eaton, Virgil E., 241–42
Eaton, Virgil F., 102
E. coli infections, 73
Eighteenth Amendment, 274
elderly opiate users, 145–46
emaciation of opiate addicts, 120–24, *122*, *123*, 185
end-of-life care for dying soldiers, 84
enslavement: and "Black superbody" myth, 46–47; and medical racism, 46–48
"epidemic," use of term, 15
eugenics, 7
Eustis, Henry Lawrence, 90

Fairbanks, Benjamin F., 71
Fallon, Patrick, 91
families: addiction as intergenerational health crisis, 143–46; domestic violence, 160; and home care of addicted persons, 156; impact of opiate addiction, 126–39; visits to asylum patients, 166–67
Family Nurse, The (Child), 32
Farber, David, 83
Ferry, Albert, 131
Fialka, Andrew, 4
fictional treatments of addiction, 102–3
First Battle of Bull Run, 64
Fisk, John, 201
Flag of Our Union (periodical), 51
Foner, Eric, 269
Foote, Lorien, 4
Fort Hamilton Inebriate Asylum, 267–68
Fort McHenry, Maryland, 229

Frank Leslie's Popular Monthly, 141, 214, 215
Franklin, Benjamin, 19, 21
Freedman Bureau hospitals, 81
French, George F., 231
Frost, Carleton P., 95

Gabriel, Joseph M., 7
Gardner, George W., 119, 121
Garfield, James, 234
gastrointestinal issues. *See* diarrhea
gendered roles, 6–7, 42–53; emasculation of male opiate addicts, 50–51; gendered conditions and medical treatment, 44–45; male dominance in medical field, 94; masculinity and male opiate addicts, 49–52; women and self-medication, 45; women as "typical" opiate addicts, 42–44; women as wartime pharmacists, 65. *See also* masculinity; women
Georgia: state asylum, Milledgeville, 152, 173
German Remedy Company, 203
Gilded Age: classist frameworks and economic inequality, 132–33; cultural context, 7, 15; government programs, growth in, 175–76; industrialization and economic context, 114; patent medicine use, 213
Gilman, Charlotte Perkins, 78
Gleason, Newell, 215
Gold Cure, 202–3, 205–6, 217–18, 223, 232, 261, 273
Gold Rush, 55
Goolrick, Charles O'Conor, 129
Goolrick, Frances B., 127–31, *128*, 133, 157–58
Goolrick, John Tackett, 127–31, *128*, 133, 144, 156–58, 169, 276
Goolrick, Nora, 129, 157–58
Goolrick, William, 129, 157–58
Gordon, Lesley J., 4
Grand Army of the Republic (GAR), 181, 183, 191; Keeley Leagues, 218; *National Tribune* (GAR publication), 71, 191, 219, 220, 239
Grant, Ulysses, 220
Gray, Elizabeth Kelly, 7, 15, 49
Gray, John P., 151–53, 174
"Great American Fraud, The" (Adams), 233

Greene, Thomas, 152
Greenville Democrat (Ohio newspaper), 95
Guiteau, Charles, 151, 234
gum opium, 23
Gunn, John C., 31–32
Gunn's Domestic Medicine, 31–32, 56, 291n72

Hall, James Ladson, 195–96, 276
Hall, Laura, 196
Halttunen, Karen, 136
Hammond, William A., 65, 170, 253
Handley-Cousins, Sarah, 4, 5, 15, 179–80, 183
Hankins, Matthew D., 91
Harding, Warren G., 127, *128*
Harmon, Cyrus, 136
Harper's New Monthly Magazine, 100, 237, 258
Harrison, Benjamin, 195
Harrisonburg, Virginia, 96
Harrison Narcotics Tax Act (1914), 49, 178, 274, 275, 277, 278, 282, 320n2
Hartshorne, Henry, 30
Hartsock, Andrew Jackson, 74
Hayden, Augustus, 91–92
Henderson, J. W., 86
Henley, Albert Wymer, 107, 110, 225
Hentz, Charles A., 229–30
heroic medicine, 23–24; backlash against, 30–31
heroin, 103, 279–80, 308n21
Herzberg, David, 7, 15, 49
Hickman, Timothy A., 7, 15, 49
Hildreth, Thaddeus, 71
historiography: author's methodology, 3–4; digitized records, 3–4; disability history, 5; medical history, 6, 7–8, 14–15; neglect of opiate addiction, 2–3; "neo-revisionism," 4
Hoare, Michael, 169
Holston, John G. F., 76
Holt, Daniel, 72–73, 87
home health guides, 31–32, 34
homelessness, 132
Hood, John Bell, 90
Horner, Arthur, 92

Index   385

"hospital courage," 85, 117
hospital expansion, Civil War era, 70
House, George, 88–89
Hubbard, Frederick Heman, 240
Hughes, William H., 203, 218
Hull, J. M., 240–41, 253–54
Humane Remedy Co., 219
Humphreys, Margaret, 6, 235
Hungerford, Allyn Merriam, 28
Hunter, David, 96
hydrocyanic acid, 252
hypodermic injections, 23, 76–77, 118, 279, 301n78; abscesses from, 118–20, *119*, 187, 247; contrasted with oral administration, 242–43; syringes, 77, *78*, *116*, 117

Imboden, John, 96
immigrants to America, 274
imports of opium, tariff records, 98
impotence, 137
independence: Gilded Age ideals of personal responsibility, 114–15
Indiana Hospital for the Insane, 155
Indiana Soldiers' Home, Indianapolis, 161
inebriety: opposition to model, 272; promotion of concept, 235–36; redefinition of addiction, 258–60; theory of, 150. *See also* inebriety clinics
inebriety clinics, 261–71; medical support for, 271; public vs. private, 269–70. *See also* inebriety
infant overdose deaths, 35
Injuries of Nerves and Their Consequences (Mitchell), 79, 247
insanity, 147–48. *See also* asylums; mental illness, addiction as
institutionalization. *See* asylum commitments; mental illness, addiction as
intemperance, 150; opiate addiction as, 180–81
Iowa Board of Health, 102, 109–10

Jackson, "Stonewall," 66, 85, 96
Jaffe, Arnold, 7
Jarvis, Edward, 44
Jefferson, Thomas, 20, 21

Jefferson Medical College, Philadelphia, 248–50
Jim Crow laws, 142–43
Jones, Amanda E., 137
Jones, Andrew J., 137
Jones, George E., 244
Jones, John, 19–20
Jordan, Brian Matthew, 4, 282
journalism: criticism of physicians, 241; exaggeration used in, 97; focus on addiction crisis, 102; muckraking, 102
Journal of the American Medical Association, 242

Kamieński, Lukasz, 8
Kane, H. H., 120, 219–20
Keeley, Leslie E., 202, 205–6, 209, 217–18, 219, 224, 232, 233, 240, 261, 273
Keeley Center, Leavenworth, Kansas, 202–3
Keeley League, 218, 232
Keen, William W., 79, 247
Keith, H. C., 220
Kentucky: legislation concerning commitment of addicts, 269
Ketchum, J. C., 123
Key, William Ogle, 144
King, James, 259
Kirk, George W., 123–24, 226
Kirkbride, Thomas, 152–53, 173
Kirkbride Plan, 152

Latham, Milton, 54
laudanum, 21, 23, 196, 197; home use of, 32; as substitute for alcohol, 45
Lazelle, Joseph A., 184
Lears, T. J. Jackson, 224
Leavenworth, Kansas, 201
LeFavour, Joseph, 132
legal frameworks: institutionalization of addicts, 170–71; legislation concerning opium distribution, 142
Letterman, Jonathan, 64, 69
Libby Prison, 121, 238
life insurance, 133
Lincoln, Abraham, 27
Linderman, Gerald, 4, 85

Little House on the Prairie (television series), 2, 280
Lobelia inflata (pukeweed), 31
Long, George W., 175
Longview Asylum, Ohio, 151
Lost Cause mythology, 85, 198
Louisville Medical News, 209
Ludlow, Fitz Hugh, 100–101, 237, 258, 259
lying, compulsive, 159–60, 262
Lynch, Barry, 93

malaria, 25, 70
manliness, concept of, 7. *See also* masculinity
Mann, Edward, 121, 125, 133, 134, 261
Mansfield, George, 81
Manual of Military Surgery (Confederate Army), 94
March, F. E., 219
Marks, Jeannette, 278–80
marriages, impact of addiction on, 137–38. *See also* families
Marshall, Orville, 102
Marten, James, 2, 4, 180, 282, 285n9
Martin, Samuel M., 161, 186–89, *188*, 255
Maryland Board of Health, 102
masculinity: and "business ability," 125–26; and culture of pain, 84–85; emaciation contrasted with, 121–24, *122*, *123*; and employment, 124–25, 126–27; impact of opiate addiction on, 110–12; and impotence, 137; male opiate addicts in pre–Civil War era, 49–52; maintained at end of life, 84; martial manhood, 50; and pain, 84–85, 117–18; and "weakness" and painkillers, 107–8, 157
Mason, George, 127
Mason, Lewis D., 256
Massachusetts: Board of Health, 102, 135, 214, 243; Boston physicians' prescription trends, 257; Joint Special Committee on Inebriation as a Disease, 268–69; legal frameworks for institutionalization of addicts, 171–72; Massachusetts General Hospital, 256, 257; Washingtonian Home, 255, 265

Matthews, Edward Sylvester, 164, *165*
Matthews, Mary, 164
Mattison, Jansen Beemer, 73, 80, 111, 214, 230–32, 255, 262, 267–70
McClurken, Jeffrey W., 4
McCoy, William K., 84
McCready, B. W. M., 52
McGuire, Hunter, 85
McIlwain, R. J., 194
McKeen, Byron, 110, 225
McPherson, James, 281
Medical and Surgical History of the War of the Rebellion, The, 64, 78, 234, 243, 256
Medical and Surgical Reporter, 271
medical education on opiate addiction, 36–37
medical history, 6; doctors' daybooks/account books, 29–30; heroic medicine, 23–24, 30–31; home health guides/domestic medicine, 31–32. *See also* physicians
medicalized concepts of addiction, 258–60, 262–63
medical prescriptions for opiates, 236–45. *See also* physicians
medical racism, 7, 46–48, 80–82
Medical Society of South Carolina, 230
Medical Society of the State of Pennsylvania, 102
men. *See* masculinity
mental illness, addiction as, 5; historical context of, 148–49; overview, 147–50; suicide, 161–66. *See also* asylums
Michaels, George W., 201
Michigan Soldiers' Home, 202, 204, 237–38
Middleton, Eliza, 45
military entitlement programs: overview, 177–79; pensions, 179–98; soldiers' homes, 198–206
Miller, Christian, 93
missionary movements, 53–57
Missouri: Confederate Home, 199
Miss Ravenel's Conversion from Secession to Loyalty (De Forest), 102–3
Mitchell, Silas Weir, 78–79, 117–18, 121, 236, 244, 246–48, *249*, 253, 257, 263
Moncure, James Dunlap, 170

Index 387

Moore, Samuel Preston, 67
Morehouse, George R., 79, 247
morphine, 75–76; and danger of addiction, 79–80; deathbed use of, 84; morphine maintenance clinics, 145; morphine sulfate, 23; "morphinomania," 150, 151, 244–45, 280; for pain, 75–80
Morris, F. Baldwin, 133
Morris, Mary A., 190
Morris, Wirt, 136, 190–91
Mrs. Winslow's Soothing Syrup, 212
"muckraking" journalism, 102
myocarditis, 129

Nailer, George W., 87
"narcotics farms," 279, 280
National Home for Disabled Volunteer Soldiers (NHDVS), 177, 200–206; in Dayton, Ohio, 190; Keeley Leagues, 218–19; and Leslie E. Keeley, 232; in Marion, Indiana, 205; in Milwaukee, Wisconsin, 202, 204; in Togus, Maine, 191
National Institute on Drug Abuse, 280
National Tribune (GAR publication), 71, 191, 219, 220, 239
nerve injuries and disorders, 247–48
neurasthenia, 139–40, 243, 262
New England Magazine, 51
New Hampshire: laws concerning institutionalization of addicts, 171–72
New York City, 35, 58; Kings County Inebriate Asylum, 267–68; Parrish Hall, 270
New York Daily News, 51
New York state: Inebriate Asylum, Binghamton, 170, 264–65, 266, 270; legal frameworks for institutionalization of addicts, 172; Lunatic Asylum, Utica, 43, 154–55, 174; Willard Asylum for the Chronic Insane, 155, 160, 167, 174, 175, 229
New York State Inebriate Asylum, Binghamton, 170, 264–65, 266, 270
New York State Lunatic Asylum, Utica, 43, 154–55, 174
New-York Times, 55, 58, 96, 98, 113, 141, 273
NHDVS. See National Home for Disabled Volunteer Soldiers

Nixon, Richard, 280
Noble, Richard J., 244
North American Review, 278
North Carolina: Confederate soldiers' home, 199; Dorothea Dix Hospital, Raleigh, 155, 167, 254; North Carolina Hospital for the Insane, Raleigh, 155
novels: fictional portrayals of opiate addiction, 102–3

Oatman, Alvah V., 202, 204–5
Ocasio-Cortez, Alexandria, 277, 283
Ogilvie, John W., 33, 47, 294n27
Ohio: Commercial Hospital of Cincinnati, 256; Dayton National Home for Disabled Volunteer Soldiers, 190; legal frameworks for institutionalization of addicts, 171
Ohio Soldier (newspaper), 118
"On Irritable Heart" (Da Costa), 248
opiate addiction: accusations and rumors of, 89–91; brain changes with long-term use, 111; among Civil War veterans, 5, 99–102, 277–78; in contemporary United States, 8–9; cowardice, appearance of, 89–93; criminality and moral failings, 135–36; deception and concealment, 97–98, 133–35; elderly users and long-term health, 145–46; increasing concern about in the nineteenth century, 33–34; as intergenerational health crisis, 143–46; medical responsibility for, 236–45; medical role in nineteenth-century concepts of, 234–36; monetary costs of, 226–29; moral blame vs. compassion for, 129, 203–4, 205; moral blame vs. personal responsibility, 113–14; opioid crisis (twenty-first century), 283; pain, endurance of, 117–18; physical appearance, 38, 109–10, 118–19, 184, 120–24, 122, 123, 310n60; and "racial decline," 139–43; racial disparities in, 82–83; relapse, 127; rising rates, post–Civil War, 98–99; side effects, 33–34; "slavery" metaphor, 113–15; stereotypes, 92, 103–4, 141–143; stigmatization of, 133–34; and unemployment, 124–25; viewed as vice, 97; and women, 99–100

—among Civil War soldiers: addiction rates among veterans, 94–104; black market for opiates, 68; blockade-runners, 67–68; cowardice, 89–93; cultural context, 6–7; diarrhea and opiate addiction, 70–74; opiates in Civil War medicine, 62–70; overview, 1–3, 60–61; pain and morphine, 75–86; physician reliance on, 68–69; stress and self-care, 86–89

—pre–Civil War, 8, 33–39; binary framework for "good" and "bad" addicts, 48–50, 293n2; clinical understanding of, 37; cultural explanations for, 39, 40–42; male addicts, 49–52; media coverage of, 58; medical training and increasing concern for, 36–37; prevalence of, 57–59; racialized contexts, 53–57; and social reform movements, 53–57; statistics, 34–35; tolerance and escalating consumption, 37–38

—treatment: custodial care vs. curative care, 168–69; home care vs. institutionalization, 155–61; inebriety clinics, 263–71; Keeley's Gold Cure, 202–3, 205–6; medicalization of, 258–63; NHDVS admission for, 202; temperance-style approaches, 218. *See also* patent medicines

opiates: alternatives to, 251–57; availability, pre–Civil War era, 32–33; biblical language and metaphors for, 57; black market, 68; as cholera remedy, 25–26; dosing guidelines, 30, 94, 108–9, 288n34; esteemed by physicians, 27–28, 28, 33; health risks, 108–10; history of, pre–Civil War era, 19–21; home use of, 31–32; intoxication and loss of control, 57; medical use, pre–Civil War era, 22–33; nineteenth-century understanding of, 6; oral vs. injection, 80; overdoses, 35; over-prescription of, 236–45; as painkillers, 26–27; prescription trends, 245–50, 256–57; self-medication by soldiers, 86–87; and suicide, 35–36; tariffs on, 64–65; utilitarian reliance on, 27–30, 62–63

opiate withdrawal. *See* withdrawal process

opium: imports and tariff records, 34; production process, 22
"opium dens," 141–43
Opium Eating (addiction narrative), 113–14, 121, 124, 238, 239–40
Opium Habit, The (Day), 99
"opium mania," 150, 151. *See also* mental illness, addiction as
Opium Wars, 22
overdose: accidental, 94, 144; of chloral hydrate, 254; concealment of, 97–98; deaths, 35, 95, 129–30; reversal of, 36; suicide, 35–36
Overland Campaign, 92
Owens, Deirdre Cooper, 46

Pacific Medical and Surgical Journal, 244
Packard, Jasper, 217
pain: endurance of, 117–18; and masculine culture, 84–85; use of morphine, 75–80; "weakness" and painkillers, 107–8, 157
Painless Opium Antidote, 123–24, 215–17, 216, 221, 225, 226, 229, 272
palliative medicine, 26–27
Panic of 1873, 269
Papaver somniferum, cultivation of, 67
Paracelsus, 19
paregoric, 23
Parker, Willard, 260, 266
Parrish, Joseph, 258–59, 260, 266
Parrish Hall, Brooklyn, 270
Parsons, William M., 33
patent medicines: advertising for, 213–14, 219, 220–21; affordability of, 226–30; clinic backlash against, 230–32; clinician use of, 229–30; and criticism of physicians, 240; decline of, 230–33; history of in Civil War era, 212–21; opiates as ingredient, 212–13, 230–31; overview, 97, 209–12; religious language used to market, 222, 224; and temperance movements, 272–73; testimonials used for marketing, 216, 221–26; *Theriaki* (advertising pamphlet), 216–17, 224
Patterson, John J., 124, 144, 223
Pearson, Susan J., 7

Index 389

Pellens, Mildred, 279–80
Pemberton, John Stith, 220
Pennsylvania: Committee on Intemperance as a Disease, 102, 134–35, 258, 260, 266; Jefferson Medical College, Philadelphia, 248–50; Medical Society, 258, 259; Turner's Lane Hospital, Philadelphia, 76, 78–79, 80, 117, 118, 246, 247
pensions: adjustments to, 186–87; denial of and moral judgment, 195–97; Dependent Pension Act (1890), 181–82; dependents' pensions, 197; federal government's search for fraud, 191–92; and moral judgments, 179–81, 182–83; opiate addictions, disguise and denial, 189–92; Pension Bureau, expansion of, 197–98, 322n13; Pension Bureau agents, 177, 182, *182*; pension examinations and "vicious habits," 182–85, 322n24; subjective criteria vs. guidelines, 179; widows' pensions, 193–97
pharmacies, federally funded, 65–66, *66*; theft from, 299n42
phenacetin, 251
Phillips, George, 88
physicians: records of prescriptions, 256–57, 290n59; responsibility for over-prescription of opiates, 236–45; shift away from opiate prescription, 245–50, 275–76, 330n4
Physician's Visiting List, The, 36
Pickett, George, 60
Pickett's Charge, Gettysburg, 60–61, 131, 237
Pinel Hospital, Richmond, Virginia, 170–71
Pomoroy, Willis B., 254
Popular Science Monthly, 241–42
Porcher, Francis Peyre, 67
post-traumatic stress disorder (PTSD). *See* PTSD
poverty: classist frameworks, 132–33; and homelessness, 132; and opiate addiction, 226–30; and public welfare, 131–32; soldiers' homes, 198–99
Pratt, Clesson, 219
Pratt, Isaac, 33
Pray, Frank E., 73–74, 190

Prohibition, 274, 279
prostitution, 45, 95, 126
Providence Journal (newspaper), 95
psychiatry, 148–49. *See also* mental illness, addiction as
PTSD (post-traumatic stress disorder), 4, 149, 248, 314n2, 314n4; and suicide, 163–64
pukeweed (*Lobelia inflata*), 31
Pure Food and Drug Act (1906), 233

Quarterly Journal of Inebriety (QJI), 263, 270
Quinones, Mark A., 282

"race suicide," 140
"racial decline," 139–43
racial issues: opiate prescriptions, differing rates, 80–82; segregation in asylums, 154; white racial decline, fear of, 7
racism: anti-Asian, 41, 54–55, 141–43; and coroners' inquests, 34–35; medical racism, 7, 46–48; among Union soldiers, 93
Reagan, Ronald, 280
religion as element of treatment for addiction, 224, 273–74
Resources of Southern Fields and Forests (Porcher), 67
"rest cure," 78, 246, 257
Richards, J. M., 115, 223
Richmond Christian Advocate (newspaper), 66
Richmond Dispatch (newspaper), 64
Richmond Medical Journal, 242
Roberts, J. D., 83
Roe, Edward Payson, 103
Rogers, Coleman, 26
Roosevelt, Franklin Delano, 22
Roosevelt, Teddy, 140
Rorabaugh, William J., 34
Rosecrans, William, 90
Rosenberg, Charles E., 15, 275
Rosenberg, Max, 91
Roundtree, L. M., 229
Rush, Benjamin, 20–21, 23, 33–34
Rutherford, William, 69

Salmonella bacteria, 73
Sanitary Commission Bulletin, 258
sanitation, poor, 71–72
Satterlee General Hospital, Philadelphia, 70
Sawyer, Benjamin F., 224
Schofield, John S., 58
Scientific American, 101, 141
Second Battle of Corinth, 76
Seeger, C. L., 49
self-advocacy by addicted veterans, 204–5
self-care, 86–89
self-medication, 45, 144, 213. *See also* patent medicines
Sell, E. M., 243
Seven Days Battles, 87–88
Seward, William, 90
Shelton, O. C., 86, 90
Shenandoah Herald (newspaper), 96
Shenandoah Valley, Virginia, 96–97
Sheridan, Philip, 96
Shigella bacteria, 73. *See also* diarrhea
Shurtleff, Albert T., 85–86
Silkenat, David, 4
Sims, James Marion, 48, 82, 295n35
Sivils, Solomon, 123
Slack, David F., 25
slavery: slave narratives, 224; slaves, access to opiates, 46
"slavery" metaphor for addiction, 53, 113–15
Smith, Clinton, 117–18
Smith, Eliza, 117
Smith, Mason, 75
Smith, William R., 92
social contagion concepts of addiction, 264
sodium salicylate, 251, 252
"soldier's disease," 2, 277–78, 338n1
soldiers' homes: Confederate soldiers' homes, 198–200; Union soldiers' homes (NHDVS), 200–206, 325n57
Sommerville, Diane Miller, 4, 15, 99, 282, 285n9
South Carolina: Confederate Infirmary, 199; Lunatic Asylum, Columbia, 155; Medical Society of South Carolina, 230
Spillane, Joseph F., 7, 49
Squire, W. B., 219

state boards of health, 102, 307n215
Staunton, Virginia, 96–97, 145; Western Lunatic Asylum, 153, 155, 173–74, 175
Staunton Spectator (newspaper), 97
Staunton Vindicator (newspaper), 97
St. Elizabeths, Washington, DC, 154, 155, 167, 175, 201
Stephens, J. L., 220, 228, 230, 233
stigmatization: of drug users, 14, 49–50; and suicide, 161–62
Stiles, Benjamin Edward, Jr., 90
St. Louis Daily Dispatch (newspaper), 166
St. Louis Daily Globe Democrat (newspaper), 101
stomach pumps, 36, 37
Stowe, Frederick, 265
Stowe, Harriet Beecher, 265
stress and self-care, 86–89
Sturgeon, Charles Y., 167, 276
suicide, 35–36, 93, 161–66, 314n160
Swann, A. F., 79, 118, 121, 247
Sweeting, Thomas, 228
Swinney, Daniel, 33
Swisher, D. Z., 161
Sydenham, Thomas, 19
syphilis, 185

Taft, William H., 104
tariff records, 98
Taylor, James, 280
Taylor, J. C., 93
temperance movements, 50, 53–57, 95, 218, 271–74; opposition to inebriety model, 272; and patent medicine sellers, 272–73
Tennessee State Soldiers Home, 199
Terry, Charles E., 279–80
Terry, William R., 131
testimonials used to market patent medicines, 221–26
Thacher, James, 26
Theriaki (advertising pamphlet), 216–17, 224
Third Battle of Winchester, 85
Thompson, Mark M., 219
Thompson cure, 203
Thomson, Samuel, 31
Thomsonian medicine, 31

Tillman, Ben, 142
Tilton, William S., 203–4, 205
tolerance, physical, 37–38, 108–9
Tracy, Sarah J., 7
trauma studies, 149. *See also* PTSD
Travers, Alice, 194–95
Travers, John T., 194–95
treatment. *See* opiate addiction: treatment
triage system, 69
Trichinella roundworms, 73
Turner, J. Edward, 264–65
Turner's Lane Hospital, Philadelphia, 76, 78–79, 80, 117, 118, 246, 247
typhus, 70

Uncle Tom's Cabin (Stowe), 265
Union Army veteran pensions, 193
United Confederate Veterans, 239
United States Colored Troops (USCT), 81
US National Commission on Marihuana and Drug Abuse, 280
US Sanitary Commission, 65, 72, 245–46, 258

Vermont Watchman and State Journal, 193
"vicious habits" and pension examinations, 182–85, 189
violence: in asylums, 174–75; domestic violence, 160
Virginia: Eastern State Lunatic Asylum, Williamsburg, 157, 170–71; legal frameworks for institutionalization of addicts, 170–71; Pinel Hospital, Richmond, 170–71; Shenandoah Valley, 96–97; Staunton, 96–97, 145; Western Lunatic Asylum, Staunton, 153, 155, 161, 163, 173–74, 175
Virginia Medical Monthly, 171
Voice of the West (Buchanan, Michigan, newspaper), 95

Walnut Hill Asylum, Hartford, Connecticut, 270
Walnut Lodge Hospital, Hartford, Connecticut, 74, 270
Walsh, Mary, 175
Walsh, Redmond, 175

Warburton, Mary, 126–27, 196
Warburton, Robert B., 126–27, 144
Warner, John Harley, 29, 256
War on Drugs, 8, 178, 280
Warren, Patrick J., 91
Washington, Bushrod, 21
Washington, George, 19, 21
Washington, Julia Ann Blackburn, 21
welfare state, 175–76
West, Royal F., 137
Western Lunatic Asylum, Staunton, Virginia, 96, 153, 155, 161, 163, 173–74, 175
Whallon, Eugene M., 196
Whallon, Jessie, 196
White, Moses Clarke, 33, 37, 38, 51, 54–55, 56, 59
white-collar workers and addiction, 125–26, 262
whiteness and "racial decline," 139–43, 170
Whites, LeeAnn, 6, 127
"white slave" trope, 103
widows' pensions, 193–97
Willard, Frances, 272
Willard Asylum for the Chronic Insane, Ovid, New York, 155, 160, 167, 174, 175, 229
Williams, Charles L., 202, 204–5, 237–38
Williams, Frank B., 163, 164
Williams, Kidada E., 15
willpower and withdrawal, 111–13, 115–17, *116*
Wilson, J. C., 244, 250, 275
Wilson, W. Stockton, 69
Wilson Chemical Company, 220
Winslow, Ferdinand Sophus, 70–71
Wirz, Henry, 73
Wishard, Milton M., 161, 164
withdrawal process, 308n21; gradual tapering of opiates, 202, 268; in inebriety clinics, 265; pre–Civil War era approaches to, 21; and relapse, 113; willpower and weakness, 111–13, 115–17, *116*
Without a Home (Roe), 103, 307n217
Wixom, Isaac, 94
Woman's Christian Temperance Union (WCTU), 272–73; Anti Opium Department, 272–73

women: asylum commitments, 43, 153–54; frailty and infirmity, as stereotypes, 42–43; as opium addicts, 99–100, 137–38; pain tolerance and opiate prescriptions, 295n35; and self-medication, 45; as "typical" opiate addicts, 42–44; as wartime pharmacists, 65; widows' pensions, 193–97

Woodbury, Frank, 244

Woodward, Joseph Janvier, 62, 234, 236, 243, 256

Woolley, Basil M., 220, 224, 225, 233

work: employment vs. unemployment and need for support, 124–25, 126–27; opiate-addicted persons' lack of ability, 124–26; white-collar work, 125–26

Wright, John J., 254

Wright, Laura, 254

Wyatt-Brown, Bertram, 282

xenophobia, 141–43. *See also* racism

yellow fever, 25

Yellow Wallpaper, The (Gilman), 78

Zell, Henry, 213–14, 215

Zion's Herald (temperance magazine), 101

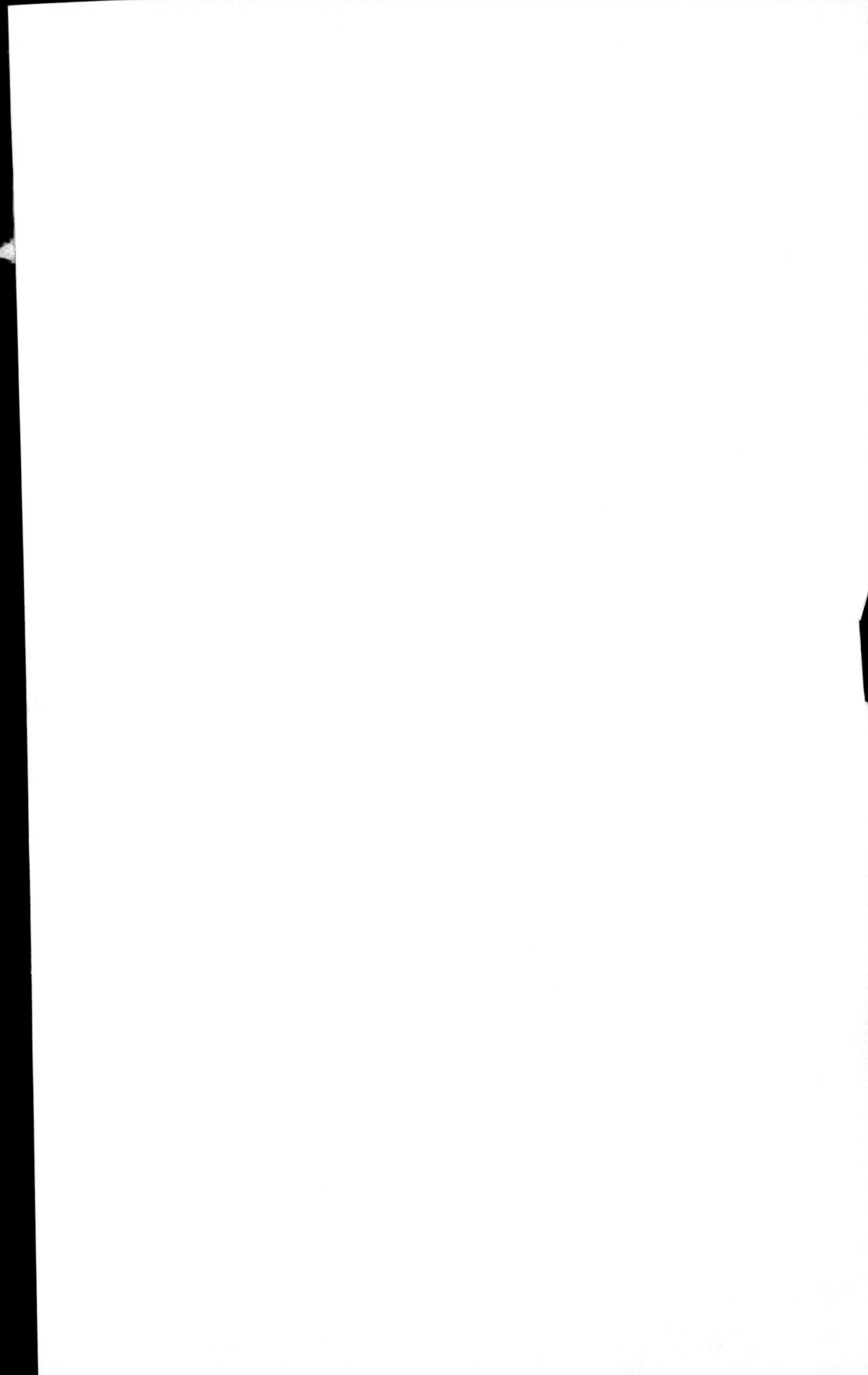

www.ingramcontent.com/pod-product-compliance
Lightning Source LLC
Chambersburg PA
CBHW032011300426
44117CB00008B/990